R. Fujita, J.R. Jass, M. Kaminishi, R.J. Schlemper (Eds.)
Early Cancer of the Gastrointestinal Tract
Endoscopy, Pathology, and Treatment

R. Fujita, J.R. Jass
M. Kaminishi, R.J. Schlemper (Eds.)

Early Cancer of the Gastrointestinal Tract

Endoscopy, Pathology, and Treatment

With 353 Figures, Including 289 in Color

Springer

Rikiya Fujita, M.D.
Chief of Endoscopy Division, Gastroenterology Center, Cancer Institute Hospital
3-10-6 Ariake, Koto-ku, Tokyo 135-8550, Japan

Jeremy R. Jass, M.D.
Department of Pathology, McGill University
Duff Medical Building, 3775 University Street, Montreal, Quebec, Canada H3A 2B4

Michio Kaminishi, M.D., Ph.D.
Department of Gastrointestinal Surgery, The University of Tokyo
7-3-1 Hongo, Bunkyo-ku, Tokyo 113-8655, Japan

Ronald J. Schlemper, M.D., Ph.D.
Specialist in Internal Medicine and
Medical Director, International Clinic Tojinmachi
1-4-6 Jigyo, Chuo-ku, Fukuoka 810-0064, Japan

ISBN 978-4-431-56085-2 Springer-Verlag Tokyo Berlin Heidelberg New York
ISBN 978-4-431-30173-8 (eBook)
DOI 10.1007/978-4-431-30173-8

Springer is a part of Springer Science+Business Media
springeronline.com

Softcover reprint of the hardcover 1st edition 2006

Typesetting: SNP Best-set Typesetter Ltd., Hong Kong
Printing and binding: Shinano, Inc., Japan

Printed on acid-free paper

Foreword

First of all, I would like to discuss two undeniable facts. One is that cancers that are malignant neoplasias of the gastrointestinal tract are epithelial in origin, so it is natural that they grow from the mucosa of the gastrointestinal tract. Another is that an early stage of the cancer invariably exists in the mucosa. Because an early diagnosis is extremely important in the initial stages of cancer in the gastrointestinal tract, the following studies in this book are indispensable to reveal the growth and extension of the disease.

For a long time there has been a decisive difference between Japanese and Western pathologists in the understanding of early cancer. That is, Japanese pathologists diagnose intramucosal neoplastic lesions that have remarkable cellular atypia and structural atypia as cancers, but most Western pathologists don't accept that and diagnose them as dysplasias. They diagnose as cancers only those lesions that show invasion. In a sense, these diagnoses are based on philosophical and conceptual differences in thinking. One Western gastroenterologist described Japanese diagnostic methodology as "Japanese fairy tales." Prof. Manfred Stolte analyzes this point of view in this book and notes that it might better be described as a "Western deficiency."

If we leave this problem untouched, however, studies of gastrointestinal cancers may be deadlocked. How to fill the gap between Japanese and Western interpretations? Is it possible to obtain a unified view or a consensus on pathological findings of cancers? I believe that if Japanese and Western pathologists were to examine full sets of biopsy and resection specimens simultaneously, including endoscopic findings, and through discussion make a mutual diagnosis, the gap might be filled. I believed that resolution of this problem was absolutely necessary, so I adopted it as the main theme when I took up my presidency of the general meeting of the Japanese Society of Gastrointestinal Endoscopy. This book is a compilation of major aspects of that meeting.

Actually, these attempts had already been made in the TNM classification and the Vienna consensus criteria for pathological diagnosis, which are mentioned in this book, but they are still incomplete in spite of remarkable progress. We hope that the information from this book may lead to a more general understanding, and may help to settle existing differences.

Dr. Ronald J. Schlemper collected biopsy and resection specimens, including specimens from 12 gastric cases, 7 colorectal cases and 5 esophageal cases, which are described at the beginning of this book. His work is admirable. By comparing these corresponding specimens readers may ascertain that resection specimens (most of them are endoscopic mucosectomy specimens of the stomach) appear to be more malignant than biopsy specimens. This may be an important key to finding intramucosal cancers. Furthermore, readers may well recognize that certain differences exist between Japanese and Western pathologists' diagnoses. The classification used to detect the existence of intramucosal signet ring cell carcinoma or poorly differentiated adenocarcinoma may be a major breakthrough. When many cases like these are collected, if Japanese and Western pathologists examine the same specimens and discuss them without prejudice, an advanced consensus may be produced and the study of gastrointestinal cancers may be improved. I am sincerely looking forward to that.

Takeshi Oohara, M.D., Ph.D.
President Emeritus, Tsuru-City Hospital
President Emeritus, Japanese Society of
Gastroenterological Carcinogenesis

Foreword

This is a thoroughly unusual book—not so much because of its title, but because 31 leading pathologists from 12 countries have compared their experiences in treating patients. They subjected the results from biopsies and resections of 24 patients with early neoplastic changes of the gastrointestinal hollow organ to a blind study and comparison. The results of this study had provided the basis of the Vienna Classification of Gastrointestinal Epithelial Neoplasia, published on the occasion of the 1998 World Congress of Gastroenterology in Vienna. It was demonstrated then that Western and Japanese pathologists had, as expected, formed different opinions based on their assessments of identical changes in the mucous membrane. Where, for example, the histological assessments of Western pathologists of case 1 (early cancer of the stomach) covered a wide range, from an adenoma with a low-level dysplasia ($n = 1$) to an intramucosal carcinoma ($n = 7$), all of their Japanese colleagues had diagnosed a carcinoma. These differences are due to the fact that many Western pathologists classify changes of the mucous tissue without any definite indication of invasion as a dysplasia, whereas the same findings will be diagnosed by Japanese doctors as well-differentiated adenocarcinomas, as long as they share their cellular and structural atypias. This problem is particularly acute for biopsy preparations from the surface of mucous tissue changes without obvious indications of infiltration into deeper-lying areas of the mucous tissue.

We cannot thank the editors enough for having compiled this complex work. The book is particularly important because it goes beyond the mere description of the problems created by differing histological diagnoses of "early" neoplasias of the digestive tract; it also interprets and explains them.

This section of the book is accompanied and further enriched by excellent descriptions of clinical images and such endoscopic diagnostic techniques as chromoendoscopy and endosonography (including their pitfalls), as well as magnificent images of the superior quality that we have come to expect from our Japanese colleagues over the years.

The term "early" tumors is, of course, not quite up-to-date, because its qualitative assessment of the time factor seems to defy any integration into the more common tumor classifications. Early stomach carcinomas, which by definition include carcinomas of the mucous tissue and the submucosa, are nowadays classified as T1(M) or T1(SM). This differentiation is important because these carcinomas require different therapies. In *The Gastric Cancer Treatment Guideline* from 2004, for instance, the Japanese Gastric Cancer Association recommended performing an endoscopic mucosal resection (EMR) for T1(M) tumors and differentiated gastrectomy variations for T1(SM) tumors. Some endoscopists, meanwhile, are performing an endoscopic submucosal dissection (ESD) for the latter. Nevertheless, these guidelines of the Japanese Gastric Cancer Association remain interesting and obligatory reading for every gastroenterologist and abdominal surgeon with an interest in digestive oncology.

Please allow me to conclude my remarks by reminding readers of the unique achievements of Rudolf Konjetzny, surgeon at the Eppendorf University Clinic in Hamburg in the early years of the previous century. By 1913 he had pointed out a connection between gastritis and stomach cancer. Later he discovered changes in the gastric mucous membrane, which he interpreted as the first stage of cancer and which he initially described as a "pre-carcinomatous state." In the face of the typical contemporary pathological definition of stomach carcinoma as "deep-reaching, destructive growth," Konjetzny emphasized the striking similarity of the mucosal syndrome with an "indubitable carcinoma which is spreading into the deeper-lying layers of the abdominal wall." In 1940, he finally described a stomach cancer "whose growth is restricted to the mucous membrane." It was also Konjetzny who provided evidence for the hypothesis that stomach carcinomas are preceded by a chronic gastritis with metaplasia and "unusual glandular growth in different shapes which originates from the upper epithelium, by multilayered dark epitheloid coronae without basal membrane and by many cell divisions." Today we know that the *Helicobacter pylori* bacterium is the culprit for acute and chronic gastritis, which may in turn cause peptic ulcers or metaplasia, dysplasia, and finally the development of carcinoma.

I hope that this book will find the wide readership it doubtlessly deserves. It will prove to be an indispensable guide and companion not only for pathologists, but also for gastroenterologists and surgeons.

Dr. med. Meinhard Classen, Dr. hc mult.
Emeritus Professor of Medicine, Second Department of Medicine, Technische Universität München, Germany

Foreword

Worldwide, in the year 2005 there were approximately 10 million new cases of cancer and 6.2 million deaths from cancer, according to the most recent data available from the World Health Organization. Digestive cancers account for the highest incidence and mortality of cancer worldwide, with 3 million new cases and 2.2 million deaths annually (colorectal, esophageal and stomach, liver and pancreas). Because of the increasing size and aging of populations in both developed and developing countries, the absolute number of many of these cancers will dramatically increase over the next few years. National health policy in every country should be concerned with the prevention of digestive cancers. The gastroenterologist, primary care physician, endoscopist, surgeon, oncologist, and other health-care providers have a major role in the prevention of digestive cancers. A critical role is in endoscopic detection of early cases and premalignant disease (e.g., Barrett's and adenomas) in asymptomatic persons. Primary prevention is also of critical importance, especially in certain cancers, such as gastric cancer where *Helicobacter pylori* infection has been shown to be responsible for approximately 50% of these cancers, in addition to such dietary factors as diets poor in fruits and vegetables and rich in salt. Genetic susceptibility also plays a role, and the effect of chemoprevention in some digestive cancers is under rigorous study.

There are worldwide differences in the detection and management of early gastrointestinal cancers, especially when one compares the Japanese and Western experiences. This book addresses those differences superbly. Its format is novel, exciting, and very informative. Cases are presented, endoscopy described, and then Western and Japanese pathologists interpret biopsy specimens. Their interpretation was compared to the pathology of resected specimens. Commentary is then made on both the endoscopic and pathologic interpretation, with a view toward arriving at an understanding of the differences. This is unique. The approach provides insight into the two contrasting viewpoints. The second part of the book enhances this format with more didactic presentations of various aspects of diagnosis and management of gastrointestinal cancers in general and also specific cancers, such as gastric and colorectal cancers. These topics include a discussion of the Vienna classification for pathological diagnosis, early cancer in Barrett's esophagus, endoscopic ultrasound, endoscopic treatment, and survival rates of early cancer. All of the cases and topics deal with the luminal gastrointestinal cancers, i.e., of the esophagus, stomach, and colorectum. The book is an ambitious undertaking in terms of its unusual clinical–endoscopic–pathological integrative format and its presentation and discussion of Japanese and Western viewpoints. It has succeeded in bringing together contrasting perspectives by some of the world's most experienced, skilled, and knowledgeable endoscopists, pathologists, and clinicians. The book is truly a remarkable learning experience and achievement. It should be read and studied by everyone involved in the detection and management of patients at risk of digestive cancers.

Sidney J. Winawer, M.D., MACG, Dr. of Sci (Hon)
Professor of Medicine, Weill Medical College
of Cornell University
Paul Sherlock Chair, Memorial
Sloan-Kettering Cancer Center
Co-Chairman, International Digestive Cancer Alliance

Foreword

It is a great pleasure to see the publication of *Early Cancer of the Gastrointestinal Tract,* compiled by Professor Fujita, Professor Jass, Professor Kaminishi, and Dr. Schlemper.

Because early cancer in the gastrointestinal tract—above all, early gastric cancer—is very common in Japan, its diagnosis is not generally considered to be very complicated, except in special cases. However, the concept of what we call early gastric cancer in Japan was not easily understood in Europe and the United States at first. The reason was that the number of early gastric cancer cases itself was very small in Europe and the United States, and if diagnosed at all, they were classified as dysplasia, not cancer.

Recently, it has gradually become known that there are early gastric cancer cases in Europe and United States as well, and the classification of early gastric cancer established by the Japan Gastroenterological Endoscopy Society has been widely acknowledged. Still, there exists a wide gap in awareness.

That gap between Japan on the one hand and Europe and the United States on the other regarding gastrointestinal tract cancer was revealed in two papers written by Dr. Ronald J. Schlemper (who also wrote a chapter in this book) and his colleagues. One was "Diagnostic criteria for gastrointestinal carcinoma in Japan and Western countries: proposal for a new classification system of gastrointestinal epithelial neoplasia," published in the *Journal of Gastroenterology and Hepatology* in 2000, and the other was "Vienna classification of gastrointestinal epithelial neoplasia," published in *Gut* the same year.

The Vienna classification of gastrointestinal epithelial neoplasia was completed by asking 31 well-known pathologists in 12 countries to examine 76 pathological specimens of mostly early neoplastic lesions, and then compiling the members' opinions in a meeting held in Vienna in September 1998.

In Chapter One of this book, many cases offered for this pathological study are presented with the views of endoscopy commentators and pathology commentators, which include many famous endoscopists and pathologists from Japan and other countries. The composition of the cases comprised 12 gastric cases, 7 colorectal cases, and 5 esophageal cases.

The correlation between the biopsied specimens and endoscopically or surgically resected specimens was intentionally concealed from the 31 pathologists in order to reveal the difference of the views among them. By examining the Tables that show those differing views, readers can see how different pathological interpretation can be from person to person, culture to culture. It seems we have a long way to go before achieving a consensus of opinions among specialists in Japan, Europe, and the United States.

In Chapter Two, the details of the Vienna consensus criteria for pathological diagnosis are presented. Although the definitions of dysplasia, neoplasia, and carcinoma in situ are agreed upon, it is stated that Japanese pathologists are more likely to make diagnoses of cancer, while European and American counterparts do not diagnose the same cases as cancer but as dysplasia. Again, we find there is still a wide gap between different cultures.

Featured in the following chapters are early cancer in Barrett's esophagus, how to detect an early cancer, the effectiveness of EUS, endoscopic treatment for early cancer in the gastrointestinal tract, the natural course of an early cancer, surgical treatment, and survival rate of early cancer. The sections on early cancer in the gastrointestinal tract are summarized concisely.

This is the first book to compile in a straightforward manner the views of leading endoscopists and pathologists in Japan, Europe, and the United States on the same early cancer cases in the gastrointestinal tract. It graphically depicts the differences of opinions between different cultures.

Efforts to exchange views will be increasingly important in the future to bridge the gap in pathological diagnosis of early cancers in the gastrointestinal tract. To know the differing views of different specialists about the same cases has significant value. This book will play a critical role in promoting global consensus on early cancer cases in the gastrointestinal tract. It is a book that every endoscopist and pathologist should read to exchange opinions on a global basis.

Hirohumi Niwa, M.D.
President, World Organization for Digestive Endoscopy
President, Japan Gastroenterological Endoscopy Society
Professor of Medicine, St. Marianna University School of Medicine

Preface

Advanced cancers of the gastrointestinal tract develop from either superficial neoplasm or early cancer, and if they could be identified in these stages by endoscopy and diagnosed pathologically as cancer by biopsy, the benefit for patients would be immeasurable. We hope that the global dissemination of this knowledge and the techniques for the diagnosis and therapy of either superficial neoplasm or early cancer will be of worldwide benefit.

Differences in the diagnostic criteria for cancer of the gastrointestinal tract, especially for early cancer, between Japanese and Western pathologists have been a long-standing issue. Surgically resected specimens of either superficial esophageal cancer, early gastric cancer, or early colon cancer have often been diagnosed as dysplasia by Western pathologists. Gastroenterologists, endoscopists, and gastrointestinal surgeons have been unable to resolve this issue. This became a topic of personal interest during a lecture and live demonstration in a Western country. In the autumn of 1996, eight pathologists from Japan, North America, and Europe gathered and reviewed the same pathological specimens during the Asian Pacific Congress in Yokohama, Japan. R.J. Schlemper, who was a visiting scientist at Showa University Fujigaoka Hospital at that time, worked as the coordinator and raised this issue. In 1997, T. Oohara, president of the 53rd Congress of the Japan Gastroenterological Endoscopy Society, chose it as a topic of the congress, addressing it in an international symposium. Publication of Dr. Schlemper's article in *Lancet* (1997;349:1725–9) eventually led to the Vienna classification. More recently, it was our great honor and pleasure for the Japanese macroscopic classification to be recognized internationally as the Paris classification (2003). In this way, M. Kaminishi, who succeeded Professor Oohara, J.R. Jass, who attended the international symposium, R.J. Schlemper, and R. Fujita were appointed as the planning editors of this book.

The main feature of this book is that it is organized in the form of contrasting the views of East and West, bringing in the opinions of world experts in both endoscopic and microscopic specialities. From Japan, where early cancer has been intensively studied, we believe we have collected important articles exploring the natural history of early cancer, which has been demonstrated to develop into advanced cancer. We have also included an article describing many cases of Barrett's cancer, though rare in Japan, from Professor Stolte. The diagnostic methods for early cancer, including chromoscopy, magnifying endoscopy, and narrow band imaging (NBI) are still developing. Even endoscopic therapies, such as endoscopic mucosal resection (EMR) and endoscopic submucosal dissection (ESD), as well as laparoscopic surgery and combination therapies, are in their developmental stages. Since more than five years have passed from the planning of this book to its publication, we asked the authors for additions and revisions immediately before publication. We would like to sincerely thank them for their cooperation.

The 12 gastric and 5 esophageal cases presented in Part 1 are from Showa University Fujigaoka Hospital, 5 of the 7 colorectal cases (13–17) are from National Cancer Center Hospital, Tokyo, and 2 colorectal cases (18 and 19) are from Niigata University School of Medicine. We would like to thank these patients and their physicians for their contribution to the clinical, endoscopic and pathological material presented. In particular we would like to thank Professor H. Watanabe, who made almost all photographs of the histological material in his office in Niigata University in 1996, and Dr. T. Shimoda, who helped to collect clinical data for the National Cancer Center Hospital cases in September 2005.

We would also like to especially acknowledge the invaluable assistance of the editorial staff at Springer-Verlag Tokyo, for their devoted efforts in the preparation and editing of this book.

September 2005
Editors
R. Fujita
J.R. Jass
M. Kaminishi
R.J. Schlemper

Contents

List of Authors

Aoki, Fumio (Chap. VII-1)
Department of Gastrointestinal Surgery, Graduate School of Medicine, The University of Tokyo, 7-3-1 Hongo, Bunkyo-ku, Tokyo 113-8655, Japan

Axon, Anthony T.R. (Chap. I-2)
Department of Gastroenterology, Room 190A Clarendon Wing, The General Infirmary at Leeds, Great George Street, Leeds LS1 3EX, UK
e-mail: anthony.axon@leedsth.nhs.uk

Chiba, Tsutomu (Chap. VI-3)
Division of Gastroenterology and Hepatology, Department of Internal Medicine, Graduate School of Medicine, Kyoto University, 54 Kawara-cho, Shogoin, Sakyo-ku, Kyoto 606-8507, Japan

Crespi, Massimo (Chap. I-4)
National Cancer Institute, Viale Regina Elena 291, Rome 00161, Italy
e-mail: mcrespi@uni.net

Dawsey, Sanford M. (Chap. I-4)
Nutritional Epidemiology Branch, Division of Cancer Epidemiology and Genetics, National Cancer Institute, 6120 Executive Boulevard, Suite 320, Rockville, MD 20852, USA
e-mail: dawseys@mail.nih.gov

Dohmoto, Matatoshi (Chap. IV-4)
Tokushukai General Hospital Yamagata, 2-89-6 Kiyosumi-cho, Yamagata 990-0834, Japan
e-mail: md2002@nifty.com

Dostler, Irina (Chap. III-1)
Institute of Pathology, Klinikum Bayreuth, Preuschwitzer Str. 101, 95445 Bayreuth, Germany

Ell, Christian (Chap. III-1)
Dr. Horst-Schmidt-Klinikum, 65199 Wiesbaden, Germany

Fujii, Shigehiko (Chap. VI-3)
Department of Surgical and Molecular Pathology, Dokkyo University School of Medicine, 880 Kitakobayashi, Mibu, Shimotsuga, Tochigi 321-0293, Japan
e-mail: s-fujii@dokkyomed.ac.jp

Fujimori, Takahiro (Chap. VI-3)
Department of Surgical and Molecular Pathology, Dokkyo University School of Medicine, 880 Kitakobayashi, Mibu, Shimotsuga, Tochigi 321-0293, Japan

Fujisaki, Junko (Chap. IV-1)
Endoscopy Division, Gastroenterology Center, Cancer Institute Hospital, 3-10-6 Ariake, Koto-ku, Tokyo 135-8550, Japan

Fujita, Rikiya (Chap. IV-1)
Chief of Endoscopy Division, Gastroenterology Center, Cancer Institute Hospital, 3-10-6 Ariake, Koto-ku, Tokyo 135-8550, Japan
e-mail: rikiya.fujita@jfcr.or.jp

Gossner, Liebwin (Chap. III-1)
Dr. Horst-Schmidt-Klinikum, 65199 Wiesbaden, Germany

Hayashi, Kazuhiko (Chap. IV-3)
Surgery, Institute of Gastroenterology, Tokyo Women's Medical University, 8-1 Kawada-cho, Shinjuku-ku, Tokyo 162-8666, Japan

Hiki, Naoki (Chap. VII-1)
Surgery Division, Gastroenterology Center, Cancer Institute Hospital, 3-10-6 Ariake, Koto-ku, Tokyo 135-8550, Japan

Hoshino, Yoko (Chap. IV-3)
Gastrointestinal Endoscopy Institute of Gastroenterology, Tokyo Women's Medical University, 8-1 Kawada-cho, Shinjuku-ku, Tokyo 162-8666, Japan

Itabashi, Masayuki (Chap. I-4)
Department of Pathology, Ibaraki Prefectural Central Hospital and Cancer Center, 6528 Koibuchi, Tomobe-machi, Nishiibaraki-gun, Ibaraki 309-1703, Japan
e-mail: m-itabashi@chubyoin.pref.ibaraki.jp

Iwashita, Akinori (Chap. I-3)
Department of Pathology, Fukuoka University Chikushi Hospital, 377-1 Zokumyoin, Chikushino, Fukuoka 818-8502, Japan
e-mail: iwa-aki@fukuoka-u.ac.jp

Jass, Jeremy R. (Chaps. I-3, II-1)
Department of Pathology, McGill University, Duff Medical Building, 3775 University Street, Montreal, Quebec, Canada H3A 2B4
e-mail: jeremy.jass@mcgill.ca

Kaminishi, Michio (Chaps. V-2, VII-1)
Department of Gastrointestinal Surgery, Graduate School of Medicine, The University of Tokyo, 7-3-1 Hongo, Bunkyo-ku, Tokyo 113-8655, Japan
e-mail: e05011@h.u-tokyo.ac.jp

Kashida, Hiroshi (Chap. VI-4)
Digestive Disease Center, Showa University, Northern Yokohama Hospital, 35-1 Chigasaki-chuo, Tsuzuki-ku, Yokohama 224-8503, Japan
e-mail: kashi-md@xf6.so-net.ne.jp

Kato, Yo (Chap. I-2)
Department of Pathology, Cancer Institute, 3-10-6 Ariake, Koto-ku, Tokyo 135-8550, Japan
e-mail: kato@jfcr.or.jp

Kawahara, Masaki (Chaps. I-3, V-2, VII-1)
Division of Surgery, Kanto Central Hospital, 6-25-1 Kamiyoga, Setagaya-ku, Tokyo 158-8531, Japan
e-mail: mkawahara-ths@umin.ac.jp

Kitajima, Kazuaki (Chap. VI-3)
The Third Department of Internal Medicine Oita University Faculty of Medicine, 1-1 Hasama-machi, Oita 879-5593, Japan
e-mail: KAZZ@med.oita-u.ac.jp

Kudo, Shin-ei (Chap. VI-4)
Digestive Disease Center, Showa University, Northern Yokohama Hospital, 35-1 Chigasaki-chuo, Tsuzuki-ku, Yokohama 224-8503, Japan
e-mail: kudos@med.showa-u.ac.jp

Lambert, René (Chap. V-4)
International Agency for Research on Cancer, 150, cours Albert-Thomas, F-69372, Lyon cedex 08, France
e-mail: lambert@iarc.fr

Mafune, Ken-ichi (Chap. VII-1)
Department of Gastrointestinal Surgery, Graduate School of Medicine, The University of Tokyo, 7-3-1 Hongo, Bunkyo-ku, Tokyo 113-8655, Japan

Makuuchi, Hiroyasu (Chap. V-5)
Department of Surgery, Tokai University School of Medicine, Boseidai, Isehara, Kanagawa 259-1193, Japan

Matsui, Toshiyuki (Chap. VI-1)
Department of Gastroenterology, Fukuoka University, Chikushi Hospital, 377-1 Zokumyoin Ooaza, Chikushino, Fukuoka 818-8502, Japan

May, Andrea (Chap. III-1)
Dr. Horst-Schmidt-Klinikum, 65199 Wiesbaden, Germany

Mimura, Toshiki (Chap. VII-1)
Department of Gastrointestinal Surgery, Graduate School of Medicine, The University of Tokyo, 7-3-1 Hongo, Bunkyo-ku, Tokyo 113-8655, Japan

Mitsunaga, Atsushi (Chap. IV-3)
Gastrointestinal Endoscopy Institute of Gastroenterology, Tokyo Women's Medical University, 8-1 Kawada-cho, Shinjuku-ku, Tokyo 162-8666, Japan

Murata, Yoko (Chap. IV-3)
Murata Clinic, Murata Bldg. 1F, 2-16-5 Nishi-Shimbashi, Minato-ku, Tokyo 105-0003, Japan
e-mail: m-yoko@terra.dti.ne.jp; murata@gi-clinic.jp

Muto, Tetsuichiro (Chap. VI-2)
Director, Cancer Institute Hospital, 3-10-6 Ariake, Koto-ku, Tokyo 135-8550, Japan
e-mail: muto@jfcr.or.jp

Nakamura, Shinichi (Chap. IV-3)
Gastrointestinal Endoscopy Institute of Gastroenterology, Tokyo Women's Medical University, 8-1 Kawada-cho, Shinjuku-ku, Tokyo 162-8666, Japan

Nomura, Sachiyo (Chap. VII-1)
Department of Gastrointestinal Surgery, Graduate School of Medicine, The University of Tokyo, 7-3-1 Hongo, Bunkyo-ku, Tokyo 113-8655, Japan

Ohta, Masahiko (Chap. IV-3)
Surgery, Institute of Gastroenterology, Tokyo Women's Medical University, 8-1 Kawada-cho, Shinjuku-ku, Tokyo 162-8666, Japan

Ohtsuka, Kazuo (Chap. VI-4)
Digestive Disease Center, Showa University, Northern Yokohama Hospital, 35-1 Chigasaki-chuo, Tsuzuki-ku, Yokohama 224-8503, Japan

Sakai, Yoshihiro (Chap. V-3)
Chief of Division of Digestive Endoscopy, Department of Medicine, Toho University, Ohashi Hospital Tokyo, 2-17-6 Ohashi, Meguro-ku, Tokyo 153-8515, Japan
e-mail: y-sakai@oha.toho-u.ac.jp

Schlemper, Ronald J. (Chaps. I-1, I-2, I-3, I-4)
Medical Director, International Clinic Tojinmachi (Internal Medicine and Gastroenterology), 1-4-6 Jigyo, Chuo-ku, Fukuoka 810-0064, Japan
e-mail: schlemper@internationalclinic.org

Seto, Yasuyuki (Chap. VII-1)
Surgery Division, Gastroenterology Center, Cancer Institute Hospital, 3-10-6 Ariake, Koto-ku, Tokyo 135-8550, Japan

Shimizu, Nobuyuki (Chap. VII-1)
Department of Gastrointestinal Surgery, Graduate School of Medicine, The University of Tokyo, 7-3-1 Hongo, Bunkyo-ku, Tokyo 113-8655, Japan

Shimizu, Seiji (Chap. IV-2)
Department of Gastroenterology, JR West General Hospital, 1-2-22 Matsuzaki-cho, Abeno-ku, Osaka 545-0053, Japan
e-mail: shimizus@oregano.ocn.ne.jp

Shimoyama, Shoji (Chap. VII-1)
Department of Gastrointestinal Surgery, Graduate School of Medicine, The University of Tokyo, 7-3-1 Hongo, Bunkyo-ku, Tokyo 113-8655, Japan

Stolte, Manfred (Chaps. I-2, I-5, III-1)
Institute of Pathology, Klinikum Bayreuth, Preuschwitzer Strasse 101, D-95445 Bayreuth, Germany
e-mail: Pathologie.Klinikum-Bayreuth@t-online.de

Tada, Masahiro (Chap. IV-2)
Tada Gastroenterological Clinic, 24 Umetada-cho, Nakagyo-ku, Kyoto 604-8136, Japan

Takahashi, Hiroshi (Chaps. IV-1, V-1)
Cancer Screening Center, Cancer Institute Hospital, 3-10-6 Ariake, Koto-ku, Tokyo 135-8550, Japan
e-mail: hiroshi.takahashi@jfcr.or.jp

Takayama, Yukiko (Chap. IV-3)
Gastrointestinal Endoscopy Institute of Gastroenterology, Tokyo Women's Medical University, 8-1 Kawada-cho, Shinjuku-ku, Tokyo 162-8666, Japan

Takeshita, Kimiya (Chap. I-4)
Department of Endoscopic Diagnostics and Therapeutics, Tokyo Medical and Dental University, 1-5-45 Yushima, Bunkyo-ku, Tokyo 113-8519, Japan
e-mail: take.srg1@tmd.ac.jp

Takeuchi, Tsukasa (Chap. VI-4)
Digestive Disease Center, Showa University, Northern Yokohama Hospital, 35-1 Chigasaki-chuo, Tsuzuki-ku, Yokohama 224-8503, Japan

Terano, Akira (Chap. VI-3)
President, Dokkyo University School of Medicine, 880 Kitakobayashi, Mibu, Shimotsuga, Tochigi 321-0293, Japan

Vieth, Michael (Chap. III-1)
Institute of Pathology, Klinikum Bayreuth, Preuschwitzer Strasse 101, D-95445 Bayreuth, Germany

Williams, Christopher B. (Chap. I-3)
St. Mark's Hospital, Watford Rd., Harrow, Middlesex, HA1 3UJ, England, UK
e-mail: christopherbwilliams@btinternet.com

Yamaguchi, Hirokazu (Chap. VII-1)
Department of Gastrointestinal Surgery, Graduate School of Medicine, The University of Tokyo, 7-3-1 Hongo, Bunkyo-ku, Tokyo 113-8655, Japan

Yasuda, Kenjiro (Chap. IV-5)
Department of Gastroenterology, Kyoto Second Red Cross Hospital, 355-5 Haruobi-cho, Marutamachi-agaru, Kamigyo-ku, Kyoto 602-8026, Japan
e-mail: yasuda-k@tim.hi-ho.ne.jp

Yoshida, Misao (Chap. VI-5)
Surgery, Metropolitan Bokutoh Hospital, 4-23-15 Kotobashi, Sumida-ku, Tokyo 130-8575, Japan
e-mail: misao-yoshida@bokutoh-hp.metro.tokyo.jp

Yoshida, Shigeaki (Chap. I-2)
National Cancer Center Hospital East, 6-5-1 Kashiwanoha, Kashiwa, Chiba 277-8577, Japan
e-mail: syoshida@east.ncc.go.jp

Yoshino, Junji (Chap. VI-1)
Department of Internal Medicine, Second Teaching Hospital, Fujita Health University, School of Medicine, 3-6-10 Otobashi, Nakagawa-ku, Nagoya 454-8509, Japan
e-mail: jyoshino@fujita-hu.ac.jp

I. Case Presentations: Clinical Data, Endoscopy, and Pathology

Contents of Part I

1. Introduction

Ronald J. Schlemper

The following 12 gastric, 7 colorectal, and 5 esophageal cases are part of the material used in previous studies [1–4]. In total, 76 histological specimens of mostly early neoplastic lesions were circulated to and individually reviewed by 31 well-known pathologists from 12 countries a few months before the "Vienna meeting," which was held on 5 and 6 September, 1998, and led to the Vienna classification of gastrointestinal epithelial neoplasia [1]. In Tables 1–24, the results of the assessments by these 31 pathologists are shown for 41 of the 76 specimens. These 41 specimens were taken from lesions in 23 Japanese patients, of which the endoscopic gross appearances are indicated by I, IIa, IIb, IIc, IIa+IIc or IIc+IIa according to the macroscopic classification of early neoplasia of the digestive tract [5].

The histological material reviewed by the 31 pathologists consisted of resection specimens, the assessments of which are indicated in the tables by circles, and biopsy specimens from the same lesions, indicated by crosses. The pathologists were not told the relationship of biopsy and resection specimens. They were asked to make a diagnosis of each histological specimen by choosing from the following items: negative for neoplasia (normal, reactive, or regenerative epithelium), indefinite for neoplasia, low-grade adenoma/dysplasia, high-grade adenoma/dysplasia, suspicious of carcinoma, and definite carcinoma, subclassified by the depth of invasion: (a) no invasion (Japanese viewpoint), (b) intramucosal invasion (into the lamina propria or muscularis mucosae), and (c) submucosal invasion [2].

In Tables 1–24, the nine Japanese specialists in gastrointestinal pathology are indicated by the red capitals "J." For each organ system, Western pathologists who diagnosed suspected or definite carcinoma in a similar percentage of cases as these Japanese specialists were considered (and most considered themselves) to have a Japanese viewpoint and are indicated by the red capitals "W;" these included pathologists from Germany, Austria, the United Kingdom, and Korea. The remaining pathologists diagnosed carcinoma in a lower percentage of cases than the Japanese specialists; these pathologists with a Western viewpoint are indicated by the blue capitals "W" and were from Finland, Sweden, Belgium, France, Germany, Austria, Italy, the United Kingdom, Korea, Canada, and the United States. There were two general pathologists from Japan who diagnosed in a manner similar to most Western pathologists and are indicated by the blue capitals "J."

The differences in diagnoses between most Western and Japanese pathologists were considerable. Suspected or definite carcinoma was diagnosed in 17%–66% of gastric, in 5%–40% of colorectal, and in 10%–67% of esophageal specimens by pathologists with a Western viewpoint, but in 77%–94% of gastric, in 45%–75% of colorectal, and in 81%–100% of esophageal specimens by pathologists with a Japanese viewpoint [1, 2]. Tables 1–24 depict the individual diagnoses of all 31 pathologists. For example, from Table 1 one can see that ten Western pathologists diagnosed both the biopsy and the resection specimen of this lesion as high-grade adenoma/dysplasia and three diagnosed the biopsy similarly but the resection specimen as suspected or intramucosal carcinoma, whereas of the nine Japanese specialists six diagnosed both specimens as noninvasive carcinoma, two diagnosed the biopsy as noninvasive but the resection specimen as intramucosal carcinoma, and one diagnosed both as intramucosal carcinoma.

Such diagnostic differences and discrepancies between biopsy-based and resection-based diagnoses can, in large part, be resolved by adopting the revised Vienna classification [2–4, 6]. In this classification, high-grade adenoma/dysplasia, suspected, noninvasive and intramucosal carcinoma are grouped together into one clinically relevant category termed "mucosal high-grade neoplasia." Endoscopic or surgical local resection is indicated for all lesions falling into this category. This is well illustrated by the following 24 cases.

References

1. Schlemper RJ, Riddell RH, Kato Y, et al (2000) The Vienna classification of gastrointestinal epithelial neoplasia. Gut 47:251–255
2. Schlemper RJ, Kato Y, Stolte M (2000) Diagnostic criteria for gastrointestinal carcinomas in Japan and Western countries: proposal for a new classification system of gastrointestinal epithelial neoplasia. J Gastroenterol Hepatol 15:G49–G57
3. Schlemper RJ, Kato Y, Stolte M (2001) Review of histological classifications of gastrointestinal epithelial neoplasia: differences in diagnosis of early carcinomas between Japanese and Western pathologists. J Gastroenterol 36:445–456
4. Schlemper RJ, Iwashita A (2004) Classification of gastrointestinal epithelial neoplasia. Current Diagn Pathol 10:128–139
5. Schlemper RJ, Hirata I, Dixon MF (2002) The macroscopic classification of early neoplasia of the digestive tract. Endoscopy 34:163–168
6. Dixon MF (2002) Gastrointestinal epithelial neoplasia: Vienna revisited. Gut 51:130–131

2. Early Cancer of the Stomach (Cases 1–12)

Case 1, IIc

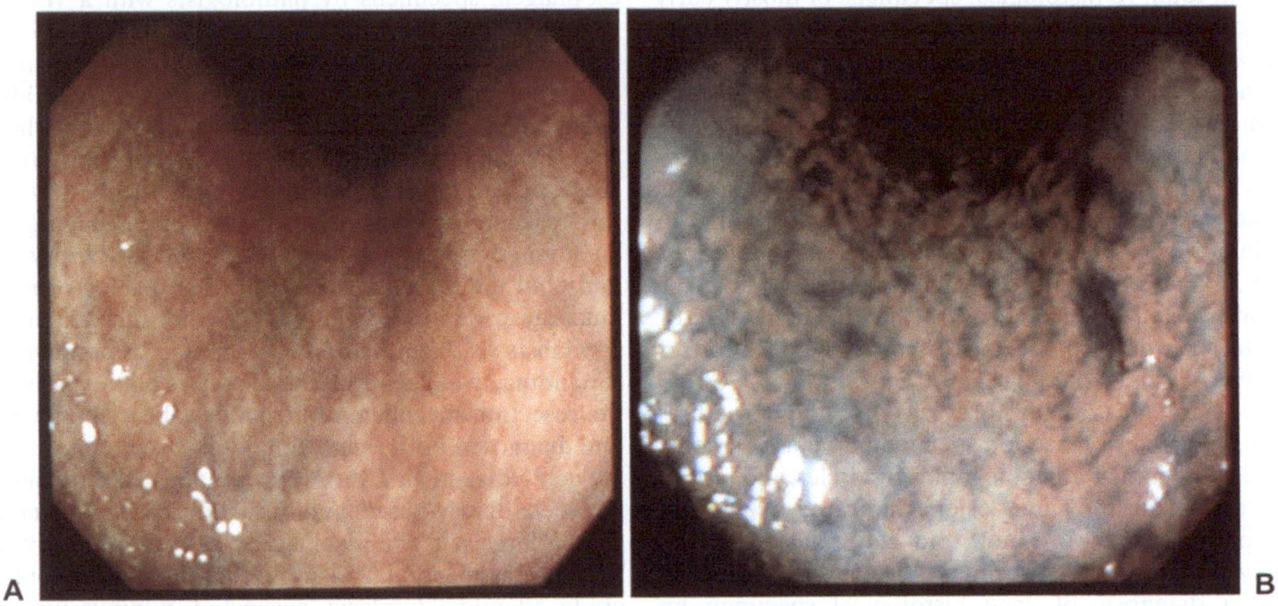

Fig. 1. **A** Corpus, lesser curvature (U-turn view). **B** Same site after spraying indigo carmine

Case Description

A man, aged 73 years, complaining of anorexia, cough, and rhinorrhea for a week, underwent a barium meal examination, which was followed up by an upper gastrointestinal (GI) endoscopic examination to rule out abnormalities. A lesion of about 5 mm in diameter was found in the corpus and was biopsied. Two months later he underwent endoscopic ultrasonographic examination and shortly thereafter endoscopic resection was performed. The resection margins were free of tumor. On follow-up endoscopic examinations, no local recurrence was found.

Endoscopy Commentary

ANTHONY T.R. AXON (UK)[1]

History

A 73-year-old man complaining of anorexia, cough, and rhinorrhea for a week would not in the United Kingdom usually be referred for a barium meal. As a general rule patients with these symptoms would be seen first by their general practitioner, who would provide symptomatic treatment and review them again after about a month. If the symptoms persisted they would be investigated according to how the patient had responded. If the symptoms had settled they would be reassured and discharged; if they were still present a specialist ear, nose, and throat opinion, a chest X-ray, or an upper digestive endoscopy would have been requested. If it

[1]The comments by Professor Axon in this chapter were based on an assessment of the cases in December 2001 and his comments relate to Western practice at that time. Since then Japanese techniques have been embraced in the West with greater enthusiasm, particularly since the Paris classification was published* which was based on the Japanese macroscopic classification of early malignancy. As a result of this, Western endoscopists use chromoscopy more frequently than they did in the past and the number of centres performing endoscopic mucosal resection has risen.

*Endoscopic Classification Review Group (2005) Update on the Paris Classification of superficial neoplastic lesions in the digestive tract. Endoscopy 37:570–578

had been an upper digestive endoscopy it is likely in the UK that there would have been some delay in undertaking the procedure.

It is unclear from the history given why following the barium meal the patient was referred for upper gastrointestinal (GI) endoscopy. In the UK it is unlikely that endoscopy would have been requested unless an abnormality had been found on barium meal examination.

Endoscopic Appearance

The appearance of the stomach without dye spray appears to show evidence of chronic atrophic gastritis with intestinal metaplasia. No focal lesion is readily apparent. It is unlikely that dye spray would have been used in the West as this is not a routine procedure. It is possible that random biopsies would have been taken from the stomach.

Following dye spray there appears to be an oval lesion with a deeply stained base and slightly elevated hypostaining mucosa surrounding it. The stained appearances suggest a small ulcer. In retrospect the lesion may be apparent on close examination of the unstained photograph. Its nature is uncertain. Was this to be an early gastric cancer, I would agree that this appearance would be a IIc.

Histopathology

The Western pathologists in this case mainly reported high-grade dysplasia on the biopsy specimen. We know from experience that high-grade dysplasia is associated with invasive cancer in the majority of cases. In the UK this histology would have been reviewed with the histopathologists and with surgical colleagues, to come to a decision as to how to proceed.

Management

There is little experience in the West of endoscopic mucosal resection, and although this is being undertaken in a number of centers it is only within the last 2 or 3 years that endoscopists have been performing this procedure, usually in specialized centers. The most likely decision, therefore, would have been for a surgeon to be involved. It is likely that further endoscopy would have been requested with additional biopsies. Had this confirmed the abnormality, it is likely that total or subtotal gastrectomy would have been performed.

Summary

In summary, it is unlikely in the West that this patient would have been referred for endoscopy. Had endoscopy been done it is unlikely that the lesion would have been identified. Random biopsies would have been unlikely to have revealed the abnormality. Had it been revealed, total or subtotal gastrectomy would probably have been undertaken.

Endoscopy Commentary

SHIGEAKI YOSHIDA (Japan)

In conventional endoscopy (Fig. 1A), a small area of redness with a minute bleeding spot can be pointed out on the lesser curvature of the lower gastric body though it is tiny and ill demarcated. Because localized redness or discoloration is a very suggestive finding of malignancy [1, 2], additional dye-spraying endoscopy using indigo carmine (contrast technique) is necessary to disclose the details of the lesion. Actually, a dye-spraying picture (Fig. 1B) clarified a minute star-shaped depression surrounded by fold-like elevation, as a pooling of dye with a partially irregular border.

According to the Japanese diagnostic criteria, the irregularity (moth-eaten appearance) at the edge of the depression is highly suggestive of superficial cancerous invasion. The depressed lesion therefore requires a biopsy. On this occasion, even if the initial biopsy results were negative for malignancy due to its minimal size, an additional biopsy should be taken because of this very suspicious finding of malignancy under chromoendoscopy. When this lesion is confirmed as malignant or there is suspicion of malignancy histologically, it should be treated with endoscopic mucosal resection (EMR), because the size is estimated as only 5 mm or less which cannot be accompanied with metastatic lymph nodes.

Many Japanese investigators have compared macroscopic and histological features of a large number of depressed early cancers resected surgically or endoscopically, to establish the endoscopic diagnosis based on the histological evidence. As a result the following relationships between the two could be clarified. In those with ulcerative change within the cancerous lesion histologically [ul(+) carcinoma], gastric wall deformity and/or converging folds are characteristic endoscopic appearances even when the finding of ulceration in itself cannot be found endoscopically. In contrast, in those without histological ulceration [ul(−) carcinoma], marginal elevation without deformities is characteristic, endoscopically.

As to the histological type, the undifferentiated type is rarely found in minute or small cancers. The reasons are explained by the following evidence: firstly, the

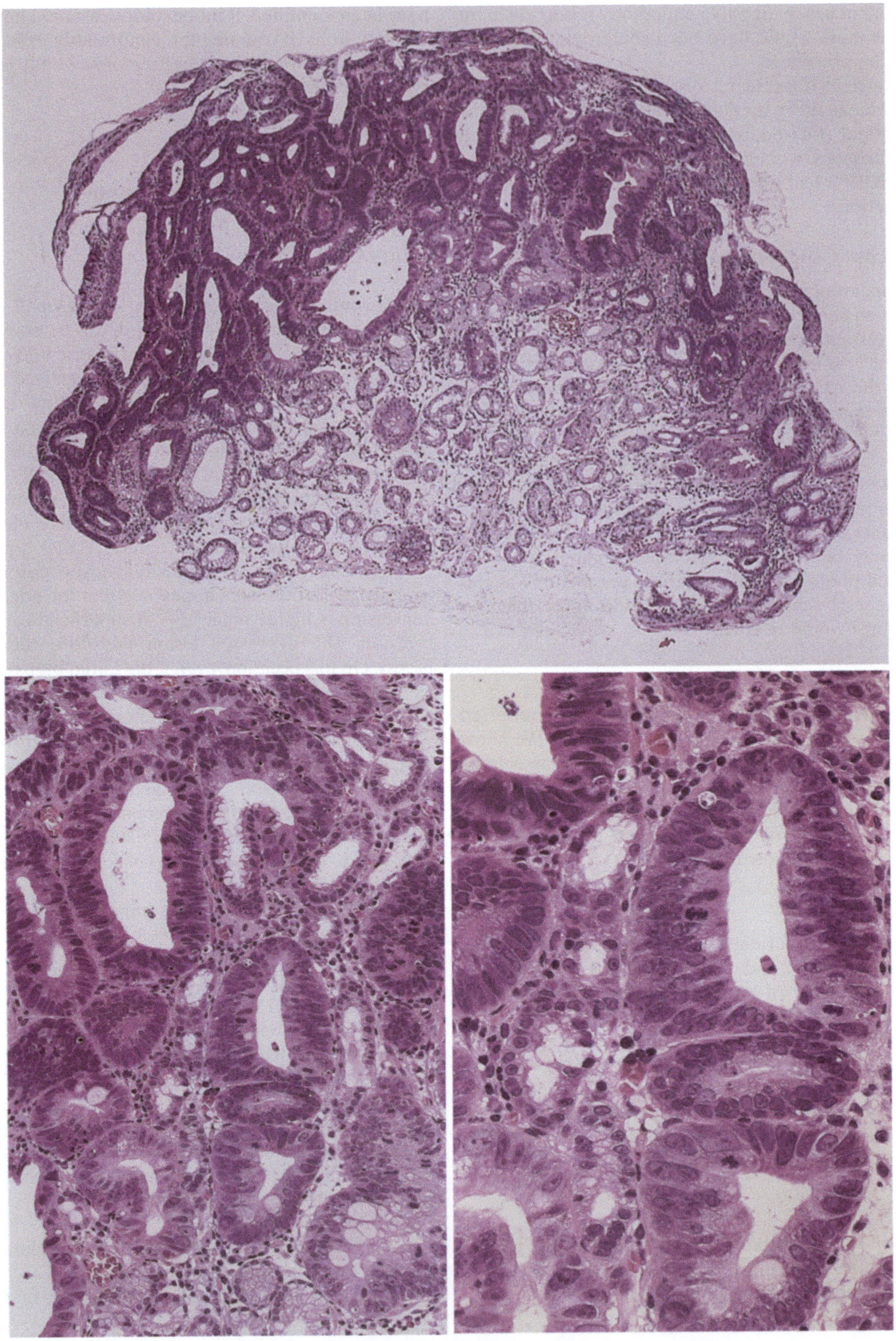

C

D

E

Fig. 1. **C** Biopsy specimen. **D** Detail of **C**. **E** Detail of **D**

Table 1. Gastric lesion 1

Biopsy: × Resection: ○	WW WW WW WW WW	W W	W	W	W	W	J J J J J W J J J	W	J J	W W J
Adenoma/dysplasia										
low-grade			×							
high-grade	⊗	×		×						
Carcinoma										
suspected		○			×	○				
non-invasive							⊗	○	×	
intramucosal			○	○	○	×		×	○	⊗

detection bias that arises because most minute cancers detected incidentally only show nonspecific findings, though several cases reveal faint monotonous discoloration endoscopically; and secondly, the histological metamorphosis from differentiated to undifferentiated types during the cancer development from a minute to conventional lesion, as shown by Saito et al [3].

In conclusion, the lesion presented can be diagnosed as a minute cancer of differentiated type without histological ulceration, and should be treated with EMR.

References

1. Yoshida S, Yamaguchi H, Tajiri H, et al (1984) Diagnosis of early gastric cancer seen as less malignant endoscopically. Jpn J Clin Oncol 14:225–241
2. Yoshida S, Yamaguchi H, Saito D, et al (1993) Endoscopic diagnosis; latest trends. In: Nishi M, Ichikawa H, Nakajima T, et al (eds) Gastric cancer. Springer, Tokyo, pp 246–262
3. Saito A, Shimoda T, Nakanishi Y, et al (2001) Histologic heterogeneity and mucin phenotypic expression in early gastric cancer. Pathol Int 51:165–171

Pathology Commentary

Manfred Stolte (Germany)

In the biopsy material obtained from the lesion, histological examination at low magnification (Fig. 1C) already clearly reveals a neoplastic rather than a regenerative change, since the normal foveolar architecture has been completely replaced by irregularly arranged, neoplastic tubuli. The diagnosis of neoplasia is confirmed under high magnification (Fig. 1D and E): the nuclei of the neoplastic epithelial cells are polymorphic and irregularly arranged, often hyperchromatic, and reveal an irregular chromatin structure, prominent nucleoli, and several abnormal mitotic figures. Based on these findings, the differential diagnosis lies between high-grade intraepithelial neoplasia (dysplasia) and well-differentiated tubular adenocarcinoma. Although no invasive tumor cells are definitely seen in the lamina propria, the highly irregular architecture of the densely packed neoplastic tubuli of varying caliber is no longer compatible with the budding and branching of a high-grade intraepithelial neoplasia. Rather, the invasive neoplastic tubuli clearly point to the histological diagnosis of a tubular adenocarcinoma.

The diagnosis of carcinoma is confirmed in the endoscopically resected specimen. At low power (Fig. 1F) the neoplastic tubuli are seen running perpendicular to the surface. On the edge of the tumor some show a parallel arrangement, suggestive of noninvasive neoplasia. However, the irregular architecture of the neoplastic tubuli, some aligned parallel to the muscularis mucosae as seen in the center of the tumor, clearly identify the lesion as an invasive carcinoma. This diagnosis is confirmed under higher magnification (Fig. 1G and H): the normal architecture of the surface structures of the gastric mucosa is completely disrupted. In high-grade intraepithelial neoplasia the architecture of the parallel arrangement of glands lined with neoplastic epithelial cells ought to be intact. However, here again we see densely packed, irregularly arranged invasive neoplastic tubuli of varying caliber. The cytological criteria for an adenocarcinoma are also met.

In conclusion, there is no doubt that the diagnosis is invasive intramucosal well-differentiated adenocarcinoma, established in both the biopsy and endoscopic mucosectomy specimens.

Western pathologists often underdiagnose intramucosal well-differentiated adenocarcinoma as high-grade dysplasia, in this particular case by ten of the Western pathologists. Four other Western pathologists then corrected their biopsy-based dysplasia diagnosis on

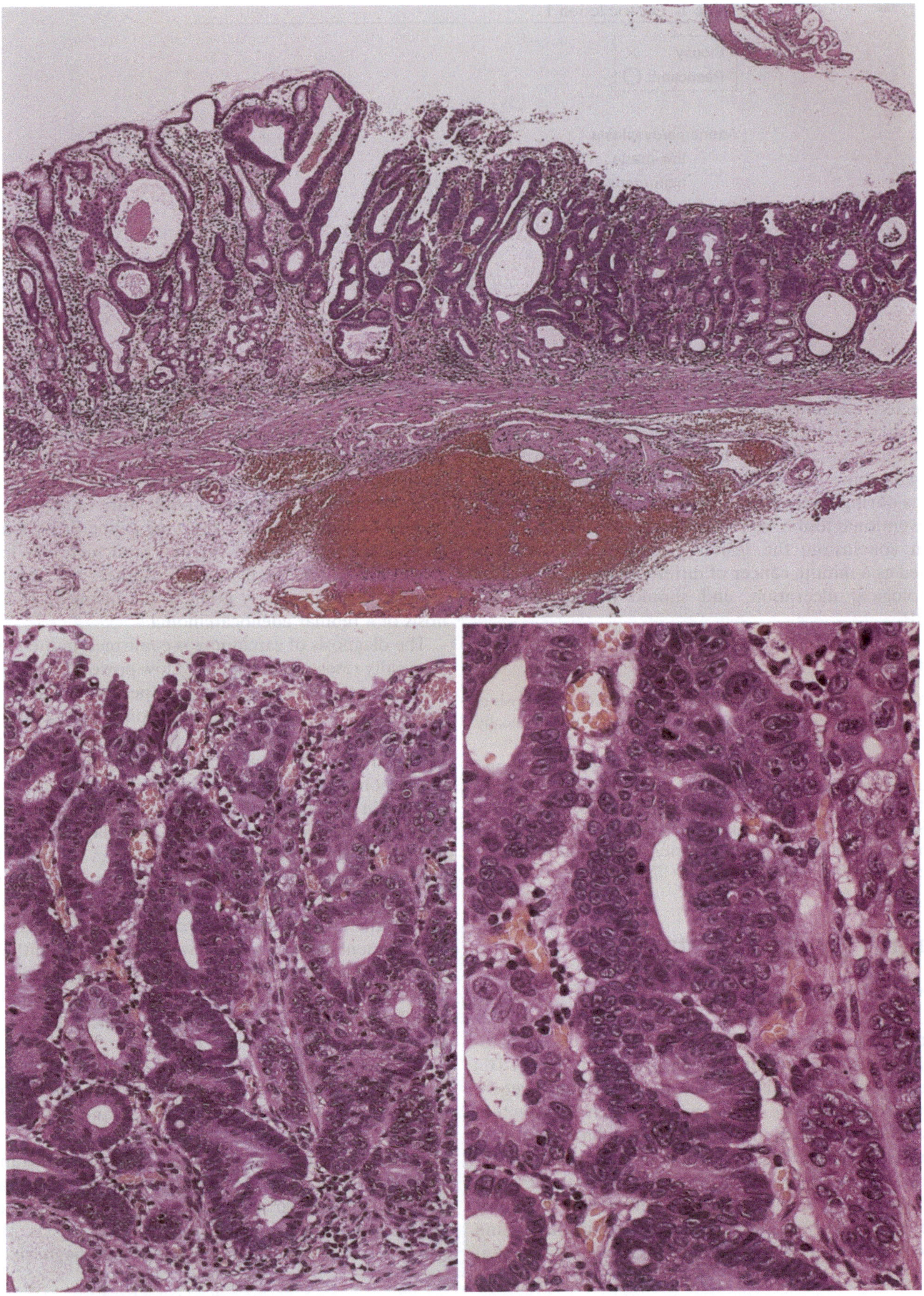

F

G

H

Fig. 1. F Endoscopically resected specimen. **G** Detail of **F**. **H** Detail of **G**

interpreting the mucosectomy specimen. In common with all the Japanese pathologists, however, six Western pathologists made the correct carcinoma diagnosis.

Pathology Commentary

Yo Kato (Japan)

The low-power view of the biopsy specimen shows an aggregate of slightly irregular-shaped round or tubular glands in the upper half of the mucosa (Fig. 1C). The glands consist of columnar cells with a swollen oval nucleus and a high N/C ratio accompanied by moderate nuclear pseudostratification (Fig. 1D). The nuclei are vesicular, containing one or two prominent nucleoli, and the mitoses are remarkable (Fig. 1E). Non-neoplastic glands with small nuclei are interspread among the neoplastic glands. Since the invasion is not clear, the change corresponds to noninvasive carcinoma from the Japanese viewpoint, to be classified as category IV in the Vienna classification (Fig. 1F).

In the endoscopic mucosal resection (EMR) specimen, the tubular tumor with occasional dilated glands is completely limited to the mucosa, occupying its full thickness in the right half of the figure (Fig. 1F). The slightly irregular tubular glands are composed more of cuboidal cells with a swollen round nucleus than in the biopsy specimen. (Fig. 1G). Round nuclei with one or two dark eosinophilic nucleoli are prominent (Fig. 1H). Similar to the biopsy specimen, the invasion is not clear, therefore noninvasive carcinoma is considered to be the proper diagnosis also for the EMR specimen, i.e., category IV by the Vienna classification (Fig. 1F).

Case 2, IIc

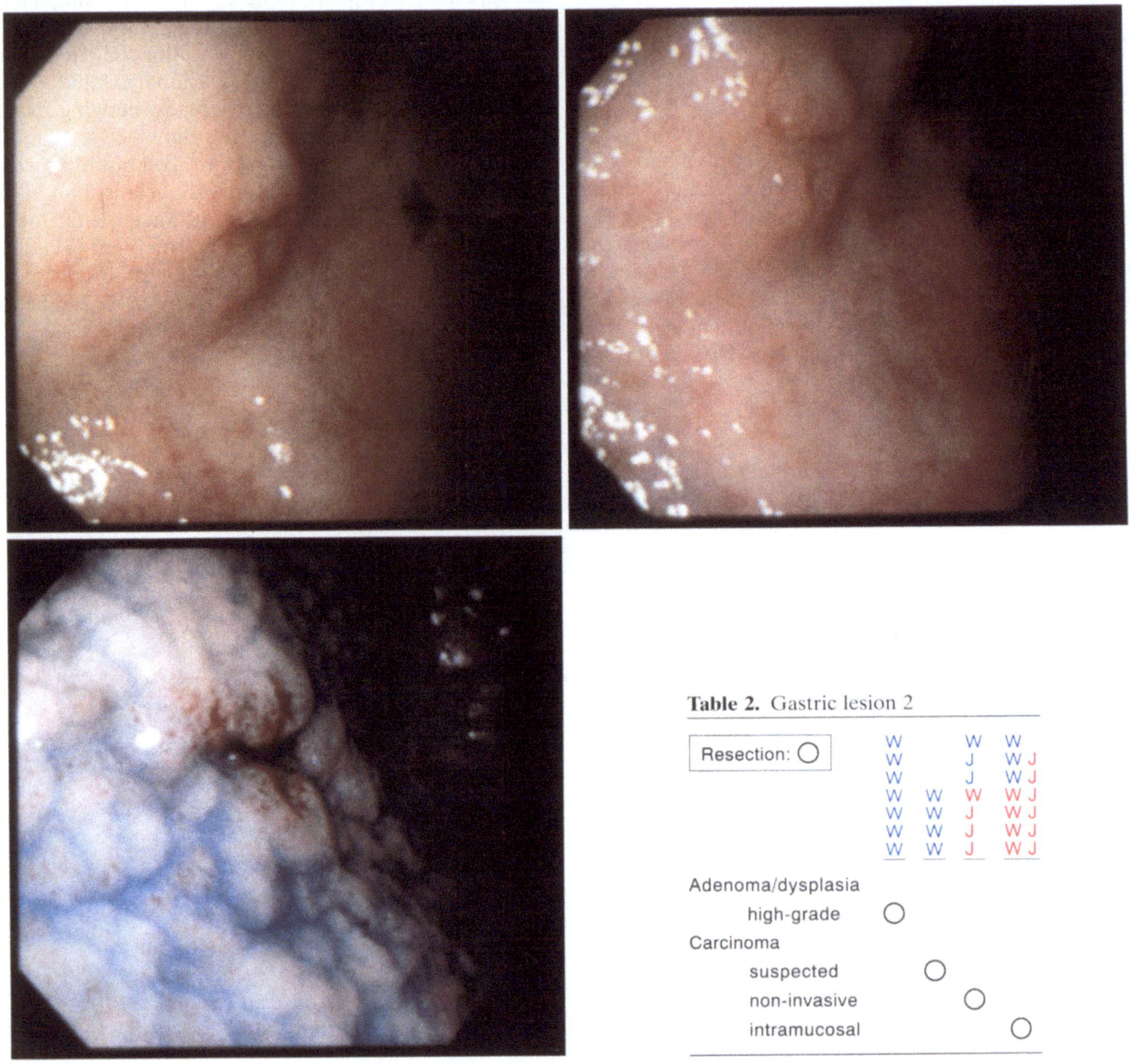

Fig. 2. A Angulus, anterior wall. **B** Same site. **C** Same site after spraying indigo carmine

Table 2. Gastric lesion 2

Resection: ○				
	W		W	W
	W		J	W J
	W		J	W J
	W	W	W	W J
	W	W	J	W J
	W	W	J	W J
	W	W	J	W J
Adenoma/dysplasia				
high-grade	○			
Carcinoma				
suspected		○		
non-invasive			○	
intramucosal				○

Case Description

A man, aged 78 years, with a history of pulmonary emphysema, complained of mild anorexia for a month and underwent an upper GI endoscopic examination. A lesion of 7 mm in diameter was found at the anterior wall side of the angulus and was biopsied. One month later, endoscopic ultrasonographic examination and, on the following day, endoscopic resection were performed. The resection margins were free of tumor. On follow-up endoscopic examinations, no local recurrence was found.

Endoscopy Commentary

Anthony T.R. Axon (UK)[1]

History

A man of 78 years with a month's history of mild anorexia would have attended his general practitioner, who would have taken a history, and would have been unlikely to have referred the patient for endoscopy unless there had been some weight loss or other reason for referring for a gastrointestinal opinion. It is likely that some blood tests and chest X-ray would have been undertaken and the patient would have been reviewed following the results of these tests. If the symptoms of anorexia had persisted he would probably have been referred for a medical opinion at the hospital, where a specialist would have undertaken further investigations and probably referred him for upper digestive endoscopy.

Endoscopic Appearance

The upper digestive endoscopy shows a protuberant lesion in the stomach close to the angulus. The stomach appears to have significant chronic gastritis and intestinal metaplasia. The appearance arouses suspicion of an early carcinoma and would, I think, have been detected by a Western endoscopist. Biopsies would have been taken from the lesion. As the lesion is protuberant it is unlikely that this would have been classified in the West as a IIc. It is more likely that a Western endoscopist would have classified it as a I, if requested to classify it. In the West, however, endoscopists do not commonly use the Japanese classification when reporting endoscopic appearance. We have little first-hand experience with early gastric cancer, the majority being identified as such only after resection of type III lesions.

Histology

The biopsy report in this case is not available, only the resection specimen; however, the appearances of the resection specimen were, according to Western pathologists, highly suggestive of high-grade dysplasia or carcinoma.

Management

It is possible that in some specialized centers endoscopic ultrasound would have been performed here; however, a combination of the macroscopic appearance with the suspicious histology would have led to surgical referral. It is likely that the final decision would have been that this was a cancer, and resection of the distal stomach would have been undertaken.

Summary

It is likely that there would have been a greater delay in the time taken for endoscopy to be performed. It is probable that the lesion would have been diagnosed as cancer and that distal gastric resection would have been performed.

[1]See footnote on p. 4.

Endoscopy Commentary

Shigeaki Yoshida (Japan)

A depressed lesion around less than 10mm in size (corresponding to the diameter of two or three granules of *areae gastricae*) is located in the anterior wall of the lower gastric body or angulus. The endoscopic finding grossly consists of a star-shaped depression and surrounding elevated components, as shown in Fig. 2A. A conventional endoscopic picture in close-up view (Fig. 2B) discloses the irregularity in the margin of the depressed area and the typical moth-eaten appearance indicating definite malignancy.

The questions raised are how to perform macroscopic typing and how to estimate the degree of vertical invasion. The answers should entirely depend on whether we consider the elevated components as a result of cancerous invasion or of benign inflammatory changes. In this respect, a dye-spraying picture (Fig. 2C) gives us useful information that the appearance of the elevated components is mostly the same as the surrounding granular lesions (boiled-rice appearance) of intestinal metaplasia, although some erosive changes are detectable at the border of the depression. In addition, since elevated early cancers usually show lustrous and hyperemic appearances under dye-spraying endoscopy, the elevated components in this case are estimated to be the result of hyperplastic changes of metaplastic mucosa, rather than neoplastic growth. Also, the surrounding elevated component is not so dominant, so that this lesion can be classified macroscopically into not IIa+IIc, but IIc type.

The target findings best known to estimate submucosal invasion in general are swelling of tips of converging folds and fusion of folds. The dye-spraying picture fails to reveal such folds. The invasion should be limited, also because the lesion presented is not accompanied with slow-sloped elevation, as in a submucosal tumor, due to deep invasion.

As to the histological type, the hyperemic appearance in the depressed area whose margin is vaguely defined

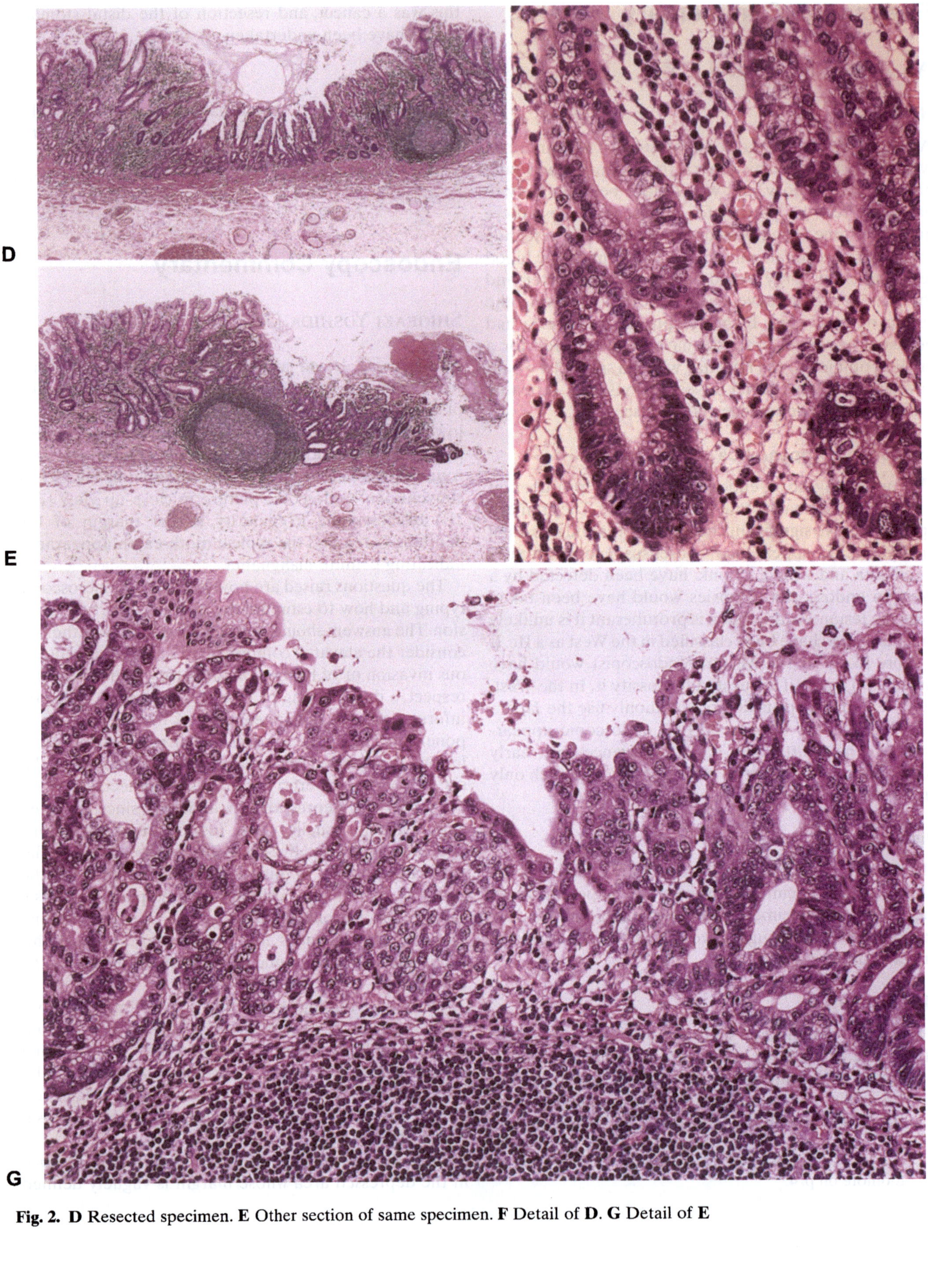

Fig. 2. **D** Resected specimen. **E** Other section of same specimen. **F** Detail of **D**. **G** Detail of **E**

is suggestive of the differentiated type, since the undifferentiated type usually shows a discolored depression with a sharply defined margin.

In conclusion, the final endoscopic diagnosis of this lesion should be a IIc type of early gastric cancer with a low probability of submucosal invasion, of the differentiated type.

Since in Japan EMR is usually indicated for mucosal cancers of the differentiated type less than 2cm without histological ulceration [1] in order to guarantee the absence of metastasis, this lesion appears to have an absolute indication for EMR. Also, when the resected specimen histologically reveals that the cancerous invasion is limited to within the mucosal layer without any components of vascular invasion, the treatment result can be regarded as curative regardless of histological type and histological ulceration, according to the criteria of Yamao et al [2].

References

1. Yoshida S (1997) Endoscopic treatment. In: Saugimura T, Sasako M (eds) Gastric cancer. Oxford University Press, Tokyo, pp 252–262
2. Yamao T, Shirao K, Ono H, et al (1996) Risk factors for lymph node metastasis from intramucosal gastric carcinoma. Cancer 77:602–606

Pathology Commentary

Manfred Stolte (Germany)

The endoscopic appearance alone (Fig. 2A–C) strongly suggests that the lesion is a type IIc early gastric carcinoma and not a benign lesion. The overview of the endoscopic mucosectomy specimen already reveals that the small lesion with its central depression is a well-differentiated intramucosal invasive tubular adenocarcinoma. The numerous densely packed, relatively small neoplastic tubuli located immediately above the muscularis mucosae are no longer compatible with a high-grade intraepithelial neoplasia, but are a result of invasion of these tubuli into the lamina propria. In the margin of the carcinoma, chronic active *Helicobacter pylori* gastritis with intestinal metaplasia and lymphoid follicles—the soil in which the early carcinoma developed—can be seen. Additional evidence for carcinoma is the superficial erosion in the center of the lesion indicating destructive growth (Fig. 2E).

The section of the lesion seen in high power view (Fig. 2F) does not permit a differentiation between an invasive carcinoma and high-grade dysplasia. Figure 2G, however, again shows the irregular pattern of the densely packed invasive tubuli and also, clearly recognizable, an invasive tumor sliver.

In conclusion this case is, without any doubt, a type IIc early carcinoma limited to the mucosa and histologically classifiable as a well-differentiated tubular adenocarcinoma.

The correct diagnosis of carcinoma was established not only by all the Japanese, but also by 13 Western pathologists. Only seven Western pathologists made the underdiagnosis of high-grade dysplasia.

Pathology Commentary

Yo Kato (Japan)

Only the resected specimen is available in this case. The erosive lesion shown in the center of Fig. 2D and in the center to right part of Fig. 2E consists of short glands and medium-sized to small glands, which are limited to the mucosa.

The glands are anastomosing irregularly in part (Fig. 2D, right and middle-left), and compacted in other parts (Fig. 2E). With these patterns, it is not difficult for Japanese pathologists to diagnose the lesion as carcinoma, moderately differentiated tubular carcinoma [tub 2 according to the Japanese Research Society for the Study of Gastric Cancer (JRSGC) classification], but for some glands included in the lesion as shown at least in Fig. 2F it is actually difficult to give a definite diagnosis.

However, the epithelia harboring relatively vesicular and swollen nuclei with a prominent nucleolus are findings suggestive of carcinoma (noninvasive carcinoma so far as the figure is concerned). As to whether the lesion is invasive or noninvasive, since small glands budding or sprouting from the medium-sized glands exist, an invasive lesion is strongly suggested (Fig. 2G). The atypical glands of Fig. 2G correspond in total to tub 2.

Here, the epithelia form a solid nest as well (Fig. 2G, center) and the lesion is generally associated with more remarkable cellular or nuclear atypias than those of atypical glands of Fig. 2F in terms of vesicular and swollen nuclei with a prominent nucleolus. These are the findings on which most Japanese pathologists base their diagnosis of carcinoma even without evident invasive patterns.

Looking at Table 2, I imagine that the differential diagnosis between invasive and noninvasive carcinoma is difficult, not only for Japanese pathologists who are not accustomed to doing it but also for Western pathologists for whom it is obligatory routinely for a diagnosis of carcinoma.

Case 3, IIc

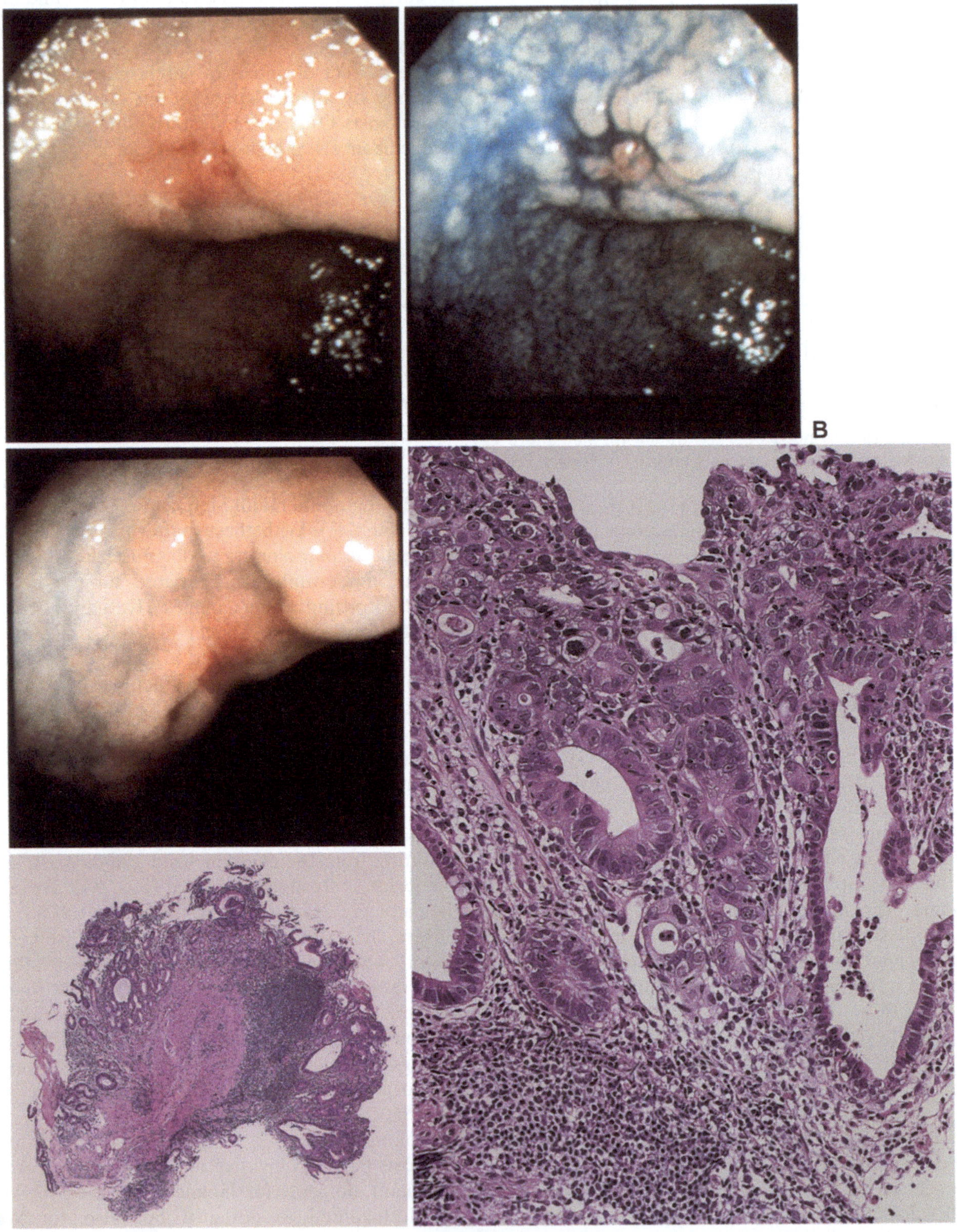

A B C D E

Fig. 3. A Angulus, anterior wall. **B** Same site after spraying indigo carmine. **C** Close-up view. **D** Biopsy specimen. **E** Detail of **D**

Case Description

A man, aged 76 years, with a history of myocardial infarction, cerebral infarction, and congestive heart failure, underwent upper GI screening by endoscopic examination. A lesion of 12 mm in diameter was found at the anterior wall side of the angulus and was biopsied. A week later endoscopic resection was performed. The resection margins were free of tumor.

Endoscopy Commentary

ANTHONY T.R. AXON (UK)[1]

History

As this was a 76-year-old man with serious general medical problems, he would not have been referred for endoscopic examination in the West unless he had complained of symptoms referable to his upper GI tract. The lesion in the stomach therefore would not have been identified.

Endoscopy

In the event that endoscopy had been carried out for some reason, the sizable lesion proximal to the angulus would have been identified. The appearances are those of an ulcer with an elevated circumferential margin, irregular in appearance and highly suspicious of cancer. It is unlikely that dye spray would have been used, but multiple biopsies would have been taken from the area.

Histology

The biopsies by Western pathologists were in agreement that there was high-grade dysplasia or worse. Only one pathologist suggested that it might be low-grade dysplasia. On this basis a diagnosis of cancer would have been made.

Management

A surgical opinion would have been requested and this would have led to a problem because the patient had sustained a myocardial infarction, a cerebral infarction, and was in congestive heart failure. So although the surgeon would have been inclined to carry out a gastric resection, the advice of an anesthetist would have been sought. If it was considered that the patient was suitable for major surgery, an operation would have been performed. If the anesthetist had felt that the patient would be unlikely to survive surgery, the implication would have been that he would be more likely to have died from his general medical condition than the carcinoma itself so, after discussion with the patient and the relatives, palliative care would have been given. With the introduction of endoscopic mucosal resection in the West, today it is possible the patient might have been sent to a tertiary referral center where endoscopic mucosal resection might have been performed.

Summary

In this case the lesion would not have been diagnosed because the patient would not have been referred for endoscopy in the first place. Had the lesion been identified it would have been resected, if the patient was fit enough to undergo the procedure; otherwise palliative

Table 3. Gastric lesion 3

Biopsy: × Resection: ○	W W W	W W	W W W	W	W W	J	W W W W	J	J	W J J	W W J W J W J	J	J J
Adenoma/dysplasia													
low-grade				×									
high-grade	⊗	○	×										
Carcinoma													
suspected		×	○		⊗	○	×						
non-invasive						×		⊗	○	×		×	
intramucosal				○			○		×	○	⊗		×
submucosal												○	○

[1]See footnote on p. 4.

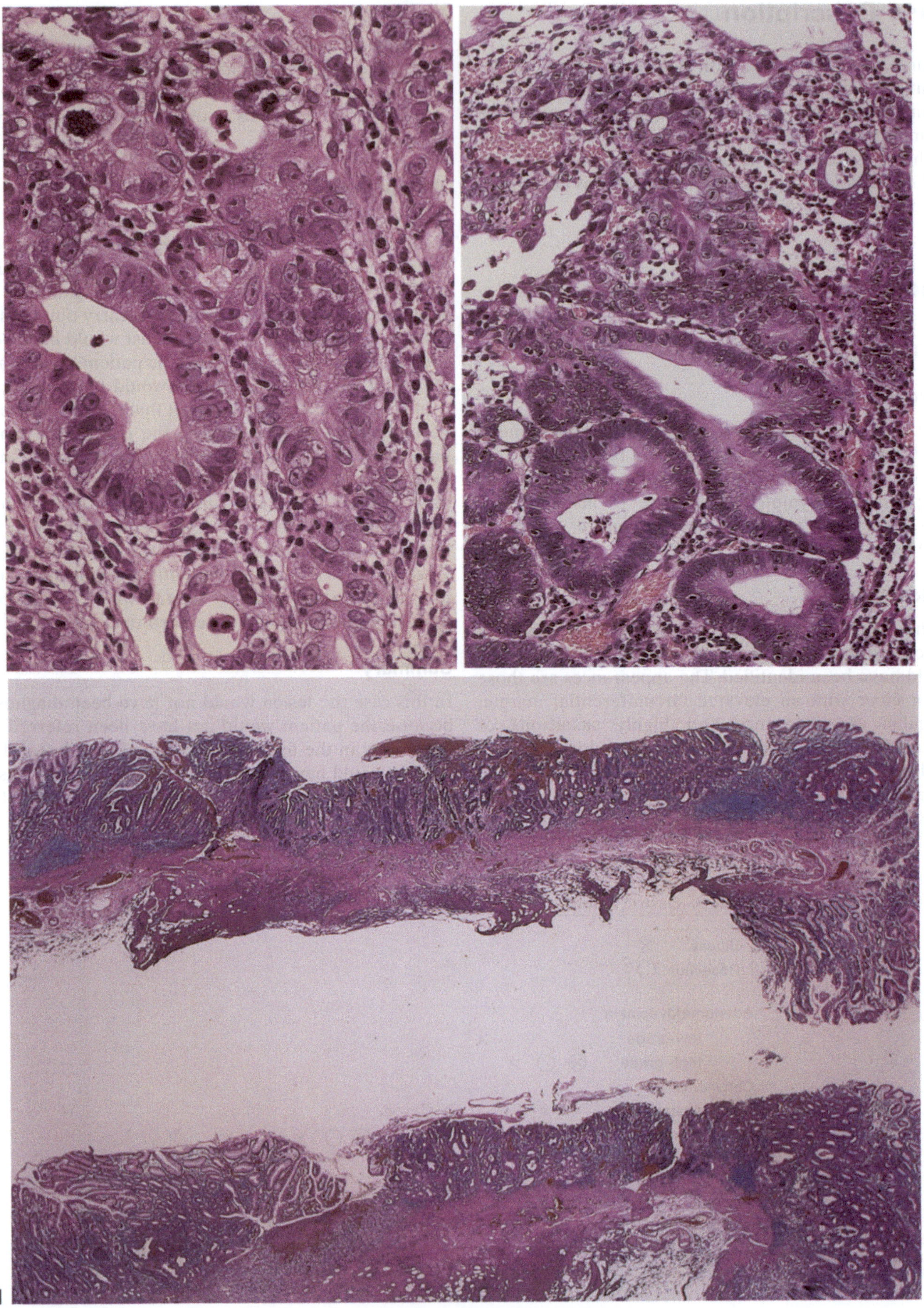

F G H

Fig. 3. **F** Detail of **E** (biopsy). **G** Detail of resected specimen. **H** Resected specimen overview care or referral to a tertiary center may have been undertaken.

Endoscopy Commentary

SHIGEAKI YOSHIDA (Japan)

A lesion of around 10–15 mm in size is located on the lesser curvature of the angulus. Endoscopically, it is seen as a superficial depression surrounded by thickened mucosa, which is actually formed by the swollen tips of converging folds (ul(+) lesion). In addition, granular lesions ("islet formation") are seen within the depressed area (Fig. 3A). The malignancy of the lesion is easily suspected from the irregularity of the depressed margin, particularly the moth-eaten appearance detected at the tip of the fold as shown in Fig. 3C, and macroscopic typing of IIc is also easy to make, because the surrounding elevated components are not remarkable macroscopically.

The question is whether the lesion has deeper invasion. Dye-spraying pictures (Fig. 3B and C) show two contradictory findings. One is that tips of folds are separated from each other, indicating little possibility of deeper invasion, and the other is the presence of a conspicuous granular lesion within the depression, indicating no small possibility of deeper invasion although it should be limited. As a preoperative diagnosis that has to assume the worst, therefore, we should accept the possibility of deeper invasion in this case.

As to the estimation of the histological type, this lesion showed characteristics of both differentiated and undifferentiated types, the former being the lustrous hyperemic appearance of the depressed area and the latter the sharply demarcated margin of the depression. Hence, it is difficult to estimate the histological type in this case.

In conclusion, this lesion can be diagnosed endoscopically as a IIc type of early cancer [ul(+) carcinoma] with possible submucosal invasion, of which the histological type is unknown.

Endoscopic mucosal resection can be indicated for this lesion as an optional choice when the depressed area is lifted up well by saline injection (negative for "nonlifting sign"), since the size is estimated to be around 10–15 mm, fold convergence is not remarkable in dye-spraying pictures, and the surrounding elevation is not suggestive of massive submucosal invasion endoscopically.

Pathology Commentary

MANFRED STOLTE (Germany)

The endoscopic appearance (Fig. 3A–C) alone shows that this lesion is not a benign lesion but must be a type IIc gastric carcinoma. This is already confirmed histologically in the biopsy specimen. The low-power view (Fig. 3D) suffices to establish the diagnosis of carcinoma on the basis of the irregular architecture of the neoplastic tubuli. This is impressively confirmed in Fig. 3E, which clearly shows aggregations of densely packed invasive tumor cells at the surface near the neoplastic tubuli. This is also confirmed under higher magnification (Fig. 3F and G). Invasive neoplastic glands with polymorphic nuclei with irregular chromatin, prominent nucleoli, and abnormal mitotic figures are seen, as well as unmistakable individual carcinoma cells that have separated from the tubuli in the adjacent lamina propria.

In the endoscopic mucosectomy specimen (Fig. 3H), the overview shows that the carcinoma is limited to the mucosa. Adjacent to the carcinoma the underlying disease, chronic active *H. pylori* gastritis, can be seen.

In this case, only three Western pathologists were of the opinion that this lesion was merely a high-grade dysplasia. Three other Western pathologists corrected their biopsy-based high-grade dysplasia diagnosis on examining the mucosectomy specimen, while all the remaining Western pathologists together with all the Japanese pathologists diagnosed carcinoma.

Pathology Commentary

YO KATO (Japan)

The biopsied mucosa is covered by atypical glands of various sizes, particularly on its right side (Fig. 3D). The atypical glands consist mostly of eosinophilic cuboidal cells with a pale, round to oval, swollen nucleus with a prominent nucleolus (Fig. 3E,F). Some small glands seem to start invading the lamina propria mucosae. The nuclear hyperchromasia seen in the right ends of the pictures (Fig. 3E,F) may be due to the artifacts related to the biopsy procedure. One nucleus corresponds clearly to mitosis. With the above findings, an invasive, moderately differentiated adenocarcinoma (tub 2) is considered, but there exists also a part corresponding to very well-differentiated carcinoma (tub 1) composed of columnar cells with a basally situated hyperchromatic round to oval nucleus (Fig. 3G, lower half).

The pathological examination of the EMR specimen revealed that the carcinoma was limited to the mucosa and was completely resected.

Case 4, IIa+IIc

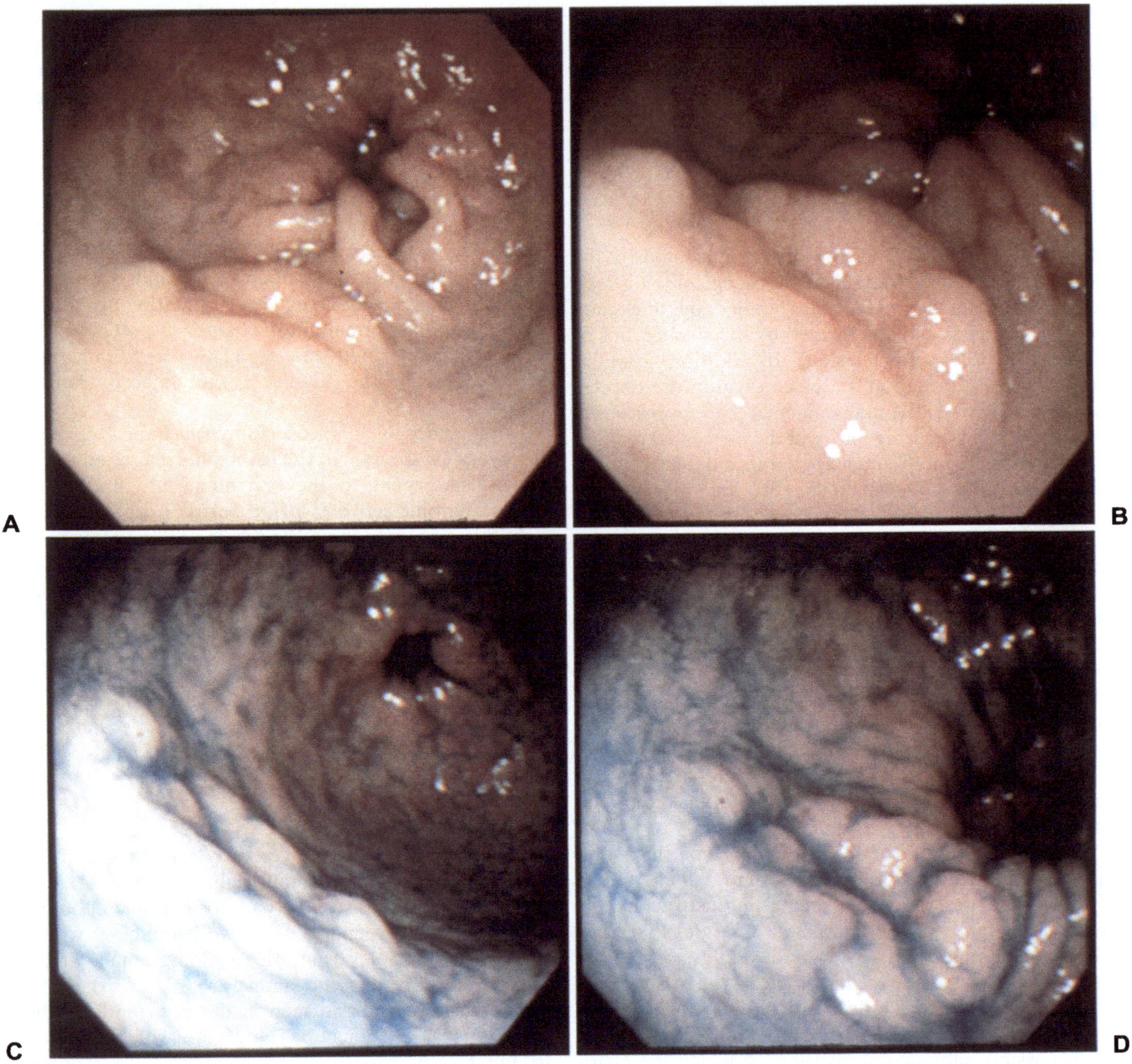

Fig. 4. **A** Antrum, anterior wall. **B** Close-up view. **C** Same site after spraying indigo carmine. **D** Close-up view

Case Description

A woman, aged 76 years, with diabetic nephropathy and normocytic anemia, had no dyspeptic symptoms but underwent upper GI screening by endoscopy. A lesion of 17 mm in diameter was found at the anterior wall of the antrum and was biopsied. Three weeks later endoscopic resection was performed. The resection margins were free of tumor.

Endoscopy Commentary

Anthony T.R. Axon (UK)[1]

History

This 76-year-old woman would not have been referred for endoscopy because GI screening for cancer is not normally undertaken in the West.

Endoscopy

Had endoscopy been undertaken, it would therefore have been for symptoms and the examination would have been orientated towards identifying a cause of the symptoms rather than seeking evidence of cancer. Had the procedure been undertaken for non-specific dyspepsia, it is probable that the lesion would not have been identified because it is set among rugosal folds. There is no abnormality of color and no ulceration. Had dye spray been used (and this is unlikely), the lesion would probably have been identified because after indigo carmine, the lumen is more distended, the folds have disappeared, and the lesion stands out more obviously. It is possible that it would have been seen without the indigo carmine if the stomach had been distended to a greater degree on the earlier photographs. Had it been recognized it would be seen to be a largish lesion, and biopsies would have been taken from it.

Histology

The Western pathologists have reported the lesion as likely to be a carcinoma and under these circumstances, a surgical referral would have been undertaken and the patient would have been subjected to total gastrectomy.

Summary

This lesion would not have been identified in the West because the patient would not have been referred for endoscopic screening for cancer. Had the lesion been identified, total gastrectomy would probably have been undertaken.

[1]See footnote on p. 4.

Endoscopy Commentary

Shigeaki Yoshida (Japan)

A depressed lesion surrounded by annular-form elevation is located in the anterior wall of the antrum. The size of the lesion is estimated to be around 20 mm. In conventional endoscopy, this is seen as a superficial depression surrounded by a worm-like elevation whose surface is smooth and lustrous, similar to gastric adenoma. The definite finding of the moth-eaten appearance can be pointed out particularly at the greater curvature side, as shown in Fig. 4A and B. Dye-spraying pictures (Fig. 4C and D) reveal fold-like components within the depressed area and, in particular, Fig. 4D demonstrates the irregular margin of the depression indicating the definite malignancy of the lesion.

The first question is which macroscopic type is more likely, IIa+IIc or IIc, because marginal elevation is not only seen in type IIa+IIc but occasionally in type IIc. In spite of this, type IIa+IIc appears to be more acceptable for the lesion presented, because the marginal elevation is obviously and constantly seen regardless of whether pictures are from conventional or dye-spraying endoscopy. In addition, fold-like elevation within the depressed area may indicate that this lesion is essentially an elevated lesion.

The second question is whether the lesion accords with submucosal (or much deeper) invasion. In the case of type IIa+IIc being deeply invasive, the following suggestive findings are usually detectable: (1) deep and destructive depression, (2) annular formation due to fusion of elevated components, (3) slow-sloped elevation surrounding the depressed area, and/or (4) converging folds due to disturbance of elasticity of the gastric wall by massive deeper invasion. In this lesion, however, the above findings are not detected at all and elevated components seen in the depressed area, meaning less destruction, should indicate a very low probability of submucosal invasion.

As to the histological type, hyperemic and smooth-surfaced appearances in the depressed area, in addition to fewer eroded components in the elevated component, are the findings being highly suggestive of the differentiated type of tubular adenocarcinoma.

In conclusion, this lesion can be diagnosed as a nonulcerative IIa+IIc type of early cancer being of differentiated type histologically, whose invasion is limited to within the mucosal layer.

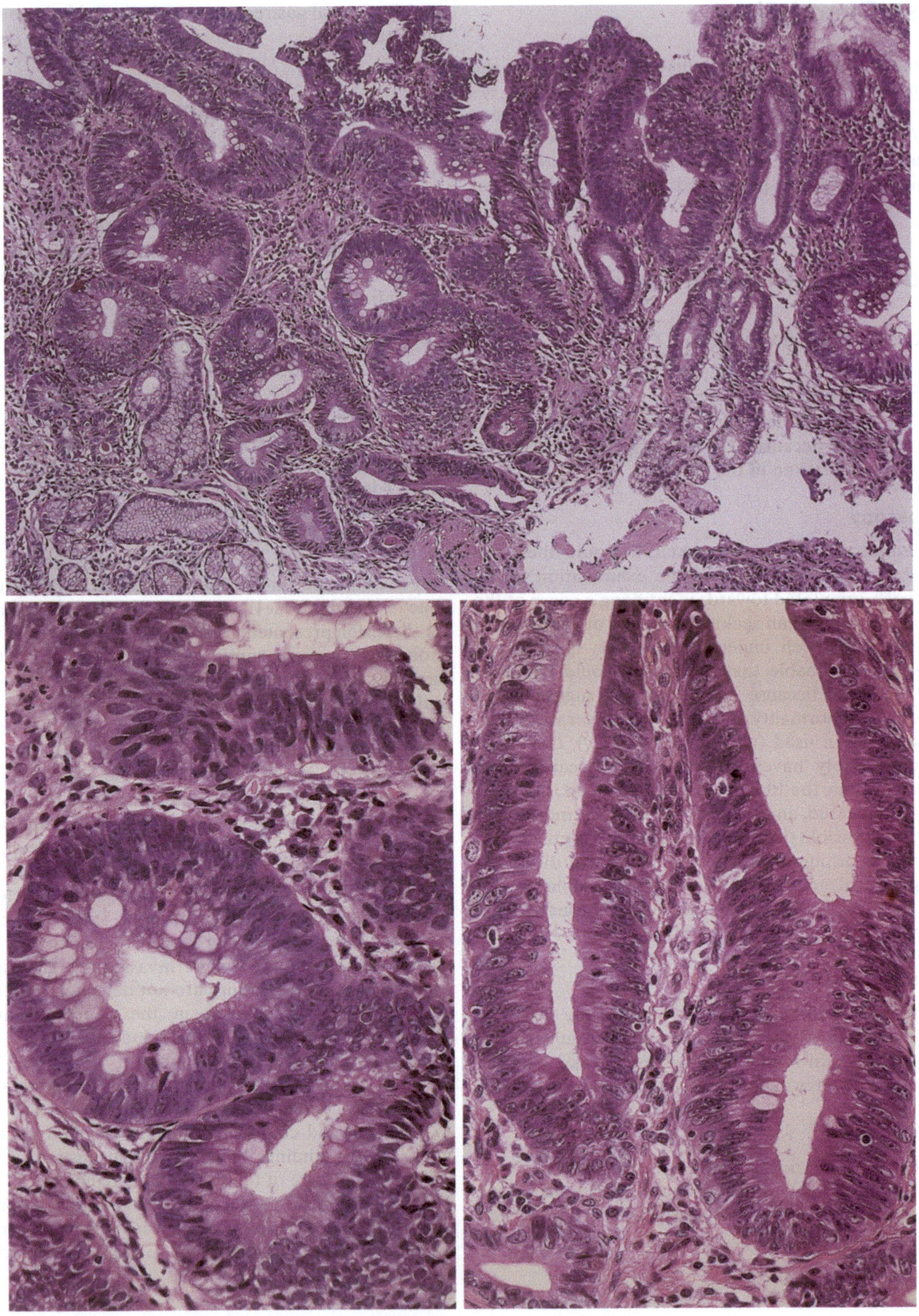

E F G

Fig. 4. **E** Biopsy specimen. **F** Detail of **E** (biopsy). **G** Detail of resected specimen

Table 4. Gastric lesion 4

Biopsy: ×
Resection: ○

	W	J	W W	WW WW WW WJ	W W	W	W	W	J	J	J JJ JJ JJ	W	W	W	W W
Regenerative changes		×													
Indefinite for neoplasia	×														
Adenoma/dysplasia															
low-grade	○		×												
high-grade		○	○	⊗	○	×	×	○							
Carcinoma															
suspected					×	○			×	○		×			
non-invasive							○		○		⊗		○	×	
intramucosal								×		×		○	×	○	⊗

Endoscopic mucosal resection can be selected for the treatment of this lesion, i.e., a differentiated type of early cancer with a very low possibility of submucosal invasion. Considering the size being around 20mm in diameter, however, conventional strip biopsy [1] appears to be a difficult approach to make a one-segment resection because of the limitation in size of the snare loop. In such cases, our newly developed EMR using an IT-knife should be useful, as previously reported [2, 3].

References

1. Tada M, Karita M, Yanai M (1987) Treatment of early gastric cancer using strip biopsy: a new technique for jumbo biopsy. In: Takemoto T, Kaeai T (eds). Recent topics of digestive endoscopy. Excerpta Medics, Tokyo, pp 137–142
2. Yoshida S (1998) Endoscopic diagnosis and treatment of early cancer in the alimentary tract. Digestion 59:502–508
3. Ono H, Kondo H, Gotoda T, et al (2001) Endoscopic mucosal resection for treatment of early gastric cancer. *Gut* 48:225–229

Pathology Commentary

Manfred Stolte (Germany)

Examination of the biopsy specimen from this lesion leaves no doubt as to the diagnosis of neoplasia. The nuclei of the tumor cells in the neoplastic tubuli manifest an irregular arrangement, contain an irregular chromatin structure and prominent nucleoli, and show abnormal mitotic figures (Fig. 4F).

The differential diagnosis includes high-grade dysplasia, noninvasive carcinoma, or an intramucosal carcinoma. In my opinion, however, clear criteria for the diagnosis of invasive intramucosal carcinoma are to be seen in Fig. 4E, which shows not only disruption of the normal glandular architecture of the antral mucosa, but also a horizontal invasive neoplastic tubule parallel to the muscularis mucosae. A further criterion for invasion is the finding of tiny glandular structures in the vicinity of this tubule.

In the endoscopic mucosectomy specimen (Fig. 4H, I, and G), the predominantly parallel arrangement of neoplastic glands running perpendicular to the surface suggests that this lesion might be "only" high-grade intraepithelial neoplasm or noninvasive carcinoma. Evidence for intramucosal carcinoma, however, is again the atypical neoplastic branches in the left margin of the lesion, and several tiny neoplastic glands that can be seen at the base of the lesion.

In conclusion I would diagnose, both in the biopsy material and the endoscopic mucosectomy specimen, a well-differentiated tubular adenocarcinoma limited to the mucosa.

The spectrum of diagnoses in this case is unusually wide. Most Western pathologists and two Japanese pathologists diagnosed only dysplasia—mostly high-grade dysplasia—while the majority of the Japanese pathologists opted for noninvasive carcinoma, and four of the other Western pathologists diagnosed an intramucosal carcinoma on the basis of the criteria mentioned above.

Pathology Commentary

Yo Kato (Japan)

The biopsy specimen indicates that the lesion consists of immature intestinal-type tubular glands, which are slightly irregularly distributed and contain a fair number of goblet cells. The lamina propria mucosae is

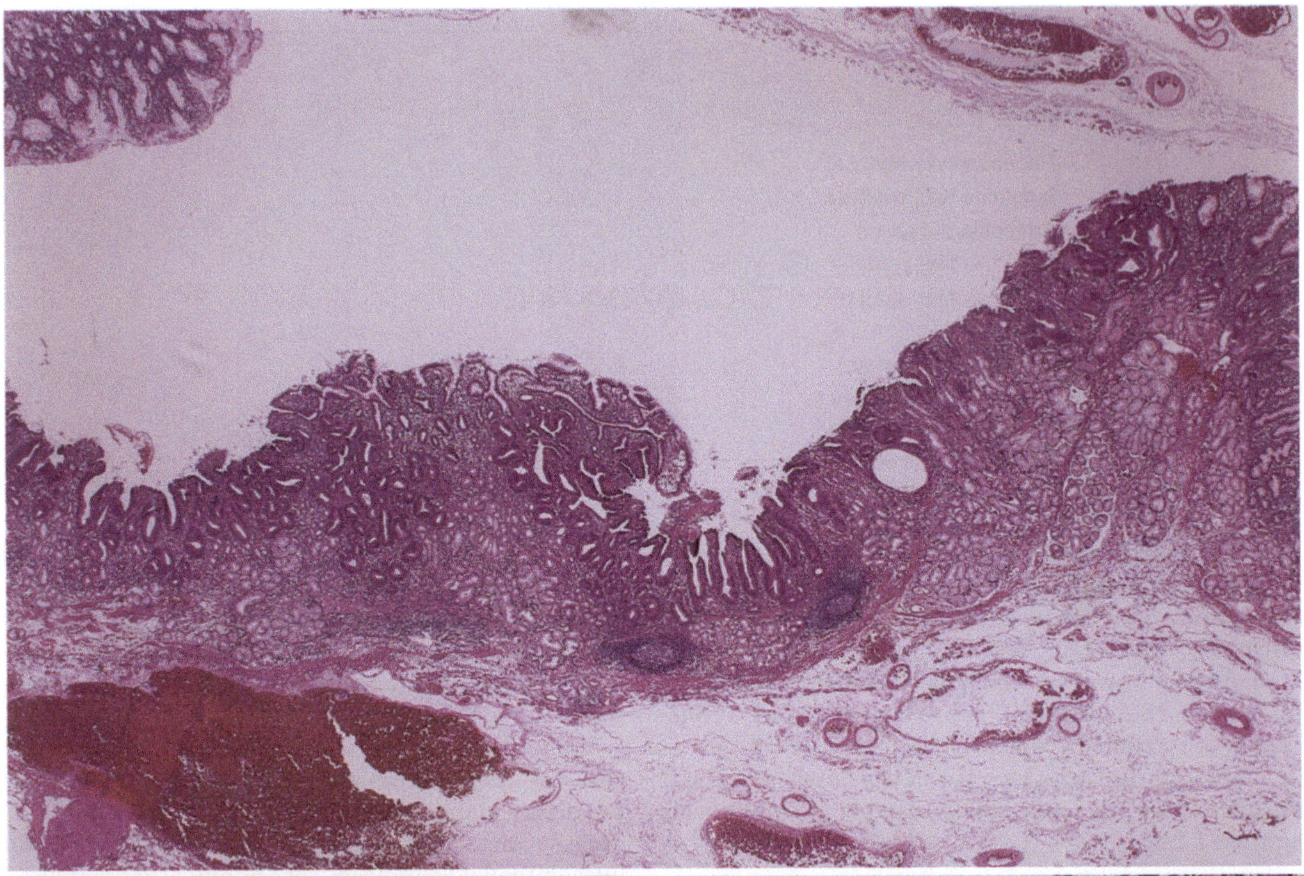

H

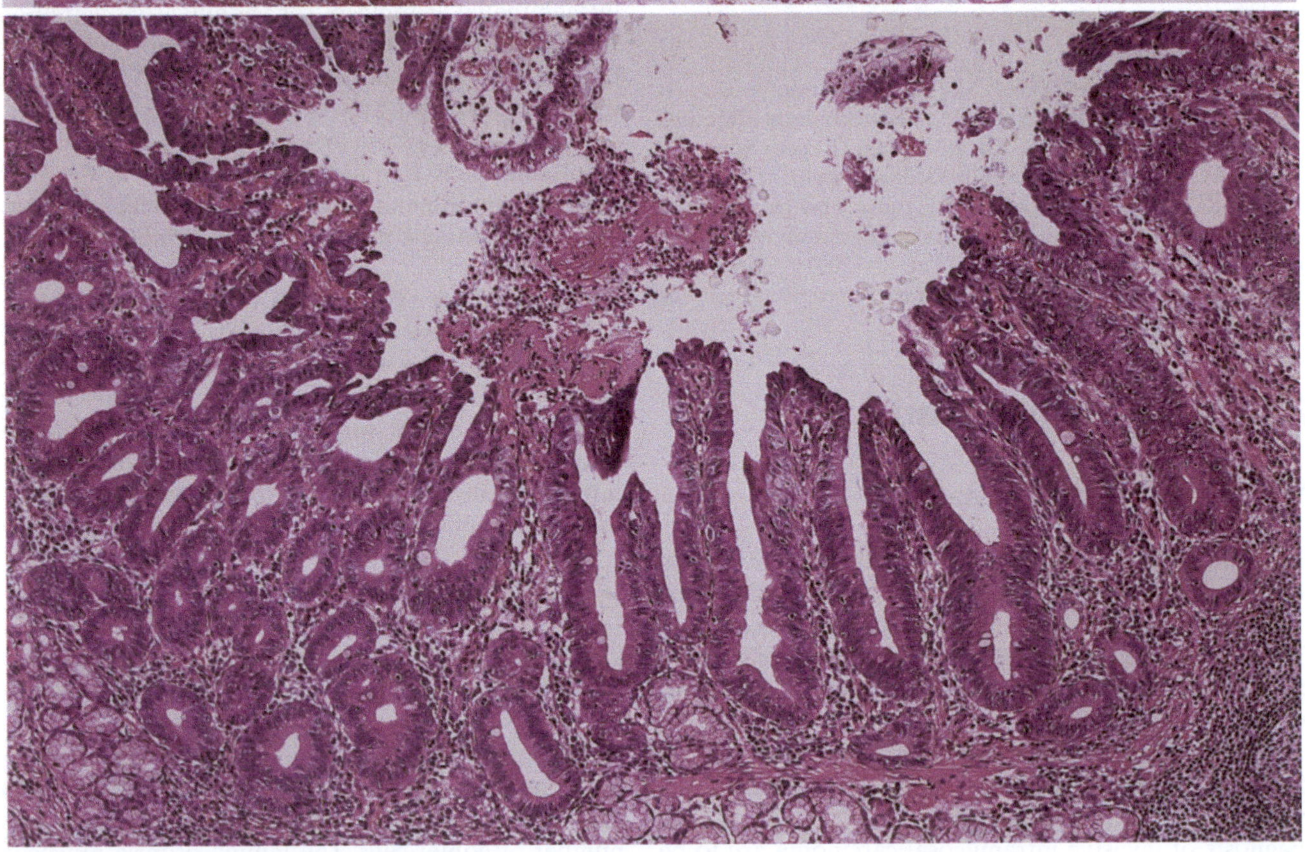

I

Fig. 4. **H** Resected specimen. **I** Detail of **H**

infiltrated with inflammatory cells. Because of the presence of slightly irregular-shaped glands with nuclear stratification in the surface of the lesion, or loss of maturation from the bottom toward the top of the glands, the change is judged as group IV, i.e., suspicion of very well-differentiated tubular carcinoma according to the Japanese classification: the change will correspond to adenoma/dysplasia of high-grade from a Western viewpoint. Figure 4F is a magnification of the center of Fig. 4E, showing round glands with crowded ovoid plump nuclei situated along the basement membrane and the epithelium, with disoriented similar nuclei in the surface of the lesion.

The EMR specimen shows a small depressed lesion (Fig. 4H), which consists of short, straight tubular or round glands (Fig. 4I). Each gland is composed of eosinophilic, tall columnar cells with an oval nucleus having a prominent nucleolus. The cells are like absorptive cells or immature cells of the small intestine. Similarly to the biopsy specimen, the nucleus is located along the basement membrane, but goblet cells are decreased in number. Since there is no tendency of the cells to differentiate from the bottom toward the surface of the glands, very well-differentiated tubular carcinoma, noninvasive, is diagnosed. The lesion was completely resected.

Case 5, IIc

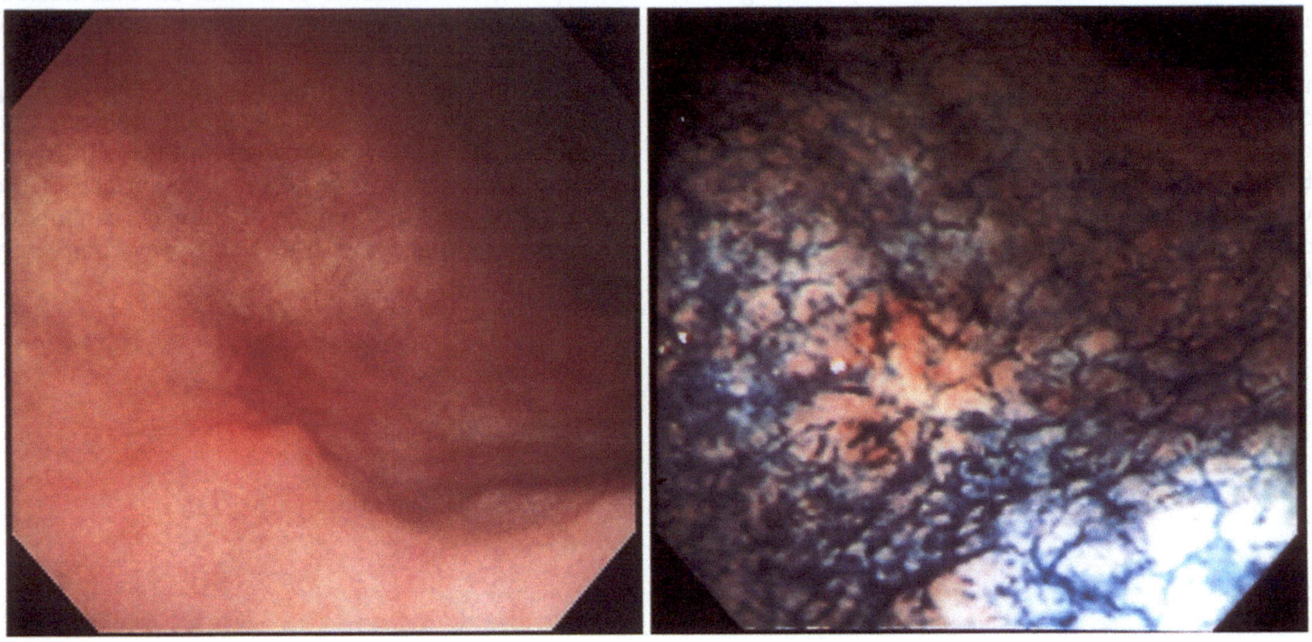

A B

Fig. 5. **A** Antrum, greater curvature. **B** Same site after spraying indigo carmine

Table 5. Gastric lesion 5

Biopsy: × Resection: ○	W W	W W	W	W W	W W	W W	W W	W W	J	W W	W J	J J J W J J J	W J J J
Regenerative changes	×												
Indefinite for neoplasia		×											
Adenoma/dysplasia													
low-grade			×	×									
high-grade					⊗	×							
Carcinoma													
suspected						○	⊗	×		×			
non-invasive			○						×			×	
intramucosal	○	○						○	○		⊗		×
submucosal				○						○		○	○

Case Description

A man, aged 67 years, with a history of recurrent gastric ulcers and ischemic heart disease, underwent upper GI screening by endoscopic examination. Apart from two gastric ulcer scars, a lesion of 7 mm in diameter at the greater curvature of the antrum and a lesion of about 15 mm in diameter at the greater curvature of the corpus were found and biopsied. Four months later endoscopic ultrasonographic examination and endoscopic resection of both lesions were performed. Histological examination revealed submucosal invasion of one of the lesions. Moreover, the resection margins were not free of tumor. Three months later subtotal gastrectomy with lymph node resection was performed. In the surgical specimen, no neoplastic changes could be observed.

Endoscopy Commentary

Anthony T.R. Axon (UK)[1]

History

It is possible that a man of 67 years with a history of recurrent gastric ulcer would have been referred for upper digestive endoscopy in the West, particularly if he was complaining of gastric symptoms.

Endoscopic Appearance

The gastric antrum shows some slight erythema and irregularity on the greater curve. There is, however, no evidence of ulceration, neither does the antrum appear atrophic nor contain intestinal metaplasia macroscopically.

Dye spraying shows slight abnormality in the areae gastricae. Dye spraying would not have been undertaken in the West in this case and had it been done, it is unlikely that it would have raised suspicion. Western endoscopists do biopsy areas of irregularity so it is possible that a biopsy might have been taken from the affected area, but in view of the past history of gastric ulcer it is probable that the irregularity would have been attributed to scarring from the previous ulcers. On balance, I think most endoscopists would probably not have specifically biopsied that area.

A Western endoscopist looking at this lesion would regard it as irregular but flat, and I think would describe it more as IIb than IIc if making an assessment; however, as indicated earlier, we have little experience of these lesions in the West.

[1]See footnote on p. 4.

Histology

Had biopsies been taken the Western pathologists would have rated the appearance as high grade or worse. As indicated earlier, the high-grade dysplasia would probably have led to further endoscopies and more biopsies and that would have confirmed a presence of high-grade dysplasia or worse. A diagnosis of indefinite for neoplasia would also have led to further endoscopic examination.

Management

The presence of high-grade dysplasia or cancer will undoubtedly have led to surgical referral and gastric resection, in this case probably partial gastrectomy.

Summary

It is possible that this patient would have been referred for endoscopy in the West, but I do not believe that the endoscopist would have diagnosed or been suspicious of cancer at endoscopy. It is possible that biopsies would have been taken from the affected area, in which case the patient would have been referred for gastric resection.

Endoscopy Commentary

Shigeaki Yoshida (Japan)

A shallow, depressed lesion can be pointed out on the greater curvature of the antrum. In conventional endoscopy (Fig. 5A), its finding is described as "faint and monotonous hyperemic appearance of which the margin is unclear." Since this is one of the representative findings in gastritis-like early cancer [1, 2], the malignancy of the lesion is highly suggestive.

The question is how to estimate the lateral extent of cancerous invasion. Actually, it is hard to trace the definite margin of the hyperemic area in the conventional endoscopic picture, but precise observation clarifies that there are two components in this area. One is the slightly elevated formation with shallow depression on the oral side and the other the shallow depression on the faint fold-like structure on the anal side. Hence, whether or not the invasion includes both components appears to be a point that needs clarifying, and a dye-spraying picture (Fig. 5B) reveals nonspecific mucosa dividing the above two components, indicating the possibility of two different lesions or the possibility that a biopsy was taken from the center of a single antral lesion. Although details are not well visualized, the

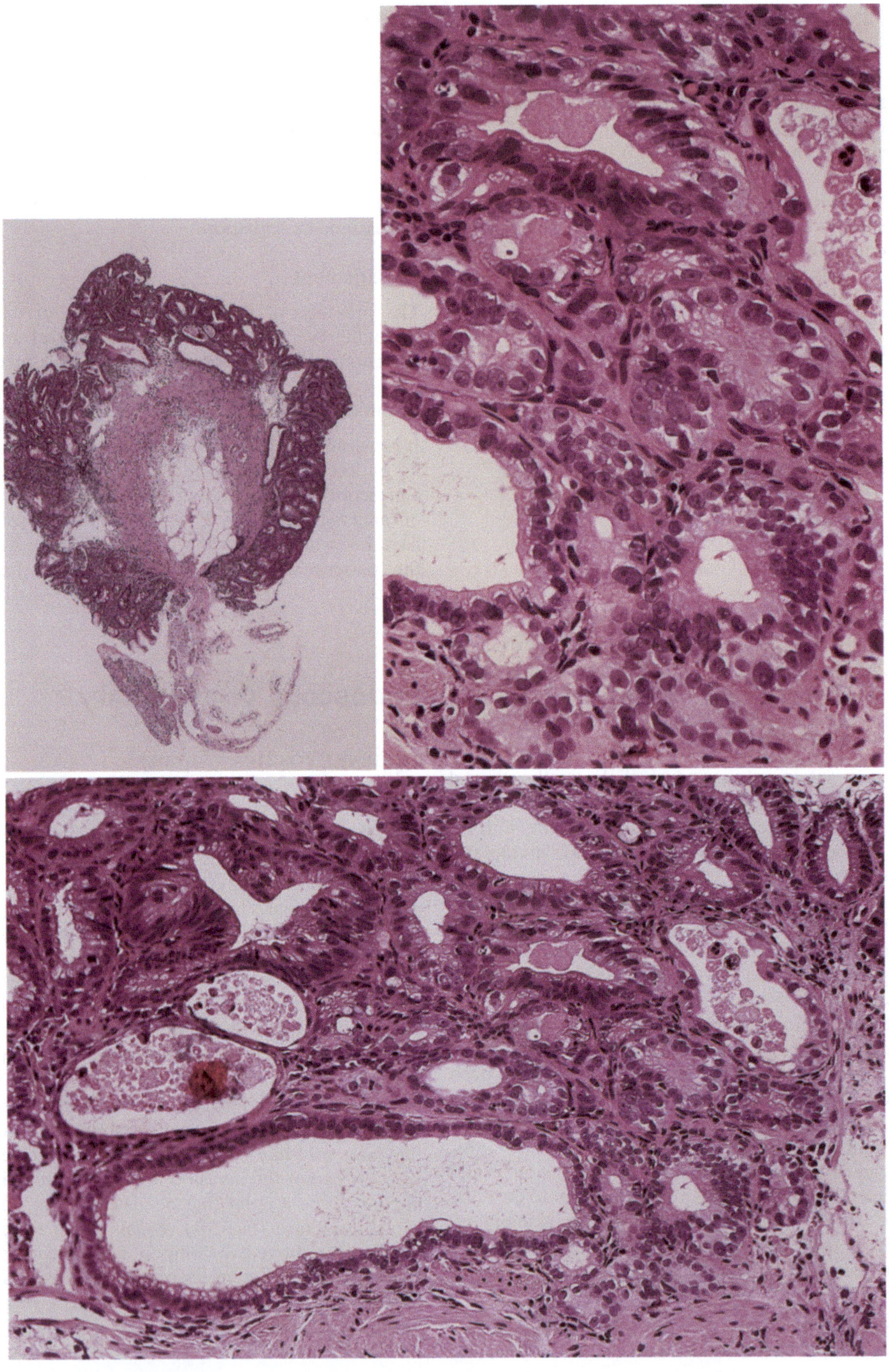
C E D

Fig. 5. **C** Biopsy specimen. **D** Detail of **C**. **E** Detail of **D**

invasive area of IIc can be estimated as limited to within the depressed area on the oral side, due to its well-demarcated marginal irregularity. Malignancy is also highly suggested in the shallow depressed area on the anal side, due to a hyperemic area whose margin is partially irregular, and a tiny star-shaped depression located at the edge of the anterior wall of this area. If the invasion includes both anal and oral areas, the size is estimated as 10–12 mm, referring to the diameter of *areae gastricae.* Otherwise, if they were separated, the oral lesion may be less than 5 mm and the anal one 8–10 mm in size, respectively.

As to the histological type, it can be said that cancerous lesions in the antrum showing a faint and monotonous hyperemic appearance are mostly of the differentiated type histologically. In the case presented here there is no finding suggesting submucosal invasion or ulcerative change within the cancerous area.

Endoscopically, therefore, the final diagnosis of this case should be two areas of nonulcerative IIc, being of the differentiated type histologically, whose sizes are estimated as less than 5 mm orally and 8–10 mm anally, respectively.

Endoscopic mucosal resection can be indicated because there is no suggestive finding of submucosal invasion.

References

1. Yoshida S, Yamaguchi H, Saito D et al (1993) Endoscopic diagnosis; latest trends. In: Nishi M, Ichikawa H, Nakajima T, et al (eds) Gastric cancer Springer, Tokyo, pp 246–262
2. Yoshida S (1998) Endoscipic diagnosis and treatment of early cancer in the alimentary tract. Digestion 59:502–508

Pathology Commentary

Manfred Stolte (Germany)

It can already be seen in the low-power overview (Fig. 5C) that the normal glands of the gastric mucosa have been replaced by a highly irregular arrangement of neoplastic tubuli. Under higher magnification (Fig. 5D and E), the tubuli that are lined by neoplastic epithelial cells are unusually densely packed and show some irregular branching of varying caliber. This finding is incompatible with the diagnosis of intraepithelial neoplasia (dysplasia). Rather, there is almost complete replacement of the original lamina propria, now hardly recognizable, by invasive neoplastic structures. In Fig. 5E, tubular formations are focally unrecognizable. In addition, the usual cytological criteria for the diagnosis of carcinoma are met.

In the overview of the endoscopic mucosectomy specimen (Fig. 5F) it is already clear that the neoplasm is not limited to the mucosa, but that irregularly branched neoplastic tubuli of varying caliber have penetrated through the muscularis mucosae and extend into the upper part of the submucosa. Under higher magnification (Fig. 5G) it becomes clear that this cannot be a pseudoinvasion, since there is no destruction of the muscularis mucosae, no fibrosis of the adjacent lamina propria, and no other evidence of a prior traumatic lesion of the mucosa and submucosa with secondary displacement of glandular components into the submucosa. In the high power views of the invasive part of the tumor in the submucosa (Fig. 5G and I), the changes in the cell nuclei and their position are not as marked as in the biopsy material. Here, many of the nuclei are located in the base of the cylindrical epithelial cells, are only mildly enlarged, and are moderately hyperchromatic. Prominent nucleoli are also seen less frequently. The lightly stained cytoplasm indicates that mucus is still being produced. These histological and cytological criteria strongly favor an adenocarcinoma with gastric differentiation, which might be confirmed by immunohistochemistry for MUC6.

In conclusion, therefore, both the biopsy and the endoscopic mucosectomy specimens reveal a well-differentiated adenocarcinoma. In the mucosectomy specimen, there is already focal invasion of the carcinoma into the upper part of the submucosa (sm1) but without invasion of lymphatic or blood vessels. The histological structure and the cytology of the tumor cells in this case indicate an adenocarcinoma with gastric differentiation.

An analysis of the diagnoses again reveals considerable variability. Nine Western pathologists diagnosed no carcinoma in the biopsy, but corrected their diagnosis in the mucosectomy specimen. However, only two of these pathologists interpreted the neoplastic glands in the submucosa as invasive submucosal carcinoma, while the majority of the Japanese pathologists and four Western pathologists who adopt the "Japanese viewpoint" interpreted the findings as clearly showing a submucosal carcinoma.

Pathology Commentary

Yo Kato (Japan)

The biopsy specimen is compacted with slightly irregular-shaped and -sized round glands, particularly in the upper half of the mucosa (Fig. 5C). In the upper part of Fig. 5D, medium-sized glands with occasional amorphous excretion or cell debris are composed of

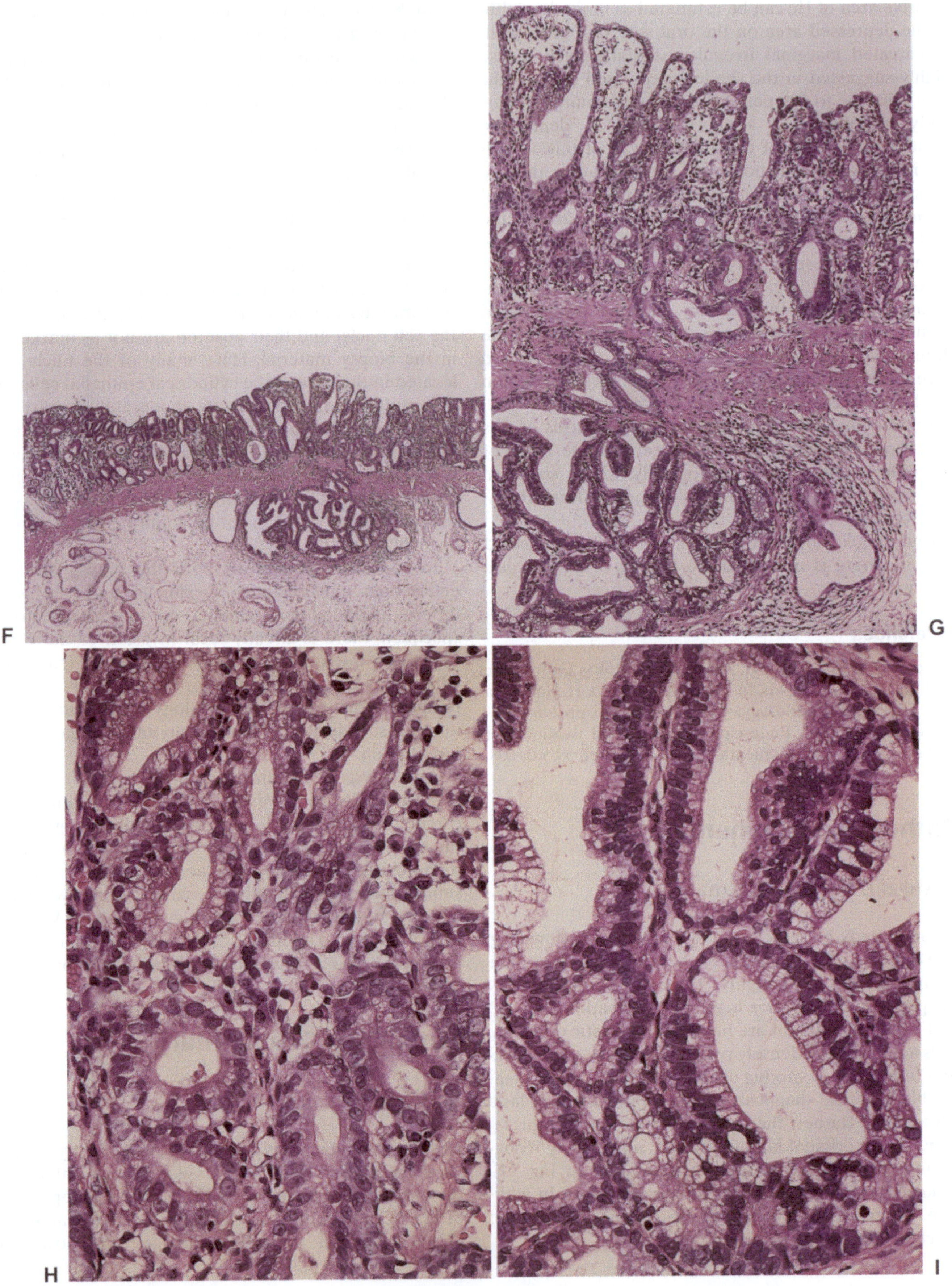

Fig. 5. **F** Resected specimen. **G** Detail of **F**. **H** Detail of **G** (mucosal portion). **I** Detail of **G** (submucosal portion)

eosinophilic columnar to cuboidal cells, i.e., intestinal-type cells, with an ovoid or spindle-shaped hyperchromatic nucleus. Here there is loss of polarity of the nuclei, and thus stratification of the nuclei is rather prominent. On the other hand, in the middle to lower part of the figure, small and large glands and a cystic-dilated gland are mixed up, and their constituent of light eosinophilic cuboidal cells is of immature gastric or pyloric gland phenotype, equally equipped with a swollen, round, pale nucleus and a prominent nucleolus. With these findings of the biopsy specimen, the atypical glands are diagnosed simply as very well-differentiated carcinoma without referring to "invasive or noninvasive" according to Japanese criteria, but will be interpreted as high-grade dysplasia/neoplasia from the Western viewpoint since there are no evident findings of invasion. Some small glands in the lower part of the figure and some parts of cystic-dilated glands, however, can be residues of non-neoplastic glands or epithelium since the nuclear sizes are smaller than those in the glands of the middle part (Fig. 5D,E). Concerning the epithelial phenotype, a mixed intestinal and gastric one is considered.

The EMR specimen shows both mucosal and submucosal lesions, consisting of slightly irregular-shaped tubular glands, and the atypical glands clearly invade the submucosa through the muscularis mucosae (Fig. 5F,G). The high-power view of the mucosal lesion as shown in Fig. 5H is more homogeneous in pattern than in the biopsy specimen (Fig. 5E), formed by round tubular glands made of cuboidal cells with a round nucleus and a prominent nucleolus. Figure 5I is a high-power view of the submucosal lesion, showing aggregates of slightly irregular-shaped glands composed of cuboidal mucinous cells with a hyperchromatic round to oval nucleus. These mucinous cells appear partly pyloric gland-like, partly goblet cell-like. It should be made clear that similar atypical glands have already appeared in the mucosa where the invasive pattern is not clear. As a whole, the lesion is diagnosed as very well-differentiated carcinoma with submucosal invasion.

Case 6, IIa

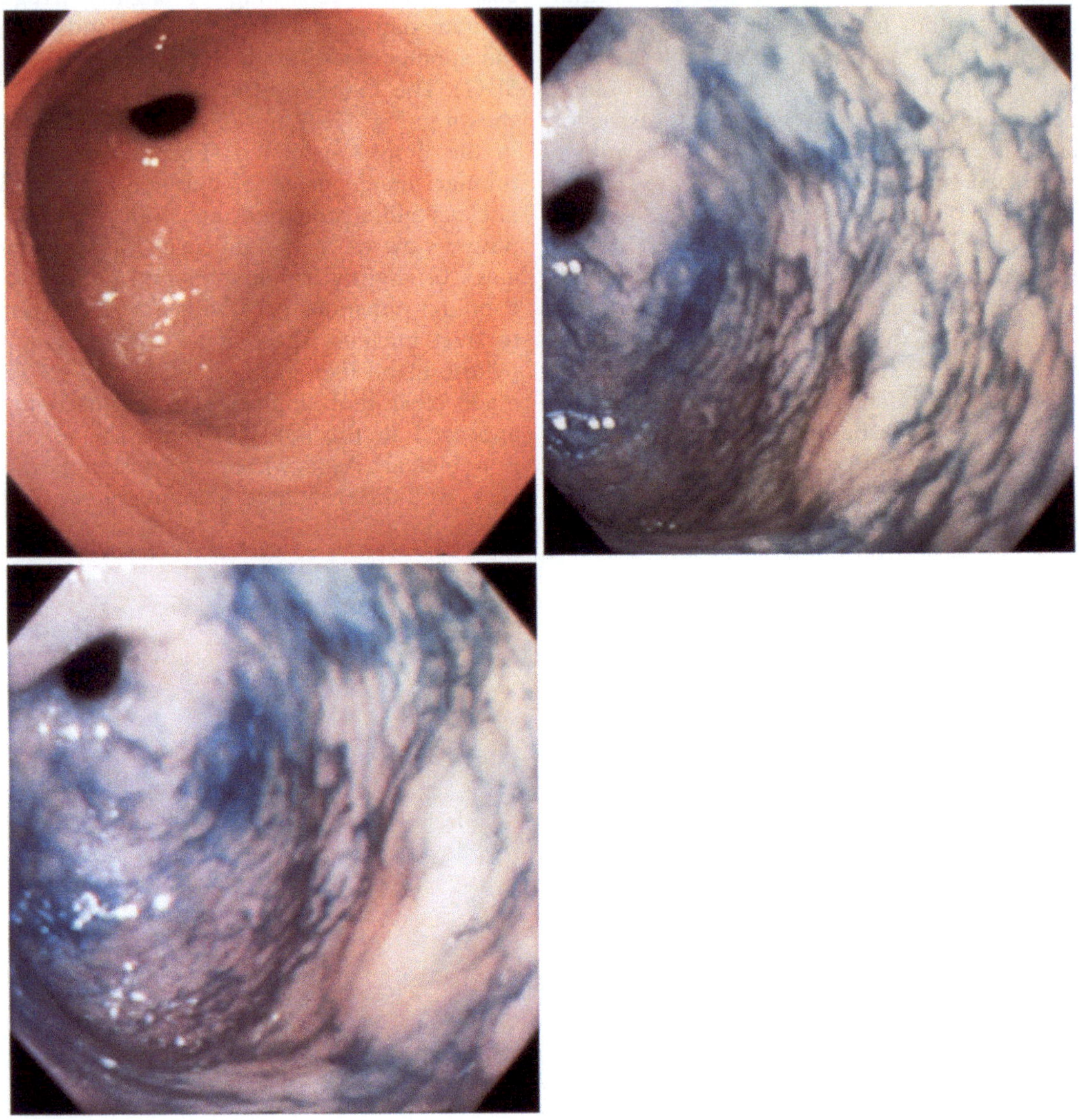

A B C

Fig. 6. **A** Antrum, posterior wall. **B** Same site after spraying indigo carmine. **C** Close-up view

Table 6. Gastric lesion 6

Biopsy: × Resection: ○	W W W W W W W W J	W W W J W W W W W J	W W	W J	J	W	J	J	J	J J J
Adenoma/dysplasia										
low-grade	⊗	○	○	○						
high-grade		×			○	○	×			
Carcinoma										
suspected			×					⊗	○	
non-invasive				×	×		○		×	⊗
intramucosal						×				

Case Description

A man, aged 69 years, known to have von Recklinghausen disease and Parkinson syndrome, underwent upper GI screening by endoscopic examination. A lesion of about 1 cm in diameter was found at the posterior wall of the antrum and was biopsied. Two months later he underwent endoscopic ultrasonographic examination and shortly thereafter, endoscopic resection was performed. The resection margins were free of tumor.

Endoscopy Commentary

Anthony T.R. Axon (UK)[1]

History

This case again is one that was referred for upper GI cancer screening and would not have occurred in the West. Endoscopy in the West is carried out only for symptoms, and Western endoscopists therefore seek a cause of the symptoms of which the patient is complaining, looking for ulcers in the duodenum or stomach, evidence of reflux esophagitis, gastric stasis, erosions, and gastritis. They do not look for slight irregularities or changes in color because these are not appearances that give rise to symptoms. This means that Western endoscopists miss these early changes of cancer. It is this difference of approach that influences the endoscopist in that you tend to "find what you are looking for." The Japanese, on the other hand, with a high incidence of cancer, search for these early cancers and find them.

Endoscopic Appearance

In this case the appearance of the antrum to a Western endoscopist appears to be normal. Dye spray, however, reveals a slightly elevated lesion on the posterior wall of the antrum with a depression in its center. As shown on the dye spray the appearance is suspicious of cancer and if this was identified by a Western endoscopist, biopsies would have been taken.

Histology

It is interesting that the Western pathologists felt that the appearance was that of low-grade, or at worst, high-grade dysplasia. A report of this nature would have led to a further endoscopy with more biopsies; the patient would then have been put into a surveillance routine that would have caused the pathologists to take a second opinion. In time, if high-grade dysplasia was again identified the patient would have been referred for gastric resection.

Summary

Again, this is a case where the patient would not have been submitted for endoscopy in the West and where the lesion would have been missed. Had it been identified, further endoscopies with biopsy would have been undertaken and eventually it is likely that it would have led to gastrectomy.

[1]See footnote on p. 4.

Endoscopy Commentary

Shigeaki Yoshida (Japan)

On the posterior wall of the antrum five or more superficial elevated lesions having a shallow central depression can be pointed out on conventional endoscopy (Fig. 6A). They are similar to each other in their gross appearance, though the most proximal lesion is larger than any of the other lesions. Because these elevated lesions show nonspecific color change and no irregularity in the depressed component, they are diagnosed as erosive gastritis in this picture. Further examination using dye-spraying endoscopy is required to make the differential diagnosis more accurate in this type of lesion.

A dye-spraying picture (Fig. 6B) reveals that only the most proximal lesion is actually solid, though the others have changed their appearance to be inconspicuous and nonspecific. In that lesion, elevated components are shown to be discolored and lustrous like gastric adenomas, but a faint hyperemic appearance in the shallow depression seen particularly in the close-up view is strongly suggestive of its malignancy (Fig. 6C).

According to the gross appearance of a plateau-like elevation involving a negligible shallow depression, the lesion can be diagnosed as type IIa early cancer, whose size is estimated to be around 1 cm, because the circumference of the prepyloric region is usually around 8 cm in the resected specimen.

In type IIa early cancer deeper invasion is generally rare, and in such a case the lesion is usually larger than 2 cm and frequently incorporates an eroded shallow depression. In addition, the undifferentiated type is rare in type IIa early cancer, and in such a case the lesion shows an eroded surface structure and/or discoloration without lustrous appearance. Hence, the lesion presented here can be estimated as mucosal cancer of the differentiated type, and EMR should be the first choice for the treatment of this lesion because of its size, histological type, and estimated depth of invasion.

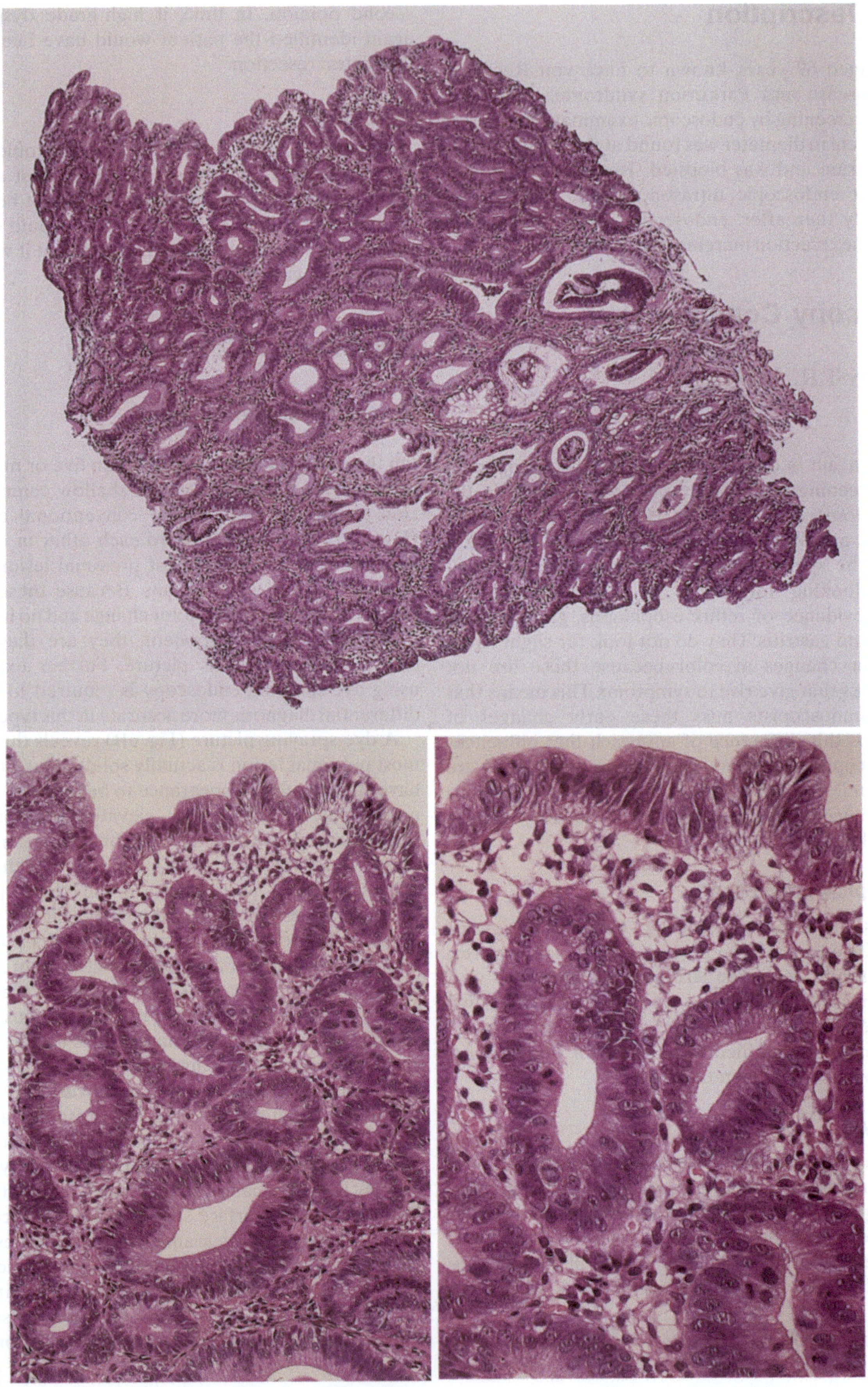

D

E

F

Fig. 6. **D** Biopsy specimen. **E** Detail of **D**. **F** Detail of **E**

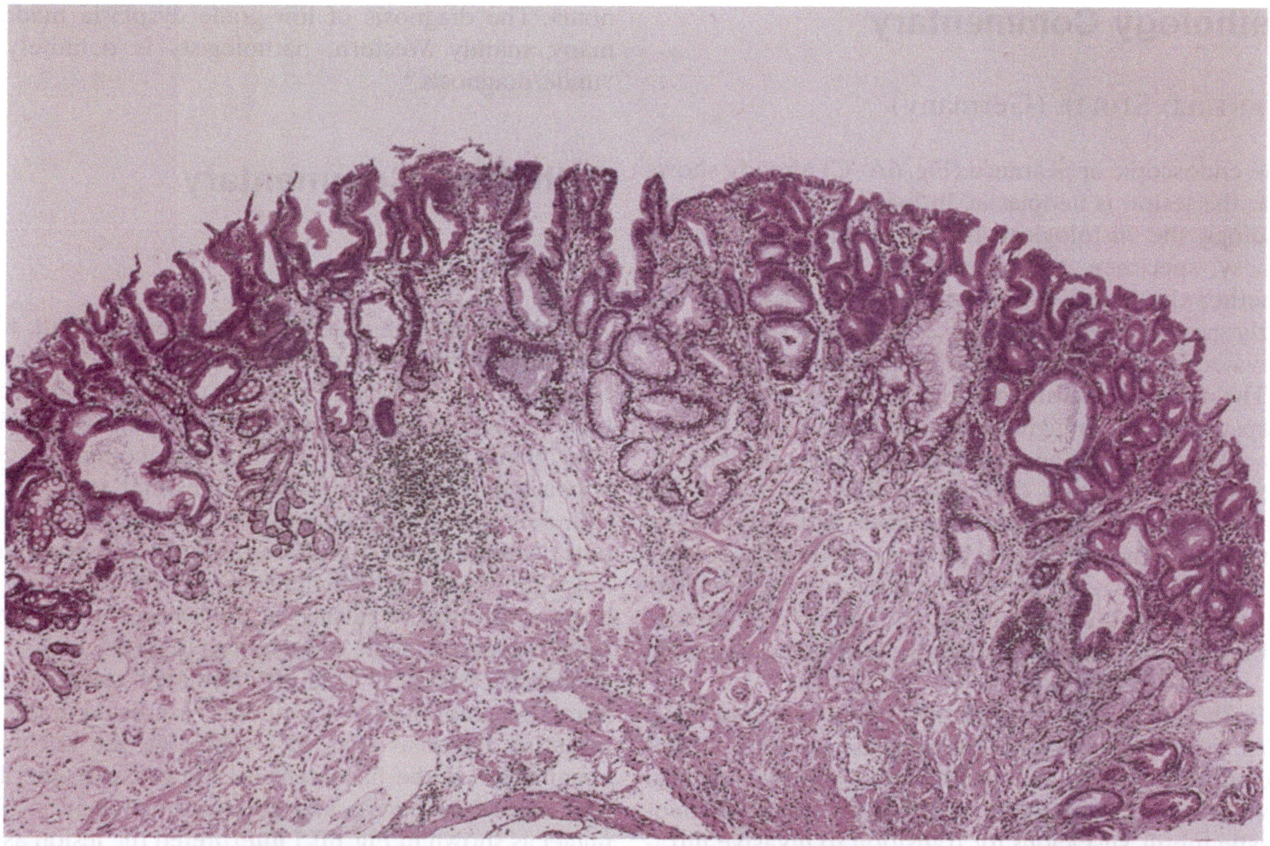

G

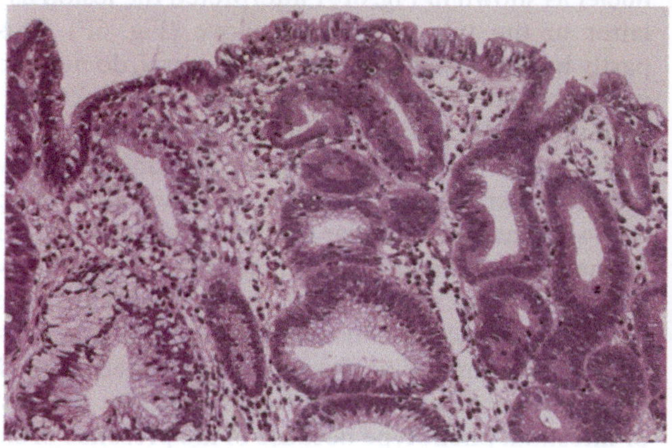

H

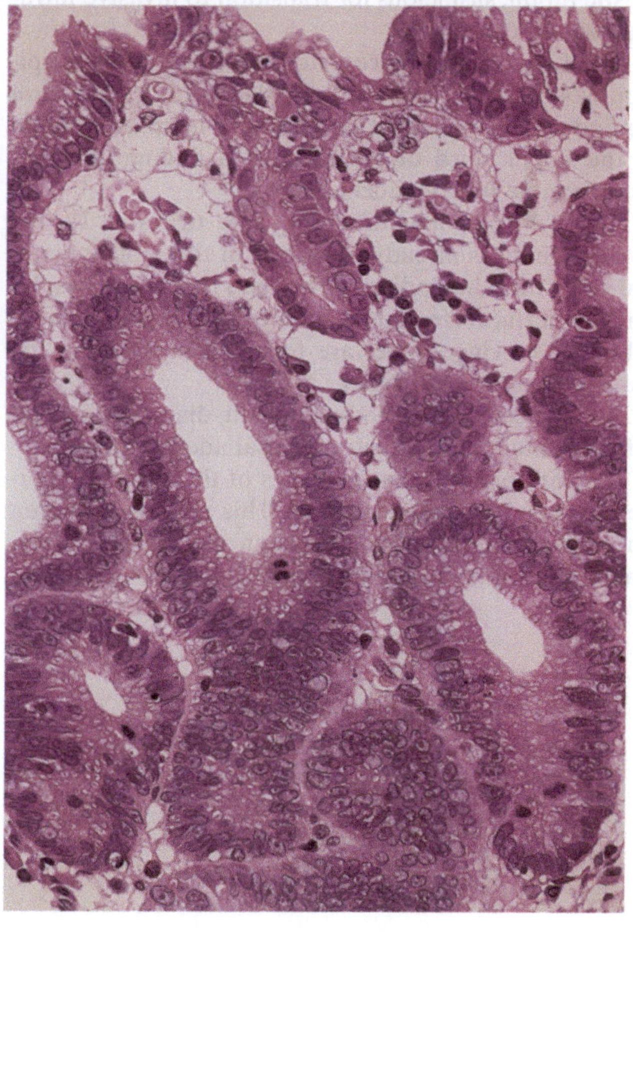

I

Fig. 6. G Resected specimen. **H** Detail of **G**. **I** Detail of **H**

Pathology Commentary

Manfred Stolte (Germany)

The endoscopic appearance (Fig. 6A–C) already shows that the lesion is neoplastic. In light of the endoscopic findings, the histological differential diagnosis of the biopsy specimen was concerned with determining whether the lesion is only an adenoma or a type IIa early gastric carcinoma. The central depression of the elevated lesion is a hint that this is a carcinoma.

The neoplastic nature of the lesion is confirmed in the biopsy material. In higher magnification (Fig. 6E and F), the architecture of the neoplastic tubuli is still relatively ordered, so that the differential diagnosis has to be made between high-grade dysplasia and noninvasive carcinoma. The cytological changes of the tumor cells with their irregular arrangement of nuclei, irregular chromatin, prominent nucleoli, and multiple pathological mitotic figures are incompatible with the diagnosis of low-grade dysplasia.

In the low-power view of the biopsy specimen (Fig. 6D), the architecture of the neoplastic glands is also incompatible with an adenoma. In addition, it also reveals irregular branches and foci of horizontal neoplastic tubuli, suspicious for transition to invasive intramucosal carcinoma.

In the endoscopic mucosectomy specimen, this suspicion would appear to be validated (Fig. 6G), since here we find a mainly parallel expansion of neoplastic tubuli in the upper third of the mucosa, a finding which is incompatible with an adenoma.

Under higher magnification (Fig. 6H and I), the nuclear changes already described in the biopsy material show that the findings go beyond low-grade dysplasia. Furthermore, foci of irregularly arranged neoplastic tubuli of varying caliber are to be seen, which in my view indicate initial invasive growth.

In conclusion, therefore, I would diagnose a well-differentiated invasive intramucosal adenocarcinoma.

The variability in the diagnoses of this difficult "borderline case" is understandable. This applies, however, only to the differentiation between high-grade dysplasia, noninvasive carcinoma, and intramucosal carcinoma. The diagnosis of low-grade dysplasia made by many, mainly Western, pathologists is definitely an "underdiagnosis."

Pathology Commentary

Yo Kato (Japan)

The biopsy specimen is, though tangentially cut, filled with many rather equal-shaped and -sized atypical tubular or round glands except for the center which contains an aggregate of non-neoplastic glands (Fig. 6D). The glands consist of eosinophilic columnar cells, appearing to be of immature intestinal type, with a round or oval plump nucleus, with a conspicuous nucleolus throughout the glands. Mitoses are also prominent. Since the tendency of the cells to differentiate from the bottom toward the surface of the lesion is not definite, both adenoma with severe atypia (i.e., high-grade adenoma) and very well-differentiated tubular carcinoma (i.e., noninvasive carcinoma) are listed in the differential diagnosis (Fig. 6E). Although the nucleus is situated along the basement membrane, with the findings described above and too conspicuously swollen nuclei as shown in Fig. 6F, I interpreted the lesion as the latter of the two mentioned above (Fig. 6F). This is partly because we pathologists, in general, do not like to make an underdiagnosis at the time of biopsy.

In the EMR specimen (Fig. 6G), the lesion is situated in the upper half of the mucosa, consisting, similarly to the biopsy specimen (Fig. 6D), of rather equal-shaped and -sized atypical tubular or round glands. Again, since no maturation tendency throughout the epithelium with generally round, plump nuclei exists, with no further evidence of invasion, I consider the lesion as noninvasive adenocarcinoma of very well-differentiated type (Fig. 6H,I). The constituent tumor cells look like the gastric or intestinal phenotype because of the presence of small mucus droplets in the cytoplasm of the tumor cells (Fig. 6H,I). Interestingly, there is a double-layered gland with many goblet cells in the figures (Fig. 6G, center and Fig. 6H, left): the gland seems to be non-neoplastic, but its significance is unknown.

Case 7, IIa

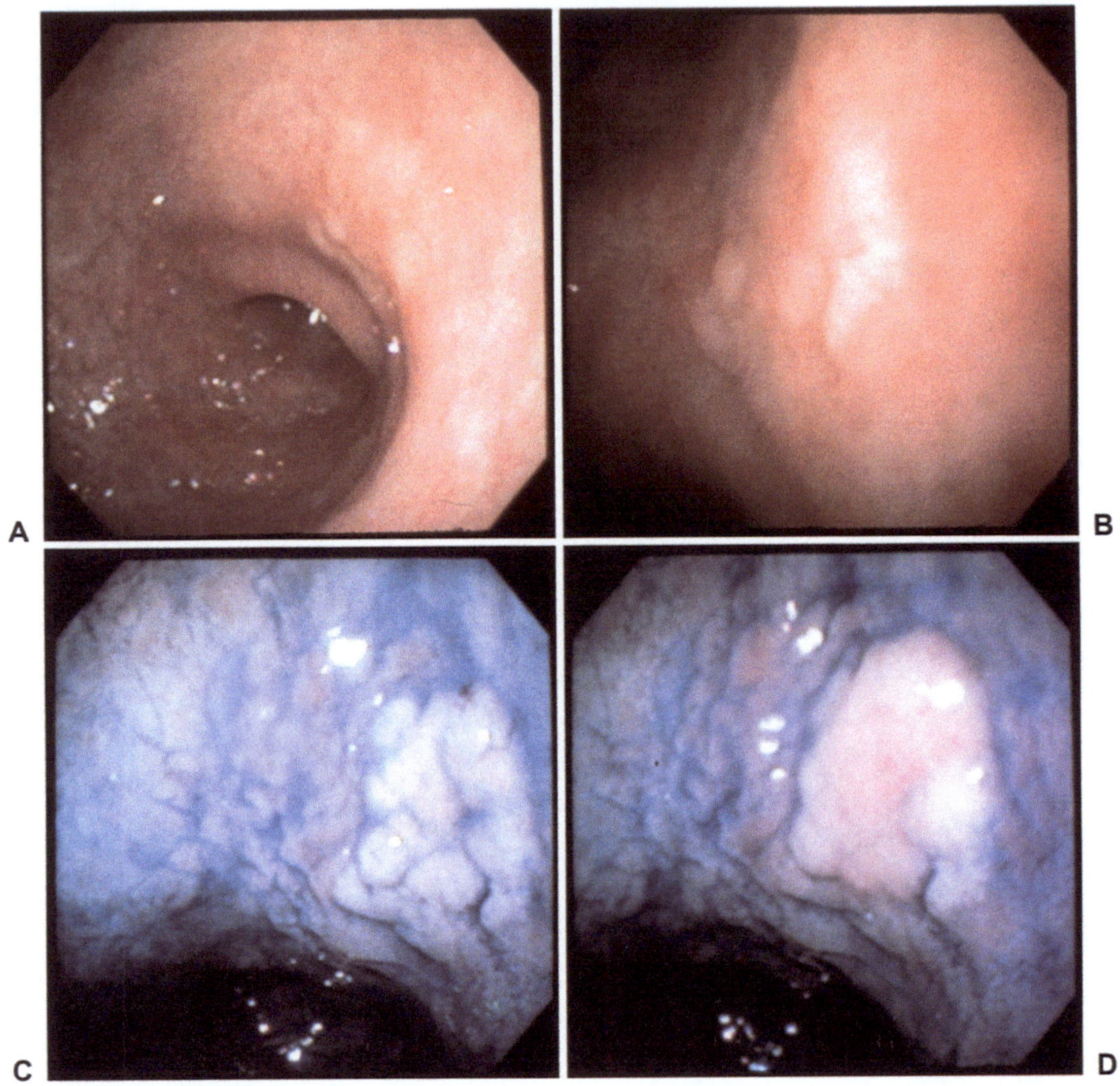

Fig. 7. A Angulus, lesser curvature. **B** Close-up view. **C** Same site immediately after spraying indigo carmine. **D** Same site a short while after spraying indigo carmine

Table 7. Gastric lesion 7

Biopsy: ×
Resection: ○

	W W J	W W W W W	W J	W W / W W / W J / W J / W J	J	J	W	W	W	W W J	J J J
Adenoma/dysplasia											
low-grade	⊗	×	○		×						
high-grade		○		⊗		○	×	○	×		
Carcinoma											
suspected			×			×	○			×	
non-invasive					○					○	⊗
intramucosal								×	○		

Case Description

A man, aged 63 years, with chronic hepatitis B and esophageal varices, regularly underwent upper GI endoscopic examinations. At the posterior wall side of the lesser curvature of the angulus a lesion was found. From a biopsy adenoma was diagnosed and it was followed up. Two years later the lesion had changed in shape. It measured 14 mm in diameter. Three weeks later endoscopic ultrasonographic examination and endoscopic resection were performed. The resection margins were free of tumor. On follow-up endoscopic examinations, no local recurrence was found.

Endoscopy Commentary

Anthony T.R. Axon (UK)[1]

History

This case is one where regular endoscopic examination would have been performed in the West in order to keep a check on the esophageal varices. Western endoscopists do examine the stomach and duodenum as a routine when checking for varices, and it is possible that the lesion on the lesser curve would have been identified. It has a plaque-like appearance that is irregular, with a color change. The appearances are distinctly unusual and not suggestive of a portal gastropathy. Although dye spray would not have been used in the West, I believe that biopsies would have been taken from this lesion.

Histology

Most of the Western pathologists diagnose either low-grade or high-grade dysplasia, and this would have led to further examinations and biopsy. A diagnosis of high-grade dysplasia would eventually have been made.

Endoscopic Appearance

Endoscopically, the flat nature of the lesion with protuberant areas would have probably been called type IIa or b in that there is no evidence of depression in the lesion and, although the patient does have significant other problems, undoubtedly a surgical opinion would have been sought.

Management

The presence of a lesion with high-grade dysplasia with these macroscopic changes would, I think, have led to surgical referral and to some form of gastric resection, but the portal hypertension and esophageal varices would have given cause for concern, and local therapy, if available, might have been considered.

I note from the history that a diagnosis of adenoma was made at an earlier stage. This is recognized to be a premalignant condition in the West, and further examinations with biopsy would have been undertaken.

Summary

This case describes a patient in whom the lesion would probably have been detected in the West. The combination of a macroscopic lesion with high-grade dysplasia would probably have led to surgical resection.

[1]See footnote on p. 4.

Endoscopy Commentary

Shigeaki Yoshida (Japan)

A whitish, elevated lesion is located on the lesser curvature of the angulus. A slightly hyperemic appearance is detectable from the center to the anal side of the lesion on conventional endoscopy (Fig. 7A and B). According to the whitish (discolored) nodular elevation indicating the possibility of adenoma and the hyperemic appearance indicating that of carcinoma, a cancerous lesion with adenoma would be a tentative diagnosis from conventional endoscopy.

A dye-spraying endoscopy picture (Fig. 7C) clarifies the construction of this elevated lesion in detail, i.e., a gathering of small nodules. The slightly hyperemic appearance noted on conventional endoscopy becomes inconspicuous in this picture. This may indicate a high probability of adenoma, rather than carcinoma, though the surface of the elevated components is not lustrous as in the typical appearance of an adenoma. In contrast, another picture (Fig. 7D) showing a close-up view of the lesion reveals hyperemic surface mucosa, indicating malignancy. Nevertheless, this picture is not suitable for making a definite diagnosis due to poor imaging caused by too much catchlight.

From the above, gastric adenoma rather than carcinoma should be the final endoscopic diagnosis. Considering that during the clinical course this lesion changed in shape, however, the diagnosis of carcinoma appears to be more likely than that of adenoma. In such a case it is difficult to make a definite endoscopic diagnosis; differentiation of carcinoma from adenoma is occasionally difficult even when assessing histological material obtained by biopsy. Endoscopic mucosal resection should be recommended to reach a definite histological diagnosis on such an occasion.

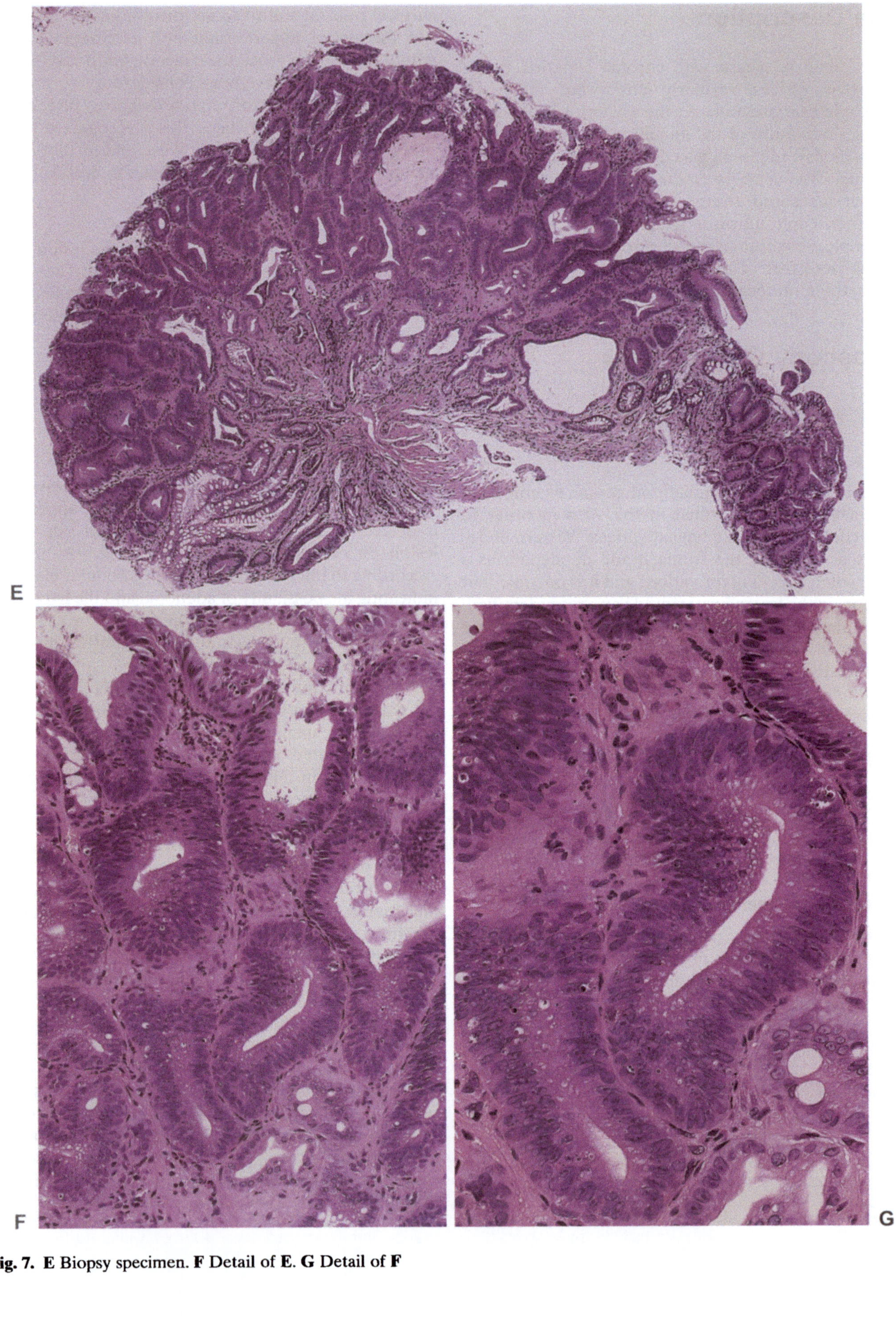

Fig. 7. **E** Biopsy specimen. **F** Detail of **E**. **G** Detail of **F**

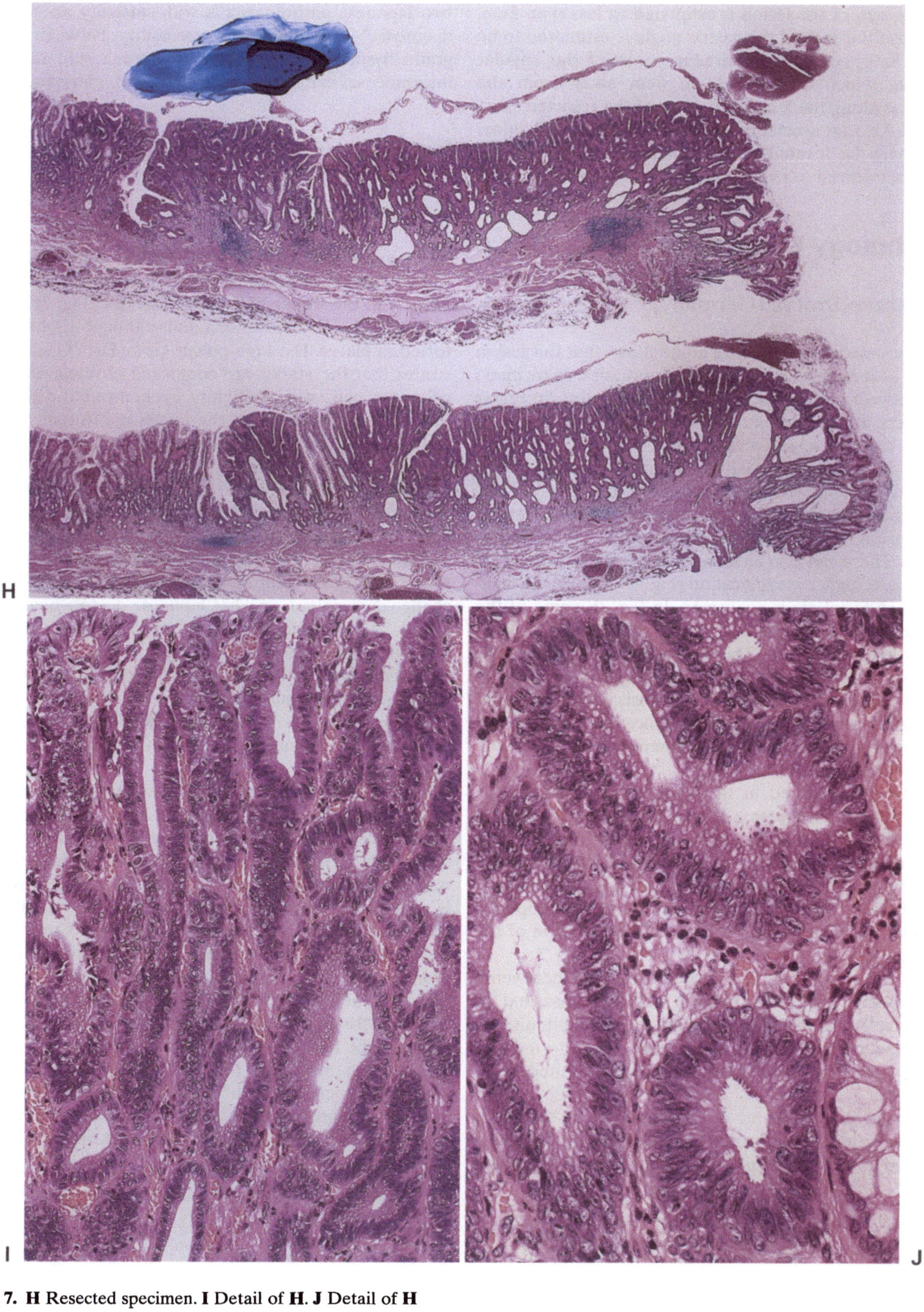

Fig. 7. **H** Resected specimen. **I** Detail of **H**. **J** Detail of **H**

The size of the lesion is estimated as less than 2cm, because the arch of the gastric angle is estimated to be 6cm long, i.e., half the circumference of the angular region, which corresponds to 6cm away from the pylorus along the lesser curvature of the resected specimen. Also, an accessory lesion of a benign peptic ulcer scar may be located on the anterior wall side of the lesion, referred to as deformity of the gastric angle.

Pathology Commentary

Manfred Stolte (Germany)

The endoscopic appearance alone shows that this lesion must be a neoplasm, and the differentiation to be made is between adenoma and carcinoma; the irregular borders at the margin, together with the tiny tumor nests, tend to suggest a carcinoma.

In the biopsy material the diagnosis of neoplasia is already quite clear at low power (Fig. 7E). Even at this low magnification, irregular architecture with lateral expansion of individual neoplastic tubuli can be recognized. These can also be seen focally in the center of the lesion. At higher magnification (Fig. 7F and G), the diagnosis of neoplasia is confirmed. In Fig. 7F, some of the nuclei are still located at the base and are only moderately hyperchromatic. The architecture of the neoplastic tubuli, however, already shows irregularity. In Fig. 7G it is clear that the differential diagnosis is between high-grade dysplasia and carcinoma, since here we can see obviously enlarged nuclei, prominent nucleoli, and irregular chromatin.

This is confirmed in the endoscopic mucosectomy specimen, in particular in Fig. 7I and J. In the low-power view (Fig. 7H) we find a number of areas of highly irregular neoplastic architecture, and this is confirmed in Fig. 7I. Despite the fact that neither individual tumor cells nor tumor cell nests are seen in the lamina propria, I would diagnose neoplastic glandular infiltration of the lamina propria.

In conclusion, this is a "borderline case" between a noninvasive carcinoma limited to the mucosa and an invasive intramucosal carcinoma. In my opinion, the architecture of this neoplasia is more likely to indicate an invasive well-differentiated carcinoma limited to the mucosa.

In this case, again, the discrepancies in the diagnoses of the various pathologists are considerable. The diagnosis of low-grade dysplasia made by three Western and two Japanese pathologists is, with certainty, an "underdiagnosis." The diagnostic variability between high-grade dysplasia, noninvasive carcinoma, and invasive intramucosal carcinoma in this case is understandable.

Pathology Commentary

Yo Kato (Japan)

The biopsy specimen shows atypical tubular glands rather equally distributed (with the same density of glands) in the upper half of the mucosa (Fig. 7E). The glands are mostly round or tubular, though slightly distorted in places. The high-power view (Fig. 7G) demonstrates that the glands are composed of intestinal-type columnar cells with a slightly hyperchromatic slender nucleus, and that most of the nuclei are situated along the basement membrane. The nucleolus is not so conspicuous. Since a tendency of the cells to differentiate from the bottom with a round nucleus toward the surface with a slender nucleus exists (Fig. 7F), the diagnosis group III "tubular adenoma, moderate atypia" will be given by most Japanese pathologists according to the group classification presented by the JRSGC: the change corresponds to what Japanese doctors have long called "ATP (abbreviation of atypical epithelium or atypical epithelial lesion)" or "IIa subtype (a superficial elevated lesion to be distinguished from adenocarcinoma of the same macroscopic type, IIa)," etc., but these days the lesion is recommended by the World Health Organization Tumor Classification to be called "tubular adenoma."

The EMR specimen demonstrates a similar pattern as in the biopsy specimen (Fig. 7H). The dilated glands found occasionally in the deeper part of the biopsy specimen (Fig. 7E) exist frequently in the lower half of the mucosa or beneath the atypical lesion (Fig. 7H), which is a finding rather common for "ATP" or tubular adenoma. The high-power view of a part of the lesion indicates glands with an equal-shaped and -sized slightly swollen nucleus. Compared with the biopsy specimen (Fig. 7F), the tendency of cell differentiation is not clear in the EMR specimen (Fig. 7I), but a faint tendency still seems to be kept in the right half of the picture as the cell nucleus becomes rather slender, with the cells reaching the surface of the lesion. Ischemic change, suggested by fibromuscular proliferation in the lamina propria mucosae, may modify the pattern typical for adenoma.

Case 8, IIa

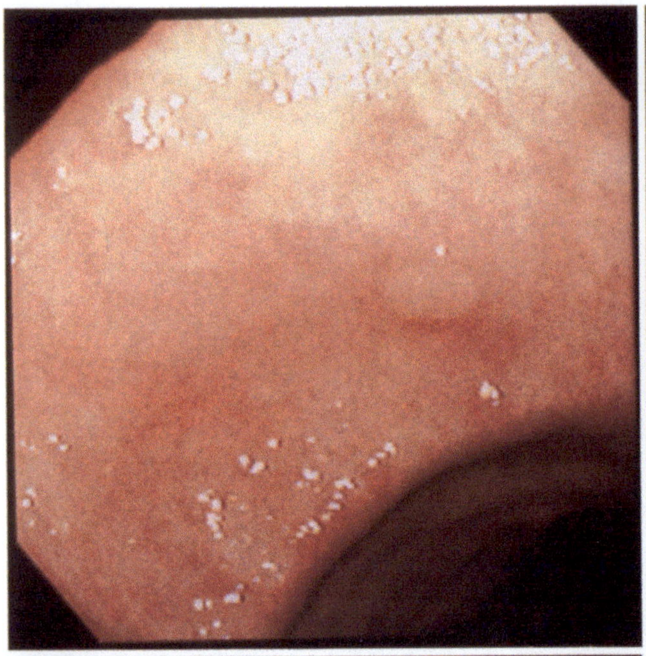

A

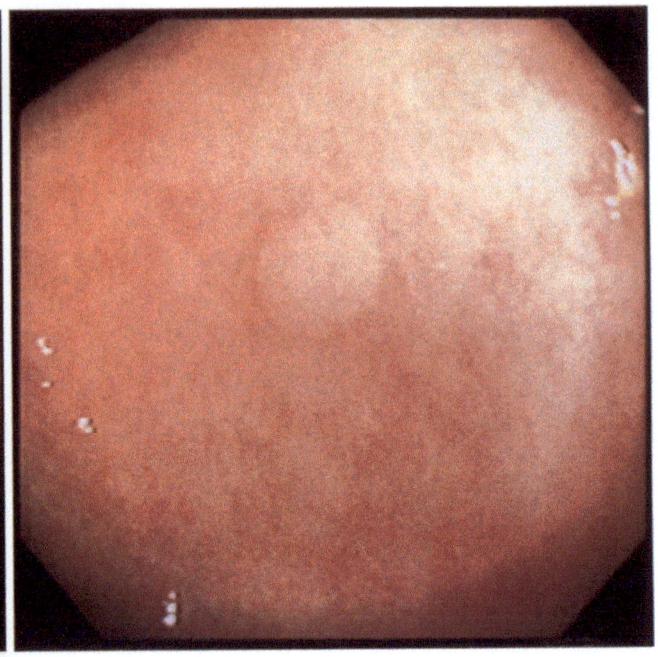

B

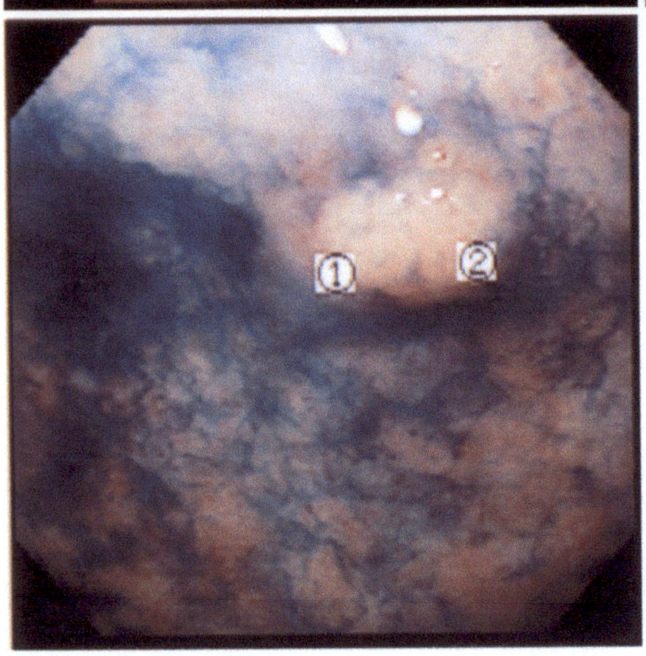

C

Fig. 8. **A** Antrum, lesser curvature. **B** Close-up view. **C** Same site after spraying indigo carmine

Table 8. Gastric lesion 8

Biopsy: ×	W W W	W W W W W W W W W W W J W J J W J J W W J	W J J	W J	J J
Regenerative changes	×				
Adenoma/dysplasia					
low-grade		×			
high-grade			×		
Carcinoma					
suspected				×	
non-invasive					×

Case Description

A man, aged 59 years, with a history of hypertension, complained of dull epigastric pain for a week and underwent an upper GI endoscopic examination. A hyperplastic polyp of 9mm in diameter was found at the greater curvature of the antrum. After polypectomy, a follow-up endoscopic examination revealed a lesion of about 3mm in diameter at the lesser curvature of the antrum. It was biopsied. On follow-up endoscopic and histological examinations, no neoplastic changes could be observed.

Endoscopy Commentary

Anthony T.R. Axon (UK)[1]

History

A man of 59 years complaining of dull epigastric pain would not have been referred for endoscopy if his symptoms had been present for only a week. Had the pain persisted then he would have been referred and the 9 mm polyp would have been identified on the greater curve of the antrum. Biopsies would probably have been taken from it and it would have shown it to be a hyperplastic polyp. Under these circumstances it is unlikely that a further procedure would have been undertaken because hyperplastic polyps are not regarded as a pre-malignant condition in the West.

Had a follow-up endoscopic examination been undertaken the interest would again have focused on the polyp, however the lesion on the lesser curve of the antrum might have been identified.

Endoscopic Appearances

The endoscopic appearance of the lesion on the lesser curve is smooth, oval and flat, it is set in atrophic mucosa, but does not appear sinister in appearance. Biopsies would have been taken from it and this probably would have shown evidence of low-grade dysplasia.

Management

The presence of low-grade dysplasia in a biopsy taken from the stomach would have caused some concern. The histology would have been reviewed with the histopathologist in a joint meeting. If the histologist confirmed the appearances to be low-grade dysplasia a further endoscopy would have been undertaken with multiple biopsies from the area in order to be certain that areas of high-grade dysplasia were not present. Further management would then have been undertaken depending upon what the new biopsies had revealed.

Summary

The lesion in the antrum would have probably been identified and biopsied. A further endoscopy would have been taken with a view to performing multiple biopsies.

Endoscopy Commentary

Shigeaki Yoshida (Japan)

A tiny, elevated lesion is located on the lesser curvature of the antrum (Fig. 8A). A close-up view under conventional endoscopy (Fig. 8B) reveals that the lesion is whitish and round-shaped without any erosive changes on the surface, which shows a similar structural pattern to that of the boiled-rice appearance of metaplastic mucosa. In other words, it is shown as an enlarged metaplastic granule.

A dye-spraying picture (Fig. 8C) reveals the discolored and lustrous surface of the lesion which is distinguishable from the surrounding mucosa, indicating that the lesion should be neoplastic. Since it is small and does not involve an eroded component, it can be diagnosed as benign adenoma.

Such a tiny, elevated lesion is occasionally removed only by conventional biopsy.

Pathology Commentary

Manfred Stole (Germany)

This superficial elevated lesion measuring only 3mm in diameter was only biopsied. Already in the low-power view (Fig. 8D) the histological work-up reveals a neoplastic lesion and no regenerative changes. The neoplasia is restricted to the upper part of the mucosa. At the margin of the lesion extensive intestinal metaplasia is seen, and in the center there are numerous densely packed neoplastic glands. The normal basic structure of the mucosa is no longer intact. At the highest magnification (Fig. 8F), however, only small irregularities in the position of the nuclei, and only moderate hyperchromasia with no prominent nucleoli, can be made out.

In conclusion, the differential diagnosis here is between high-grade dysplasia, suspected adenocarcinoma, noninvasive carcinoma, and invasive carcinoma.

[1]See footnote on p. 4.

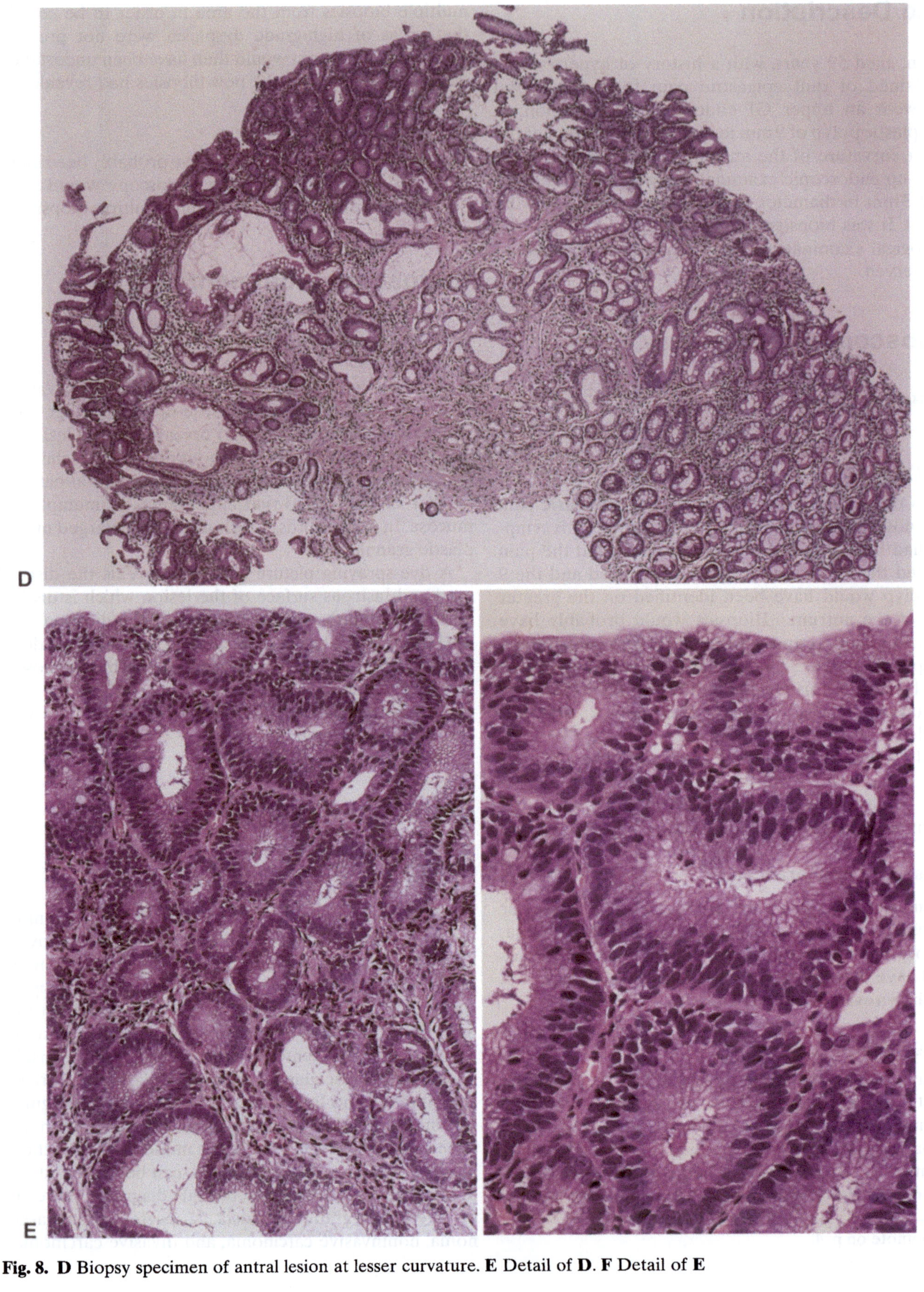

Fig. 8. D Biopsy specimen of antral lesion at lesser curvature. **E** Detail of **D**. **F** Detail of **E**

On the basis of the architecture of the neoplasia, I would diagnose a lesion that is suspicious for carcinoma and recommend endoscopic mucosectomy.

Here, again, there is considerable variability in the diagnoses of the pathologists. The diagnosis of regenerative changes made by three Western pathologists is certainly incorrect, and I consider the diagnosis of low-grade dysplasia established by most Western pathologists in the biopsy material to be an "underdiagnosis."

Pathology Commentary

Yo Kato (Japan)

Only the biopsy specimen is available, showing proliferation of atypical round tubular glands on the surface of the mucosa (Fig. 8A, center to left). The glands are uniformly round, consisting of slightly vesicular or rather mucinous columnar cells with a uniformly oval to round small nucleus. Further, the nucleus is located along the basement membrane and the tendency of the cell to differentiate from the bottom to the surface of the lesion is, though mild, apparent (Fig. 8E,F). Slight stratification of the nucleus as shown in Fig. 8F is due to cutting. The nature of the epithelium is more or less of the intestinal type, or perhaps of the intermediate type between gastric and intestinal types.

From the above findings, the lesion is interpreted as tubular adenoma, mild atypia, based on the Japanese viewpoint, corresponding to low-grade dysplasia/neoplasia by the Vienna classification.

Case 9, IIa

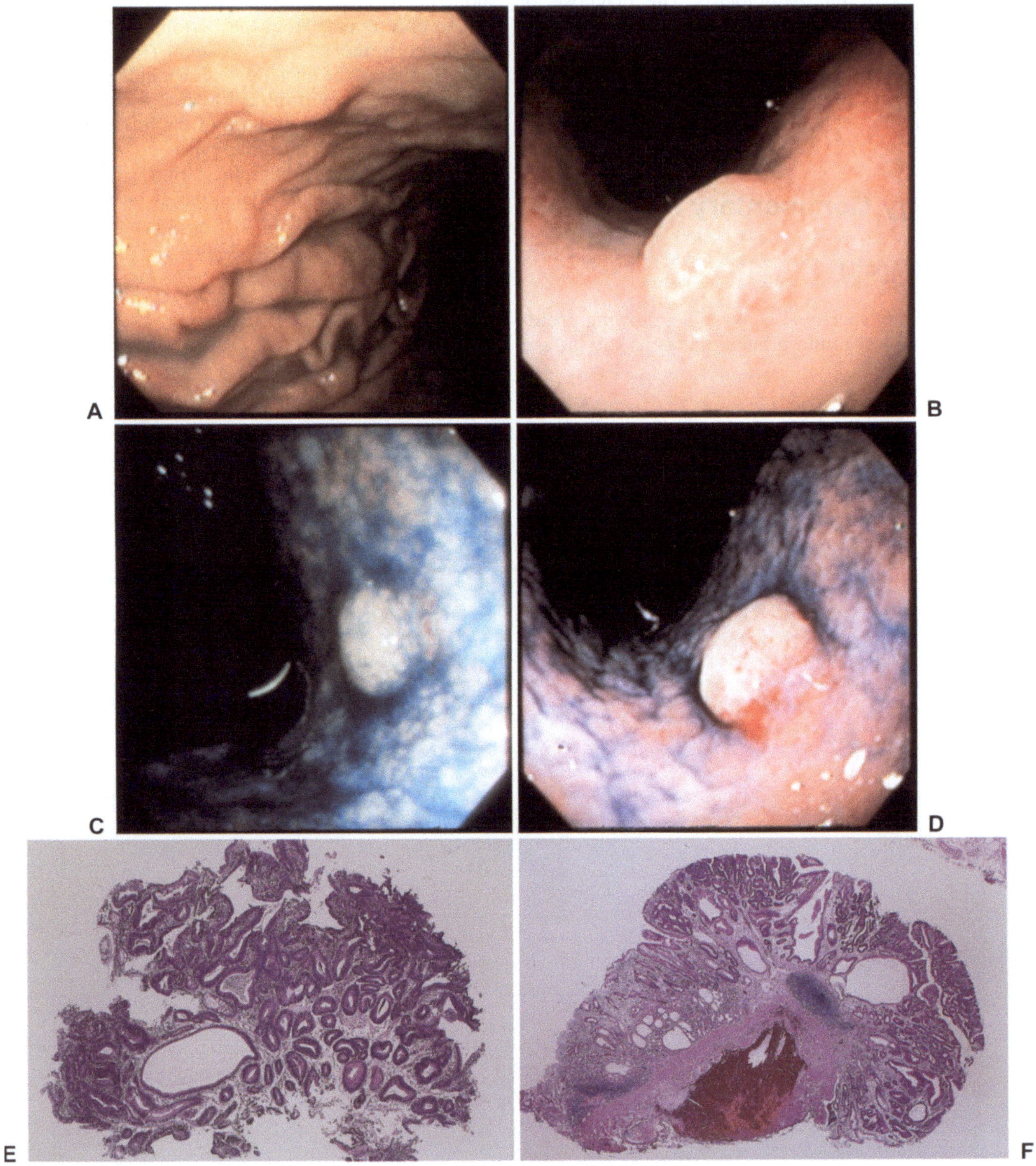

Fig. 9. **A** Corpus, lesser curvature and anterior wall. **B** Same site, U-turn view. **C** Same site after spraying indigo carmine. **D** Same site. **E** Biopsy specimen. **F** Endoscopically resected specimen

Case Description

A woman, aged 67 years, with a history of cholelithiasis and hypertension, had undergone upper GI endoscopic examinations for recurrent epigastric pain 2 years and 1 year previously. At a follow-up examination, a lesion of about 7 mm in diameter was found at the anterior wall side of the lesser curvature of the corpus (Fig. 9A–D). After endoscopic ultrasonographic examination, endoscopic resection was performed. On follow-up, 9 months later, mucosal irregularities were found at the posterior wall side of the angulus. Carcinoma was diagnosed from biopsies. Two months thereafter a subtotal gastrectomy was performed; histologically, mucosal carcinoma at the angulus and an ulcer scar without neoplastic changes in the corpus were confirmed.

Endoscopy Commentary

Anthony T.R. Axon (UK)[1]

History

This patient had undergone upper digestive endoscopy for recurrent epigastric pain. It is unclear why a follow-up examination was performed. It is not usual in the West to undertake a second endoscopy if the first one is negative. In this particular case, however, a 7-mm lesion on the lesser curve of the corpus was found at follow-up examination. Lesions of this size in the corpus would not normally lead to concern with an endoscopist because fundal polyps are common. A biopsy may or may not have been undertaken and if this showed a simple fundal polyp, no further procedure would be done. In this case, however, endoscopic ultrasonography was performed and resection undertaken.

Endoscopic Appearance

Figure 9A, showing the lesser curvature of the corpus, is difficult to interpret. There is some irregularity of the mucosa, but there is no change in color and the lesion is close to the mucosal folds. I think this lesion would have been overlooked by a Western endoscopist. On the other hand Fig. 9B, which is the retroverted view, shows a definite polyp and one that would have been identified and would have been biopsied. The retrograde view also shows considerable gastric mucosal inflammation. It is interesting in these cases that the degree of inflammatory change in the stomach of Japanese patients is considerably more obvious than that seen in most of our patients in the West.

Histopathology and Management

The biopsies are agreed by most pathologists to show, at the very least, high-grade dysplasia. This, taken in conjunction with the polypoid nature of the lesion, would have led to further endoscopies and if these continued to show abnormality, the patient would have been referred to surgery and gastric resection would have been undertaken.

Summary

It is unlikely that this patient would have been referred for a second or third endoscopy; however, had that been done it is likely that the lesion would have been identified and biopsies taken. This would have led to resection.

Table 9. Gastric lesion 9

Biopsy: ×
Resection: ○

	W W W W W W	W W W	W W W	J	J	W W	J J J J J J	W	W W J	W' W' W' J J
Adenoma/dysplasia										
low-grade		×								
high-grade	⊗		×		×					
Carcinoma										
suspected		○	○	×		×				
non-invasive				○			⊗	○	×	
intramucosal					○	○		×	○	⊗

[1]See footnote on p. 4.

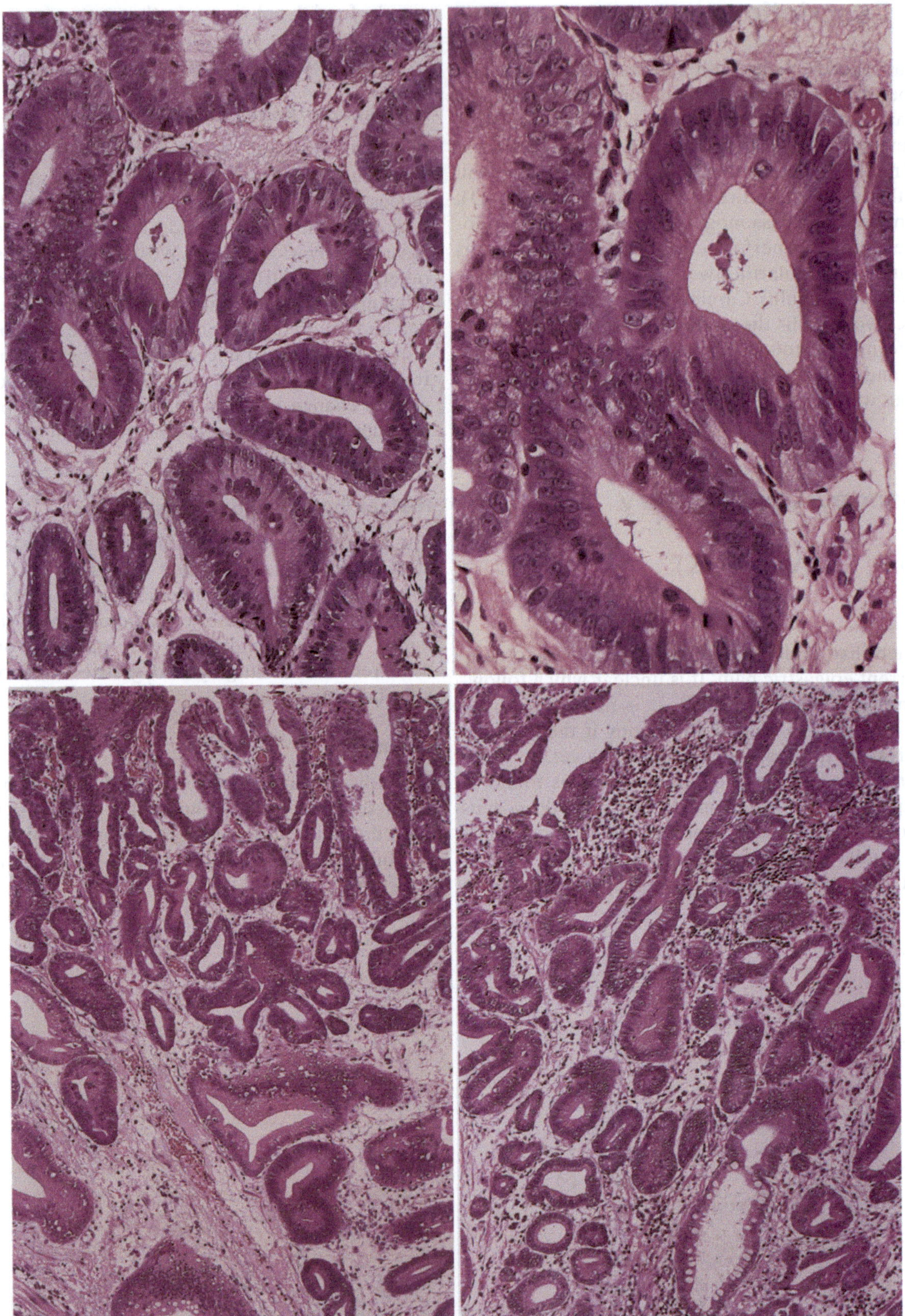

G H I J

Fig. 9. **G** Detail of **E** (biopsy). **H** Detail of **G**. **I** Detail of **F** (resected specimen). **J** Detail of **F**

Endoscopy Commentary

Shigeaki Yoshida (Japan)

A superficial elevated lesion is located in the anterior wall of the upper gastric body near the mucous lake (Fig. 9A). In close-up view (Fig. 9B), it shows a hemispherical appearance with a smooth surface. The color of the lesion is nonspecific and the size is estimated to be around 5–7 mm (less than 10 mm) by referring to the width of folds in the gastric body.

Dye-spraying endoscopy reveals its nonspecific changes on the surface (Fig. 9C), with no eroded component (Fig. 9D), though these pictures show only the anal side of the lesion.

It appears that the lesion is actually larger than that of Case 8 but is still small, at less than 1 cm. In addition, the lesion shows only a nonspecific surface pattern. This may indicate that it can be a benign lesion such as gastric adenoma or hyperplastic polyp. The final endoscopic diagnosis, therefore, is "an elevated lesion showing no definite findings suggesting malignancy."

Endoscopic mucosal resection is indicated to make a definite diagnosis if the biopsy specimens reveal neoplastic findings histologically, because we have encountered IIa type early cancer showing a nonspecific surface pattern endoscopically, though the actual number of such lesions is very limited.

Pathology Commentary

Manfred Stole (Germany)

In this 7-mm large broad-based polypoid lesion, the differential diagnosis of the endoscopic findings is between an adenoma and a very small type IIa early gastric carcinoma. Already in the biopsy specimen (Fig. 9E), the diagnosis of glandular neoplasia is quite clear even at low magnification. The architecture of a tubular adenoma is absent. Already at low power, several foci showing a highly irregular neoplastic tubular structure with densely packed, irregularly branched tubuli can be seen. At higher magnification (Fig. 9G and H) the criteria of high-grade intra-epithelial neoplasia or a noninvasive carcinoma are met. The nuclei of the tumor cells manifest an irregular arrangement, and they all contain prominent nucleoli.

In the two views showing details of the endoscopic mucosectomy specimen, lateral budding of the tubuli and a number of tiny neoplastic tubuli showing an irregular arrangement are also visible.

In conclusion, I would diagnose the above-mentioned features to be those of a well-differentiated adenocarcinoma.

In this borderline case, too, the variability of the diagnoses established by the various pathologists is understandable. Most of the Western pathologists diagnosed high-grade dysplasia, most Japanese pathologists a noninvasive carcinoma. On the basis of the above criteria, however, seven Western pathologists and four Japanese pathologists go on to diagnose an intramucosal carcinoma.

Pathology Commentary

Yo Kato (Japan)

The biopsy specimen is filled with slightly distorted atypical tubular glands having a somewhat papillary configuration on the surface (Fig. 9E). There is no evident pattern of invasion, The high-power views (Fig. 9G,H) show several round to oval or triangular glands composed of eosinophilic columnar cells, intestinal type, with a round to oval swollen nucleus with a prominent nucleolus. The nuclei in each gland are often detached from the basement membrane side, giving a pattern of nuclear stratification.

The EMR specimen indicates a slightly elevated lesion as shown in Fig. 9F. Similarly to the biopsy specimen, the lesion consists of irregular-shaped round or tubular glands with a trend of papillary configuration at the surface. The eosinophilic cells forming atypical glands are in general cuboidal, equipped with a swollen round nucleus mostly at the basement membrane side. However, the nucleus is often shifted toward the luminal side particularly in the surface papillary area of the lesion (Fig. 9I). Several glands shown in the lower half of the figure are non-neoplastic ones in a hyperplastic or regenerative process. The atypical glands shown in Fig. 9J include small glands in several places, thus the lesion is suggested to be an invasive one. My final diagnosis is well-differentiated tubular adenocarcinoma, invasive, which corresponds to intramucosal carcinoma by the Vienna classification.

Case 10, IIa

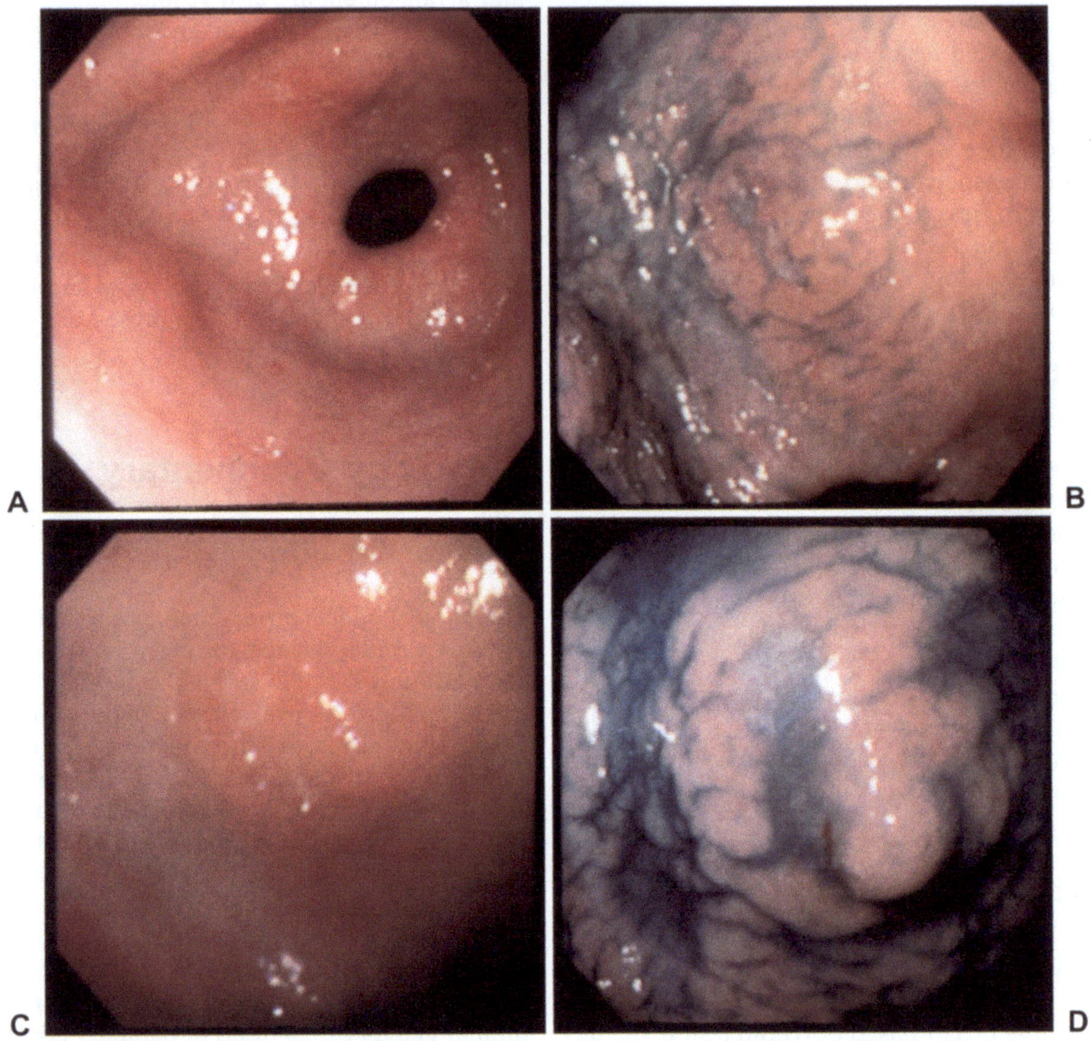

Fig. 10. **A** Antrum, lesser curvature. **B** Same site after spraying indigo carmine. **C** Antrum, lesser curvature, 4 months later. **D** Same site (4 months later) after spraying indigo carmine

Table 10. Gastric lesion 10

Biopsy: ×
Resection: ○

	W	W	W W	J	W W W W W	J	W	W	W	W W W	W	W J J J J J	J J	J	W W W J
Regenerative changes	×														
Indefinite for neoplasia				×											
Adenoma/dysplasia															
low-grade	○	○	×			×		×							
high-grade		×	○		⊗		○		○						
Carcinoma															
suspected				○		○	×			⊗	○				
non-invasive								○				⊗	○	×	
intramucosal									×		×		×	○	⊗

Case Description

A woman, aged 80 years, with pulmonary emphysema, complained of epigastric discomfort and underwent an upper GI endoscopic examination. A lesion was found at the lesser curvature of the antrum near the pylorus. Adenoma was diagnosed from a biopsy and it was followed up. Four months later the lesion had changed in shape and was about 14 mm in diameter. It was biopsied once more. Two months thereafter it was endoscopically resected. The resection margins were tumor-free.

Endoscopy Commentary

ANTHONY T.R. AXON (UK)[1]

History

This 80-year-old woman with pulmonary emphysema would have undergone endoscopy in the West had she been complaining of epigastric discomfort if significantly distressful. Had an endoscopy been performed, the endoscopist would have reported the antrum of the stomach as being congested and erythematous. Just above the pylorus there is an area of irregularity, a somewhat protuberant area that would have invited biopsy. Indigo carmine is unlikely to have been used, but had it been, I do not believe it would have influenced the decision taken to biopsy the lesion.

Management

Most diagnoses of the biopsy are highly suspicious of invasive cancer. Subject to the woman's fitness for an operation she would have been referred for gastric resection. Had it been felt that she would not have tolerated the procedure, it is possible that a more conservative approach would have been adopted, perhaps involving long-term surveillance, endoscopic mucosal resection (if a suitable tertiary referral center with this expertise was at hand), or Argon plasma coagulation.

Endoscopy Commentary

SHIGEAKI YOSHIDA (Japan)

A tiny, elevated lesion accompanied with a spotty erosion on the surface is located on the lesser curvature of the antrum near the pyloric ring (Fig. 10A). A dye-spraying picture (Fig. 10B) reveals that the erosive change pointed out on conventional endoscopy is actually a shallow central depression having an irregular margin, which is highly suggestive of malignancy, despite the nonspecific appearance of the elevated component.

In Fig. 10C the lesion is obviously enlarged compared with that shown in Fig. 10A. The central depression is also enlarged and includes a whitish exudate particularly on its oral side, indicating that erosive changes have become deeper than before. The margin of the depression is slightly irregular, particularly on the anterior wall side.

A dye-spraying picture (Fig. 10D) clearly demonstrates that the depressed area has certainly changed to become deeper and more enlarged than before, and shows the distinctly irregular margin of the depression, enforcing the definite endoscopic diagnosis of epithelial malignancy.

The first question is whether the cancerous invasion is limited within the depressed area or includes an elevated component beyond the depression. In this respect, the greater part of the elevated component is still fundamentally nonspecific even in a dye-spraying picture (Fig. 10D), indicating that the former is more likely than the latter. On precise observation, however, the lustrous appearance of the nodular formation on the posterior wall side of the lesion may suggest a neoplastic feature endoscopically, and the faint hyperemic appearance on its surface may also suggest that the lesion is cancerous rather than adenomatous.

The second question is whether the lesion should be classified into the IIa or IIa+IIc type. Definite macroscopic typing is difficult using only the two pictures presented.

Estimating the size of lesion is also difficult in this case, because both pictures of the latest examination presented give us only a close-up view of the lesion. In spite of this, it can be roughly estimated as 1–2 cm by referring to the size of areae gastricae shown in Fig. 10D, and being less than 2 cm it may indicate a low probability of deeper invasion, when the lesion is classified as type IIa. As to the histological type, there is no endoscopic finding suggesting undifferentiated type in this case.

Endoscopic mucosal resection is indicated for this lesion as the first choice of treatment, since it is easily done in cases of elevated cancer as compared with depressed cancer.

Pathology Commentary

MANFRED STOLTE (Germany)

The endoscopic pictures of this superficial elevated lesion measuring 14 mm in diameter clearly reveal it to

[1]See footnote on p. 4.

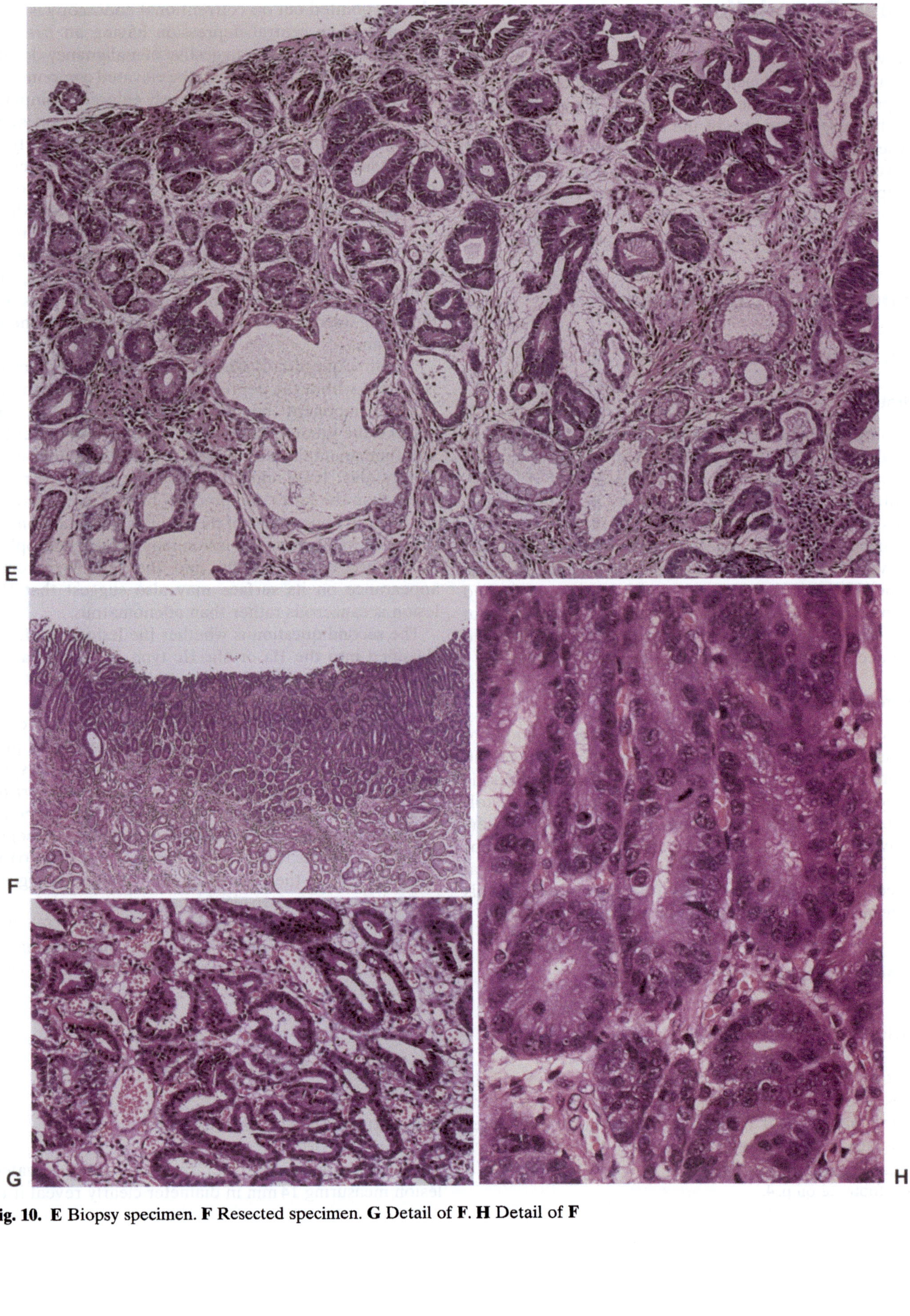

Fig. 10. **E** Biopsy specimen. **F** Resected specimen. **G** Detail of **F**. **H** Detail of **F**

be neoplastic and not a regenerative change. The central depression and the irregular margins seen in Fig. 10D suggest a carcinoma rather than an adenoma.

This is confirmed in the biopsy specimen, in which the normal architecture of the parallel arrangement of foveolae has been completely replaced by irregularly structured and irregularly arranged neoplastic glands of varying caliber showing laterally growing invasive buds, but no evidence of individual tumor cells in the lamina propria (Fig. 10E).

These findings are also confirmed in the endoscopic mucosectomy specimen. Already in the low-power view (Fig. 10F), the normal architecture of the antral mucosa can again be seen to have been replaced by densely packed, mainly small-caliber neoplastic glands. Low-grade dysplasia can be excluded in the high-power view (Fig. 10H), in which all the cytological criteria for high-grade neoplasia are seen again. The invasive character of this neoplasm is then clearly shown in Fig. 10G: here, irregularly branched neoplastic tubuli invading the lamina propria are clearly seen. A particularly impressive finding in this view is the marked neoangiogenesis in this carcinoma.

In conclusion I would diagnose, both in the biopsy and in the endoscopic mucosectomy specimen, a well-differentiated invasive intramucosal tubular adenocarcinoma.

Here, once again, there is considerable variability in the diagnoses of the pathologists. Most Western pathologists waver between low-grade/high-grade dysplasia and suspected carcinoma, while most of the Japanese pathologists and five Western pathologists favor a diagnosis of carcinoma.

Pathology Commentary

Yo Kato (Japan)

The biopsy specimen shows a proliferation of medium-sized to small round glands. The glands are, however, not always completely round and equally distributed. In some glands intraglandular papillary growth is seen. In other words, pleomorphism in the shape and size of glands exists. In addition, the constituent cuboidal cells harbor small but hyperchromatic nuclei. The nucleolus is, however, not conspicuous so far as the specimen as shown in Fig. 10E is concerned. As invasive patterns are not evident with these findings I would diagnose tubular adenocarcinoma of well-differentiated type, noninvasive, for the lesion. The glands of various sizes shown in the lower half of Fig. 10E are non-neoplastic.

The resected specimen demonstrates a lesion with compact tubular glands (Fig. 10F). The glands are more compact and more equal in shape and size than in the biopsy specimen. There is, however, a part with similar histology to Fig. 10E, where glandular pleomorphism is more pronounced than in the biopsy specimen (Fig. 10G). Figure 10H is a high-power view of a part in the right half of Fig. 10F. Compared with the histology of Fig. 10G, the eosinophilic cuboidal cells are equipped more with a swollen round nucleus with a prominent nucleolus.

Case 11, IIa

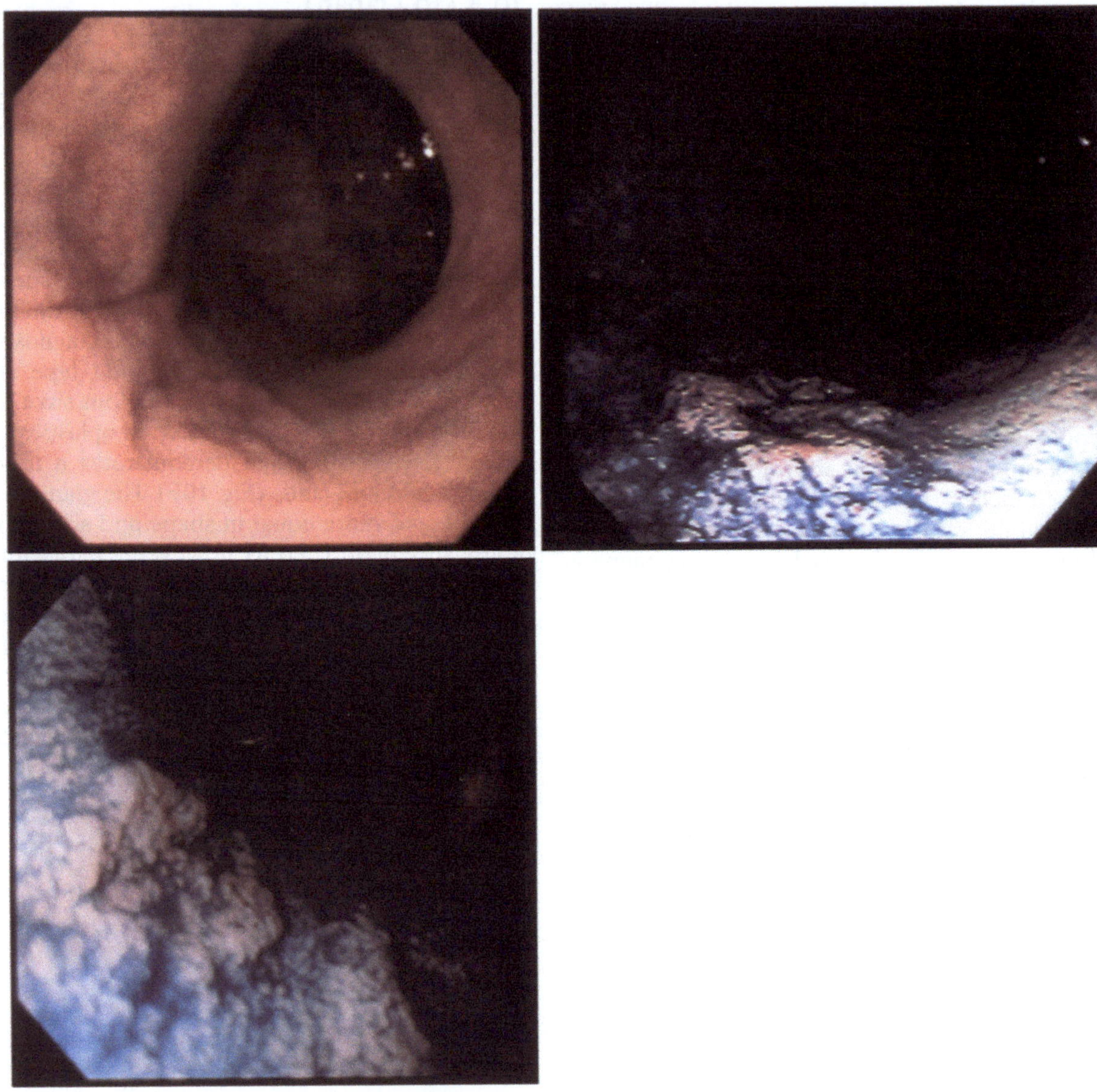

Fig. 11. **A** Corpus, greater curvature. **B** Same site after spraying indigo carmine. **C** Same site (U-turn view)

Table 11. Gastric lesion 11

Biopsy: × Resection: ○	W	W	W W W W W W J	W W W W W J	W W	W J	W W	W W	J	J	J J J J J J
Indefinite for neoplasia	×										
Adenoma/dysplasia											
low-grade		⊗	×		×	×	×				
high-grade	○		○	⊗				×			
Carcinoma											
suspected					○				×	×	
non-invasive						○			○		⊗
intramucosal							○	○		○	

Case Description

A man, aged 67 years, with a history of recurrent gastric ulcers and ischemic heart disease, underwent upper GI screening by endoscopic examination. This is the same patient as presented in Case 5. Apart from two gastric ulcer scars, a lesion of about 15 mm in diameter at the greater curvature of the corpus and a lesion of 7 mm in diameter at the greater curvature of the antrum were found and biopsied. Four months later, endoscopic ultrasonographic examination and endoscopic resection of both lesions were performed. The resection margins were not free of tumor. Subtotal gastrectomy with lymph node resection was performed 3 months later, but in the surgical specimen no neoplastic changes could be detected.

Endoscopy Commentary

Anthony T.R. Axon (UK)[1]

History

This 67-year-old patient who had had previous gastric ulcers might have undergone further endoscopies in the West had he been complaining of symptoms. In the West, however, the usual approach with gastric ulcer is for the patient to be re-endoscoped following *Helicobacter* eradication or proton pump inhibition and at that stage, if the ulcer has healed well and the patient is asymptomatic, further tests are not undertaken. If the scar appears suspicious or the ulcer is not completely healed then further endoscopies are undertaken with biopsy until the lesion is satisfactory healed. Provided that there are no further symptoms, it is unlikely that a patient with gastric ulcer would undergo further endoscopy in the West. In this case, therefore, it is not clear whether a further endoscopy would have been undertaken.

Endoscopic Appearance

Had the patient been submitted to further endoscopy, the endoscopist would have reported the corpus of the stomach as showing some erythema and irregularity compatible with previous gastric ulceration. It is unlikely that any other concerns would have been expressed. However, close examination (and to some extent with hindsight) shows an irregular area. The mucosa is heaped up with some depression in the center. The appearance is therefore suspicious; dye spray accentuates the abnormality and if undertaken (unlikely), would have caused greater concern. Had this abnormality been identified by the endoscopist, biopsies would have been taken.

Management

The pathological diagnosis here was clearly in favor of a neoplastic lesion which in turn would have led to further biopsies and referral for a surgical opinion.

Summary

It is unlikely that this patient would have been referred for further endoscopy in the West if he was not complaining of gastric symptoms. Had it been done, it is possible that the lesion in the corpus would have been overlooked. Had it been identified biopsies would have been taken, and this would have led to a gastric resection.

[1]See footnote on p. 4.

Endoscopy Commentary

Shigeaki Yoshida (Japan)

Several folds are converging toward the greater curvature of the middle gastric body where gastric wall deformity exists, indicating the presence of an ulcer scar in this area. On the posterior wall side of this ulcer scar, a slightly elevated lesion with a shallow central depression is detectable on conventional endoscopy (Fig. 11A). The margin of the lesion appears to be irregular, but the details cannot be discussed from this picture.

Dye-spraying pictures (Fig. 11B and C) clearly reveal the irregular margin of the lesion. An endoscopic diagnosis of cancer is easily made. These pictures also reveal that there is no suggestive finding of deeper invasion in both the depressed area and the surrounding mucosa.

The size of the lesion is estimated to be around 10–15 mm by referring to the width of a prominent fold on the greater curvature. Estimation of the histological type is difficult to make in this case, because the pictures presented are all poorly informative. No combination with the converging folds indicates that the cancerous lesion does not involve histological ulceration [ul(−) cancer].

Endoscopic mucosal resection is indicated for this lesion, though it is located in a difficult area for endoscopic manipulation.

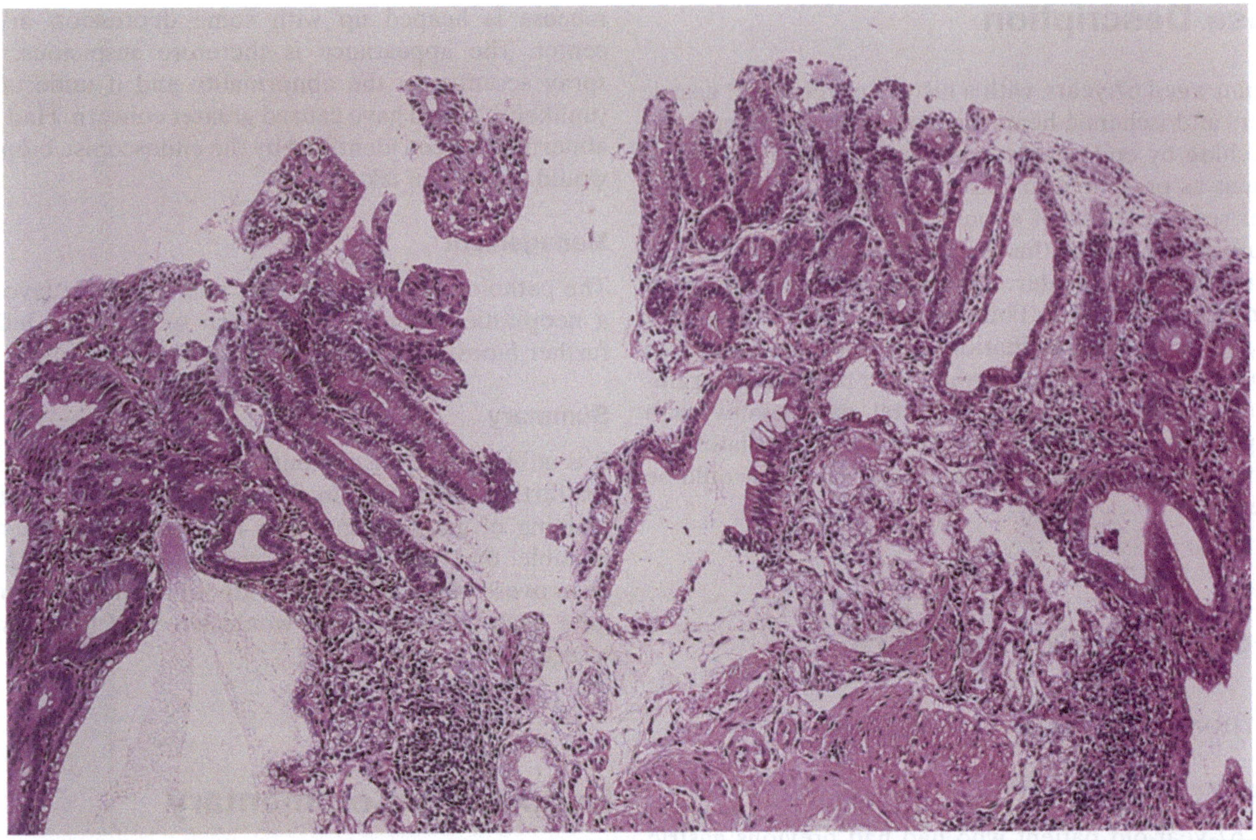

D

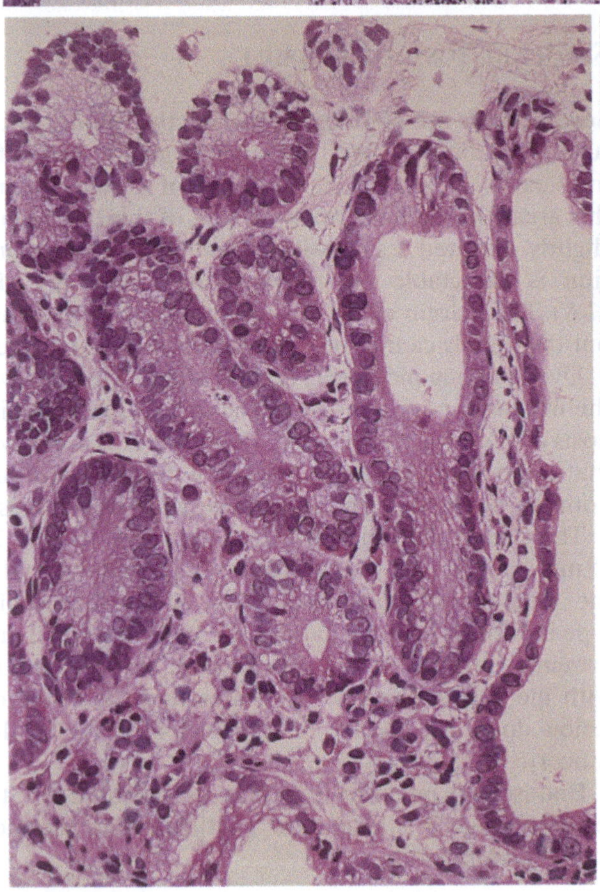

E

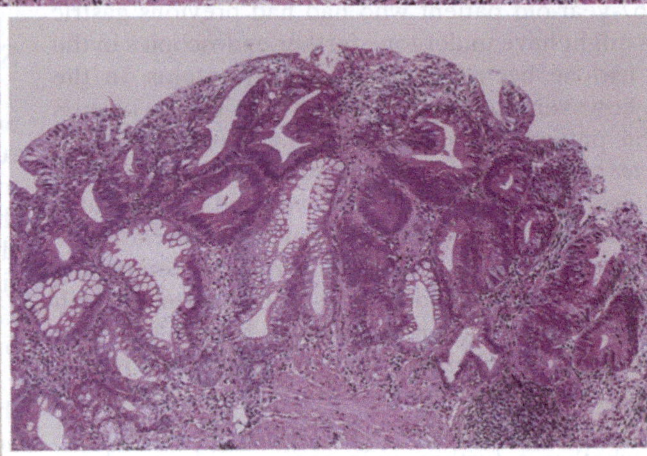

F

Fig. 11. **D** Biopsy specimen. **E** Detail of **D**. **F** Other biopsy specimen of the same lesion

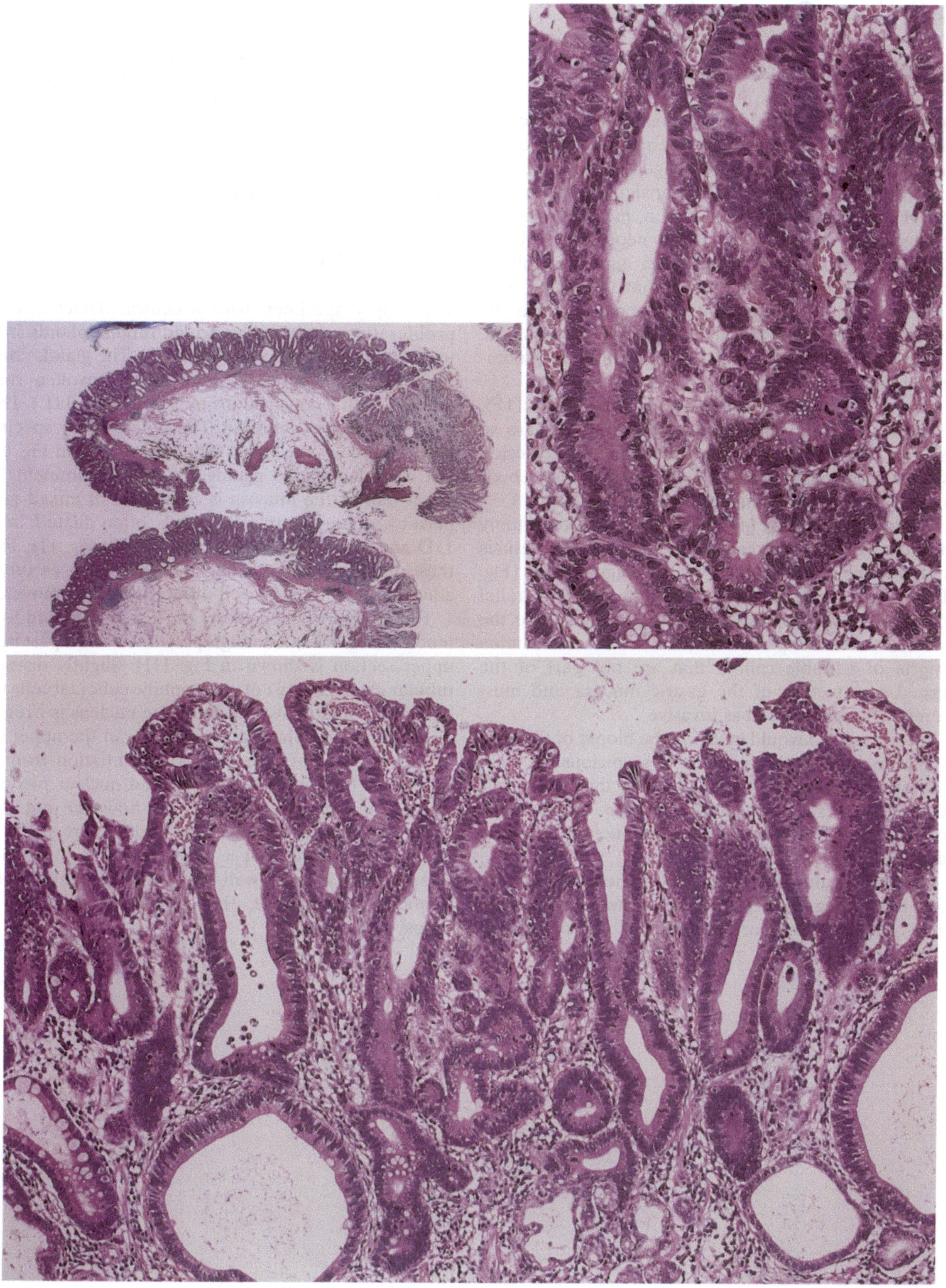

G

I

H

Fig. 11. G Resected specimen. **H** Detail of resected specimen. **I** Detail of **H**

Pathology Commentary

Manfred Stolte (Germany)

In this case, the endoscopic appearance alone indicates, with a high level of probability, a neoplastic lesion of the early gastric carcinoma type (irregular border, central depression). It is all the more surprising then to find, in one of the biopsies from this lesion, merely a parallel arrangement of mostly vertical neoplastic tubular glands, in the low-power view. Under higher magnification (Fig. 11E), it becomes clear that the lesion is at least a high-grade intraepithelial neoplasia, since the rounded nuclei are arranged in mildly irregular fashion, and show mildly irregular chromatin content and, occasionally, prominent nucleoli.

In the second biopsy from this area (Fig. 11F), neoplastic tubuli are found in several foci that are so irregular that we can no longer diagnose the lesion as intraepithelial neoplasia. Incipient neoplastic buds invading the lateral lamina propria are also seen.

The low-power view of the endoscopic mucosectomy specimen (Fig. 11G) already shows that the neoplasia is limited to the mucosa. Under higher magnification (Fig. 11H) we can clearly see, in addition to the parallel arrangement of neoplastic tubuli perpendicular to the surface, other neoplastic formations in the lamina propria of variable caliber that are not part of the normal architecture of the gastric mucosa and must therefore be interpreted as invasive.

In conclusion, I would interpret the biopsy of this case as at least high-grade dysplasia or suspicious for well-differentiated adenocarcinoma, and in the endoscopic mucosectomy specimen I would then diagnose an invasive well-differentiated intramucosal tubular adenocarcinoma.

In this difficult-to-diagnose borderline case, the variation in the diagnoses established by the pathologists is again considerable. Once more, the majority of Western pathologists are of the opinion that the lesion is only an intraepithelial neoplasia (dysplasia), while most Japanese pathologists diagnose a noninvasive carcinoma. The five Western pathologists, who adopt the Japanese viewpoint, revised their biopsy-based dysplasia diagnosis to carcinoma on the basis of the mucosectomy specimen.

Pathology Commentary

Yo Kato (Japan)

The biopsy specimen with a central defect discloses proliferation of straight or round tubular glands, in the upper half of the mucosa (Fig. 11D). The glands consist of eosinophilic cuboidal cells with a swollen round nucleus, with a conspicuous nucleolus (Fig. 11E). There is no evidence of invasion. The other biopsy specimen shows basically the same histology as that in Fig. 11D, but irregular-shaped glands are more prominent. The lower half of the mucosa is composed of mixed metaplastic and nonmetaplastic glands, often dilated, in Fig. 11D and of solely metaplastic glands in Fig. 11F. From these findings I would diagnose the lesion as tubular adenocarcinoma, very well-differentiated, noninvasive.

The EMR specimen shows the lesion is limited to the mucosa (Fig. 11G). The high-power view of a part in the upper section is shown in Fig. 11H. Slightly distorted tubular glands consist of eosinophilic cuboidal cells with a hyperchromatic oval nucleus. The nucleus is irregular in position and enlarged, particularly in the upper part of the glands: loss of cellular differentiation from the bottom to the top of the glands and nuclear pleomorphism are prominent. Invasion is, however, not clear. Small glands found in the right middle part of Fig. 11I are due to cutting, not a pattern of invasion. Thus, I interpret the case as well-differentiated tubular carcinoma, noninvasive, i.e., the same diagnosis as for the biopsy specimens.

Case 12, IIa+IIc-like

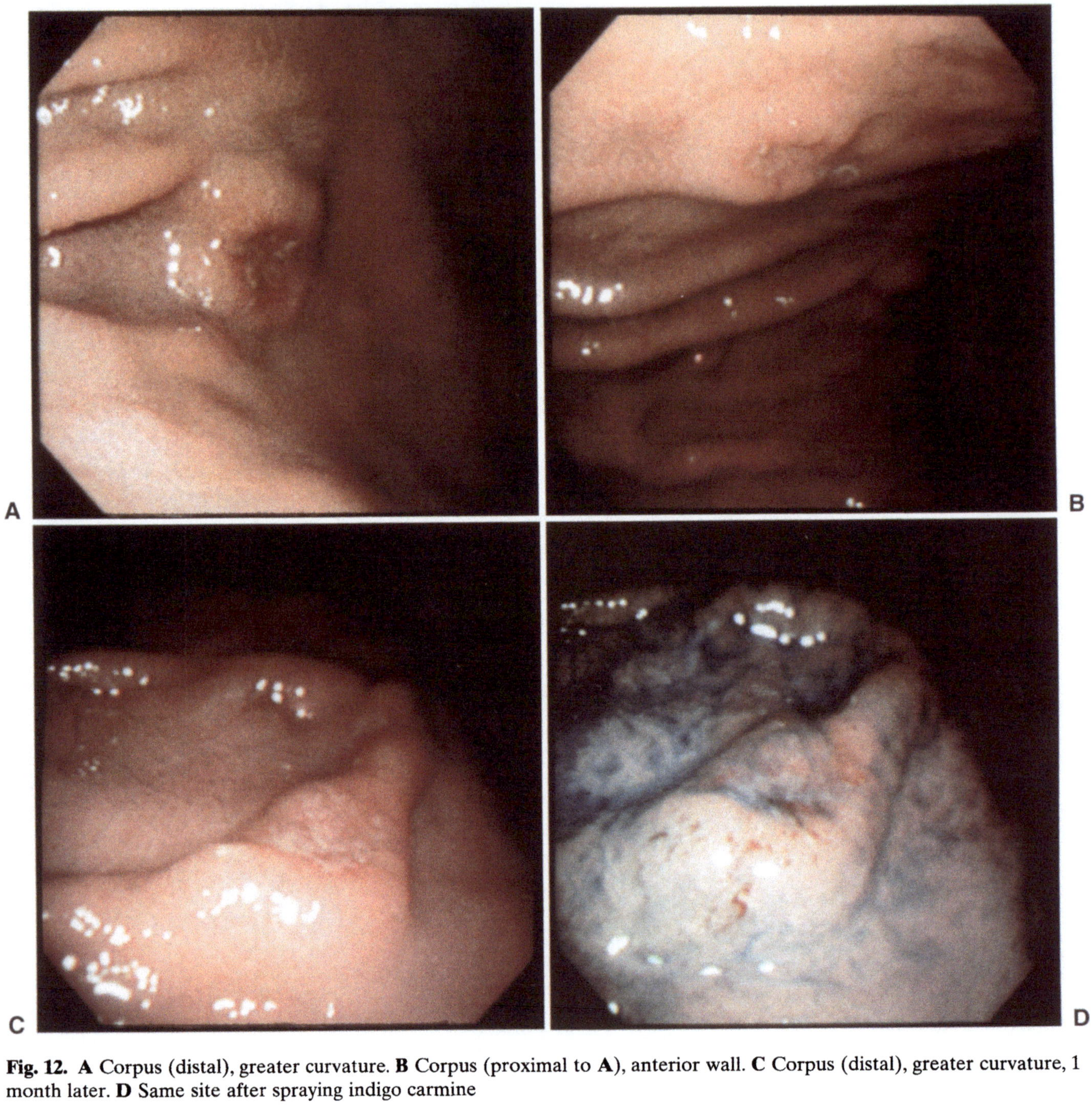

Fig. 12. **A** Corpus (distal), greater curvature. **B** Corpus (proximal to **A**), anterior wall. **C** Corpus (distal), greater curvature, 1 month later. **D** Same site after spraying indigo carmine

Case Description

A man, aged 49 years, with a history of gastric ulceration and major depression, complained of dysphagia for a month and underwent an upper GI endoscopic examination. Several lesions of 5–10mm in diameter were found in the corpus and biopsied (Fig. 12A,B). At follow-up endoscopy 1 month later, the most distal lesion at the greater curvature of the corpus (Fig. 12C, D) was endoscopically resected and a proton pump inhibitor was prescribed. Four weeks thereafter endoscopy was repeated, but no lesions were seen.

Endoscopy Commentary

Anthony T.R. Axon (UK)[1]

History

This 49-year-old man who was complaining of dysphagia for a month would undoubtedly have been submitted to upper digestive endoscopy in the West.

Endoscopic Appearance

It is unclear exactly what lesions were identified in the corpus, but if they had attracted suspicion it is probable that the endoscopy would have been repeated.

To the Western endoscopist the lesion shown in Fig. 12A would be highly suspicious if identified because although it is a small lesion, it is heaped up and is ulcerated in its center. It would have been biopsied. Similarly, the lesion in Fig. 12B also has a suspicious appearance. It is difficult to assess which of these lesions would have been found in a Western endoscopy unit. Those on the greater curve of the corpus could be missed if insufficient inflation had been used.

Histology and Management

The lesion shown in Fig. 12A reported as showing cancer would have raised considerable concern in the West. It is possible that re-endoscopy would have been undertaken, but more likely that the appearance and the pathology report would have been sufficient to warrant surgical intervention. Had the endoscopy been undertaken again a month later, as was the case in Japan, the lesion demonstrated in Fig. 12C and D would continue to cause concern. As these lesions endoscopically appear both to be protuberant rather than flat or depressed, they would most likely have been called either I or IIa.

Summary

This patient certainly would have been endoscoped. It is probable that in the West the lesions would have been found, biopsies would have confirmed potential malignancy, and total gastrectomy would have been undertaken.

Endoscopy Commentary

Shigeaki Yoshida (Japan)

Multiple depressed lesions surrounded by fold-like elevations are located on the greater curvature of the gastric body. The distal lesion (Fig. 12A) shows a well-demarcated depression surrounded by an annular-form

Table 12. Gastric lesion 12

Biopsy: × / Resection: ○	W W	W	W	W	W	W W W W W W W J	J W J	W J	W	W W W W	J J J J J J J
Regenerative changes						○	○	○	○	○	⊗
Indefinite for neoplasia					○					×	
Adenoma/dysplasia											
low-grade				○							
high-grade		○	⊗						×		
Carcinoma											
suspected		×			×			×			
non-invasive							×				
intramucosal	⊗			×		×					

[1]See footnote on p. 4.

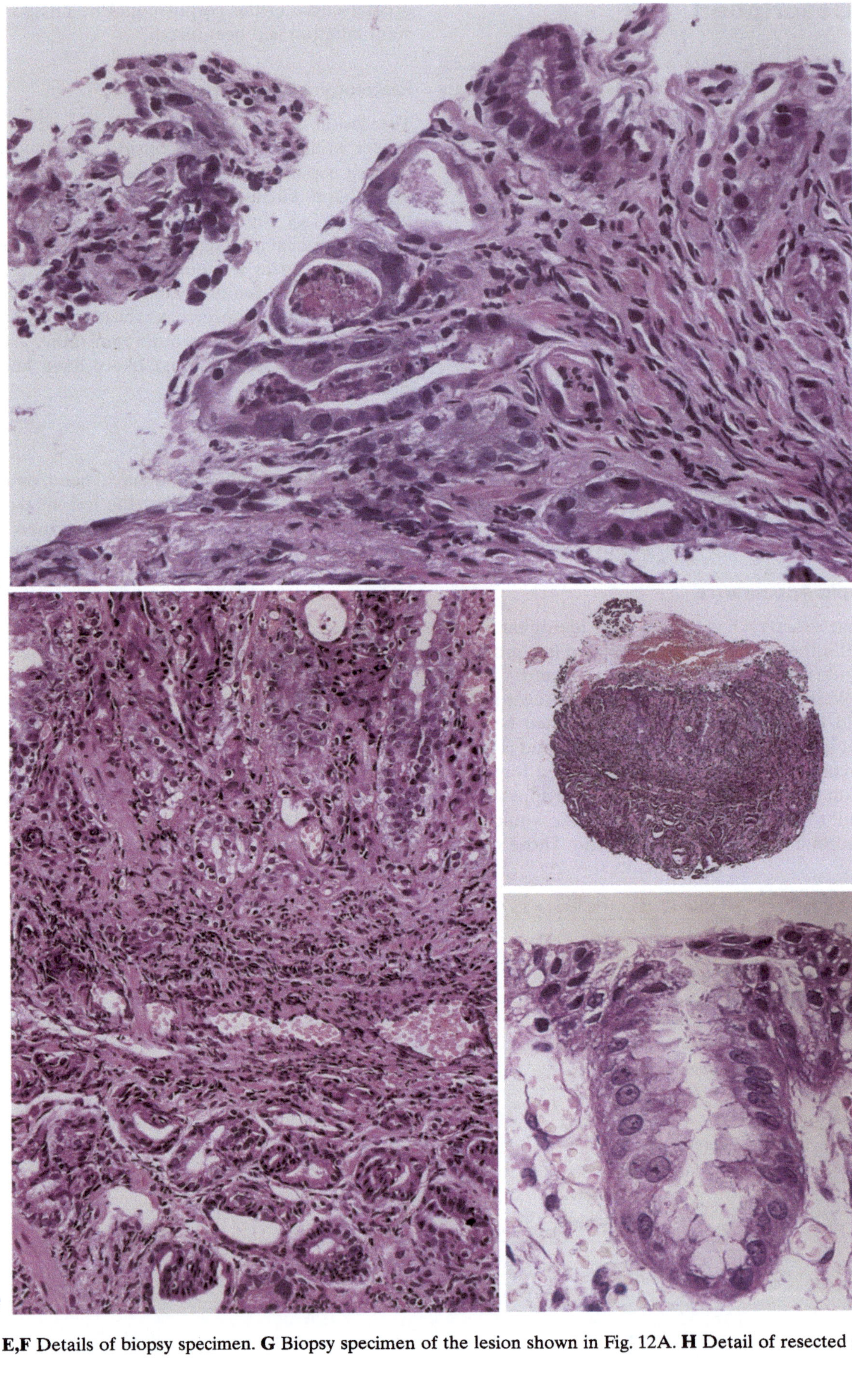

E

F

G

H

Fig. 12. **E,F** Details of biopsy specimen. **G** Biopsy specimen of the lesion shown in Fig. 12A. **H** Detail of resected specimen elevation. Deepness of the depression and nodularity in the annular elevation suggest malignancy. In contrast, a fresh hyperemic appearance in the depressed area may indicate benign inflammatory changes.

Another lesion is located in the anterior wall near the greater curvature of the gastric body (Fig. 12B). It also shows a depression surrounded by an annular-form elevation. Nevertheless, the depressed area covered with whitish exudate is shallow and has a regular margin. In addition, the elevated component is flat and fold-like. These features indicate a benign ulcerative or erosive change with swelling of surrounding mucosa, due to edema or small round cell infiltration accompanying inflammation.

A picture of the distal lesion taken at follow-up examination (Fig. 12C) demonstrates that the depressed component has become shallower than before and shows peptic ulcerative features such as hyperemic mucosa covered with a whitish exudate. In addition, the elevated component has changed its appearance from being nodular to fold-like. A dye-spraying picture (Fig. 12D) backs up these findings and reveals no definite irregularities at the margin of depression, indicating that this lesion is benign ulcerative rather than cancerous.

Apart from the endoscopic appearance in detail, a multiplicity of similar lesions generally is not a suggestive finding of cancerous but of benign peptic or lymphomatous lesions. From this point of view, the possibility of malignant lymphoma cannot be excluded.[1] Nevertheless, there are no destructive findings such as superficial erosive change or a discolored area elsewhere in the gastric mucosa, indicating a very low probability of lymphoma.

In conclusion, the two lesions presented in Case 12 should be diagnosed as benign nonspecific erosive or ulcerative.

Reference

1. Yoshida S, Yamaguchi H, Mitsushima T (1988) The early stages of primary malignant lymphoma of the stomach; its diagnosis by radiography and endoscopy. In: Maruyama M, Kimura K (eds) Review of clinical research in gastroenterology. Igakushoin, Tokyo, pp 69–81

Pathology Commentary

MANFRED STOLTE (Germany)

The endoscopic appearance of several lesions of 5–10mm in diameter in the corpus initially mitigates against neoplasia. In the presence of several such elevated lesions with central erosion, the pathologist must always consider the differential diagnosis of healing erosions, mainly induced by nonsteroidal anti-inflammatory drugs + aspirin (NSAID/ASA). Although such erosions are usually located in the antrum, they may also occur in the corpus. In this latter case, the pathologist must also give thought to the differential diagnosis of lymphocytic gastritis of the gastritis varioloformis type.

In the forceps biopsy material, on the basis of the findings shown in Fig. 12E, an adenocarcinoma might also be suspected. Since, however, most of the cells show dense hyperchromatic nuclei, I would diagnose this slide as indefinite and would, at most, suspect carcinoma.

In Fig. 12F we again find areas with compact, hyperchromatic nuclei with infranuclear vacuoles. This would suggest NSAID/ASA-induced regenerative changes rather than carcinoma. Unfortunately, the center of the lesion was not included in the biopsy specimen, so that the type of necrosis in the center of the lesion could not be determined with any degree of certainty. In Fig. 12H, under higher magnification, we again have indefinite findings with a number of the cell nuclei showing prominent nucleoli.

In this case, and on the basis of the histological changes in the biopsy material, I would initially have recommended discontinuation of NSAID/ASA medication followed by proton-pump inhibitor therapy and then endoscopy/biopsy follow-up.

However, this lesion was in fact treated with endoscopic mucosectomy. In the mucosectomy specimen, the histological findings in the low-power view (Fig. 12I) were more suggestive of regenerative changes than of carcinoma, since the architectural irregularities typical of carcinoma of the mucosa cannot be found. In addition, the homogeneous eosinophilic necrosis in the region of the surface erosion is more likely to indicate an NSAID/ASA-induced lesion than a carcinoma. This also applies to Fig. 12J. In Fig. 12K, however, we again see cell nuclei with irregular chromatin and prominent nucleoli. This renders the diagnosis of regenerative changes uncertain again. If, however, we then consider the perinuclear vacuoles, the findings do indeed suggest regenerative changes rather than a carcinoma.

In conclusion, on the basis of the biopsy material I would have diagnosed this case as indefinite, and tended to favor an NSAID/ASA-induced lesion, recommending merely endoscopy/biopsy follow-up after appropriate treatment. In the endoscopic mucosectomy specimen, the histological architectural changes typical of neoplasia are absent. Signs of an NSAID/ASA-induced erosion with corresponding regenerative changes predominate.

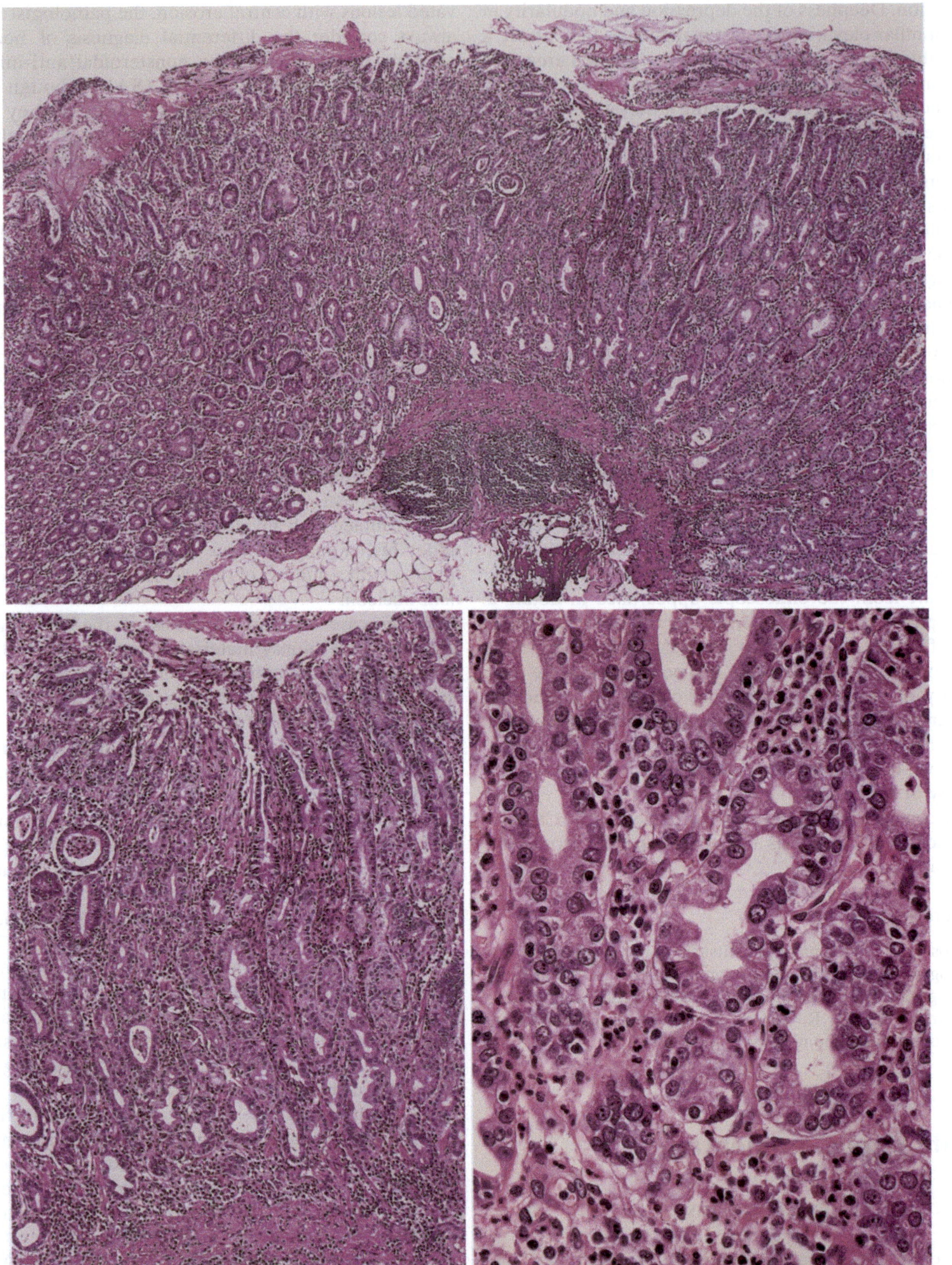

Fig. 12. **I** Resected specimen. **J** Detail of **I**. **K** Detail of **J**

The evaluation of the histological diagnoses shows that such cases represent a pitfall for the overdiagnosis of carcinoma. A positive aspect of this evaluation, however, is the fact that most pathologists diagnosed only regenerative changes in the endoscopic mucosectomy specimen.

Pathology Commentary

Yo Kato (Japan)

The biopsy specimen is a severely inflamed two-folded mucosa covered by hemorrhages and exudates, containing basophilic straight or round tubular glands on both sides of the specimen (Fig. 12G). The basic structure of the mucosa in terms of gland distribution and shape is preserved. Figure 12F is a magnification of the center of Fig. 12G, showing the deeper parts of the mucosa, consisting of degenerative or atrophic fundic glands. The slightly dilated deformed glands and occasional intraglandular epithelial infolding in the lower half of the figure are due to inflammation and biopsy procedure. The stroma is obliterated by a fibrinous or fibrous substance with dilated capillaries and inflammatory cells. The high-power view (Fig. 12E) indicates basophilic, rather dilated or small atrophied glands, with hyperchromatic nuclei. The nucleus, however, is round and basally situated along the basement membrane in a normal-looking gland in the upper part of the figure. Next to this gland, a severely atrophied gland comprised of thin epithelium is present. Since the fibrosis is remarkable in the stroma and some polymorphonuclear exudate is recognized in a small tissue over the mucosa (Fig. 12E, left), the deformity in gland structure is considered to be due to severe inflammation. Thus, I would diagnose the lesion as regenerative or degenerative change due to inflammation.

In the resected specimen (Fig. 12I), the mucosa is covered by thick inflammatory exudate and the glands appear, in general, basophilic. The glands are, however, regularly distributed, with slightly distended ones in several places (Fig. 12J,K). Although inflammatory cell infiltration in the stroma is strong enough to involve the glandular epithelium, the basic structure of the mucosa is preserved. The nucleus is slightly swollen, but round and regular in size, within a reactive change. *Helicobacter pylori* infection is clear on the surface of or between the foveolar epithelia, or inside a gland, as shown in Fig. 12H. As a whole, the lesion is concluded to be an inflammatory change caused by *H. pylori* infection.

3. Early Cancer of the Colorectum (Cases 13–19)

Case 13, IIa

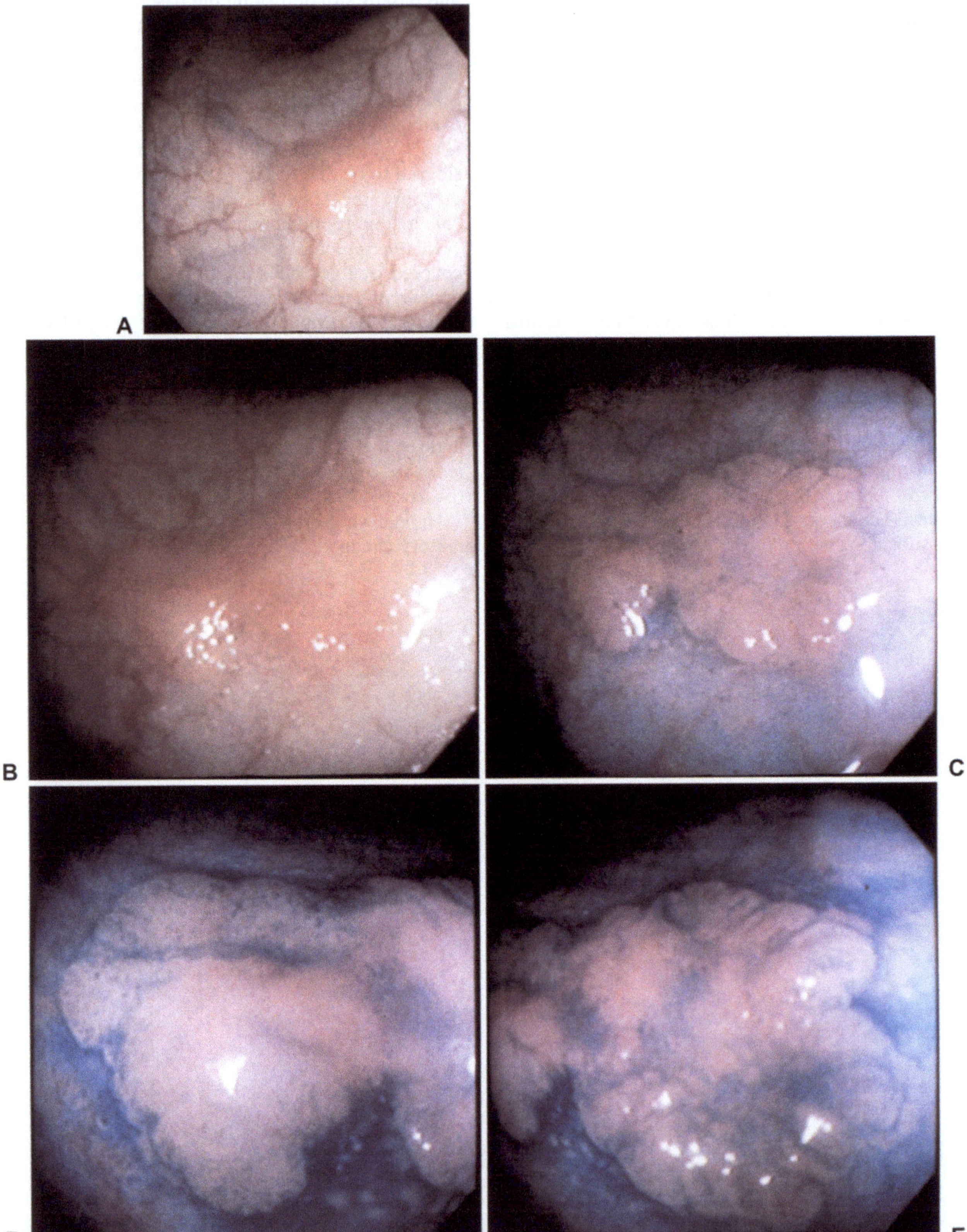

Fig. 13. **A** Descending colon. **B** Close-up view. **C** Same site after spraying indigo carmine. **D** Detail of **C**. **E** Detail of **C**

Case Description

A woman, aged 54 years, with a history of gastric ulcer and endometriosis, had no recent abdominal symptoms, but because a fecal occult blood test had turned out to be positive she underwent a barium enema examination, which was followed up by colonoscopy. A lesion of about 13 mm in diameter was found in the descending colon. Endoscopic resection was performed. The resection margins were free of tumor. On follow-up endoscopic examinations no local recurrence was found.

Endoscopy Commentary

Christopher B. Williams (UK)

This 13-mm lesion is of rather unusual shape, but endoscopically appears likely to be benign, in spite of the slightly depressed central parts. It is ideal for "injection polypectomy" or EMR (endoscopic mucosal resection). Depending on how effectively submucosal injection (2–5 cc of saline, saline/adrenaline, or other iso- or hypertonic solution) lifts the lesion above the mucosal surface, the endoscopist can decide whether to snare in one or two portions; a single specimen is clearly preferable histologically but the realities of difficult access or other practical problems in snaring sometimes forces compromise on the endoscopist. In the unlikely circumstance of there being the "no-lifting sign" or if the lesion seemed fixed or indurated, the endoscopist would be warned to be extra careful, and to mark the site with an India ink tattoo. Safety of the patient has to be paramount (over the requirements of the histopathologist), because perforation is an ever-present possibility during overaggressive electrosurgery. In all probability this lesion would have been uneventfully managed in 2–3 minutes.

After snaring, retrieval of the histological specimen would only present a problem if other polyps were also present. Aspiration of the snared portion(s) (if possible through the 3.7-mm channel of the colonoscope) would fragment the specimen and cause difficulty in interpretation. Ideally the Roth net, an ingenious atraumatic nylon bag ideal for bringing one or more specimens out of the colon; would be used for retrieval; most endoscopists would probably gently grasp the snared specimen in the snare and pull it out.

Endoscopy Commentary

Masaki Kawahara (Japan)

The endoscopic views (Fig. 13A and B) of this lesion show a small, superficial elevation (type IIa) with a reddish color, polygonal shape, and with a convex margin. The vascular network pattern (visibility of transparent capillaries) is not visible, so the border between the lesion and the surrounding normal mucosa can be clearly recognized. This observation is very important for the initial detection of superficial lesions.

No deformity or rigidity of the bowel wall is visible around the lesion. No converging folds, twitching, or white spots are visible. The lesion also has no stiffness or expansiveness. Therefore, this lesion is considered to be a mucosal lesion whose depth is limited to within the mucosal layer. The dye-scattering pictures (Fig. 13C–E), which are important for evaluating such superficial elevated lesions, clearly demonstrate the margin of the lesion and the character of the surface. The central area of the lesion has an irregular surface with a smooth convex (left part) and a small granular unevenness with very shallow depression (right part), but no ulceration or erosion on the surface is visible. These findings suggest that this superficial lesion may be a mucosal cancer (carcinoma in situ). Endoscopic treatment (EMR: endoscopic mucosal resection) is recommended for this lesion to check the pathology. A biopsy should not be performed because this procedure would cause fibrosis in the lesion, making endoscopic resection difficult by preventing the lifting of the lesion by the injection of physiologic saline during the EMR procedure.

Pathology Commentary

Jeremy R. Jass (Canada)

This lesion removed from the descending colon is small (13 mm) and slightly raised. Despite its small size, the lesion shows high-grade cytology evidenced by nuclear enlargement and pleomorphism, loss of nuclear polarity, and nucleolar prominence (Fig. 13H and I). Architecturally the lesion is composed of simple tubules with little branching. There are no features suggestive of invasion of the lamina propria.

The case is interesting for several reasons. It illustrates a small but high-grade lesion that could be missed endoscopically and subsequently present as an interval cancer. The importance of such neoplasms is only just beginning to be acknowledged in the West [1–3]. The diagnostic opinion amongst Western pathologists is

Table 13. Colorectal lesion 13

Diagnosis	Resection	Pathologists
Adenoma/dysplasia		
low-grade	○	W W W W
high-grade	○	W W J; W W J; W W W; W W W; W W J; W W J
Carcinoma		
suspected	○	W J J J
non-invasive	○	J J J J
intramucosal	○	W

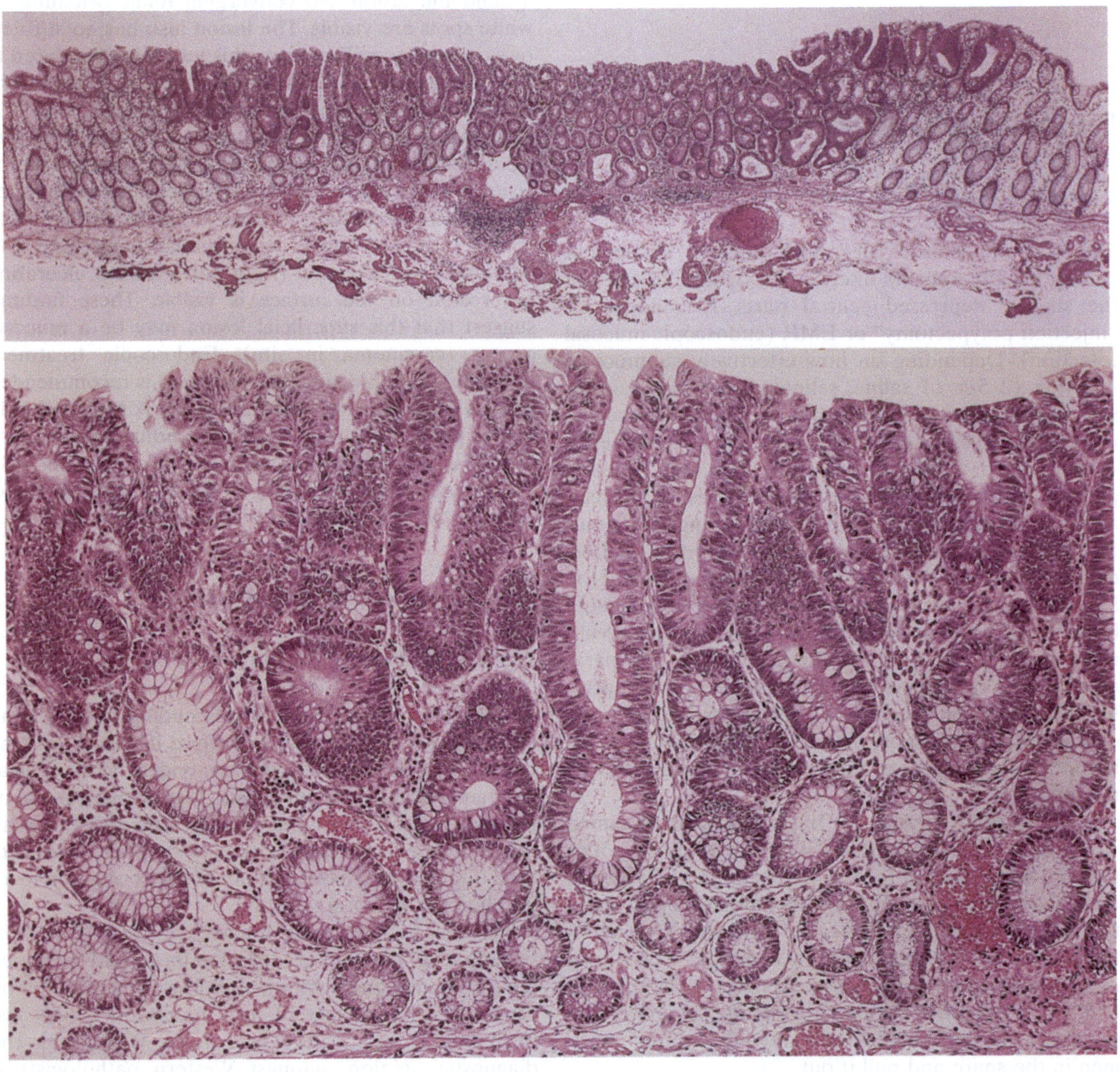
F
G

Fig. 13. **F** Resected specimen. **G** Detail of **F**

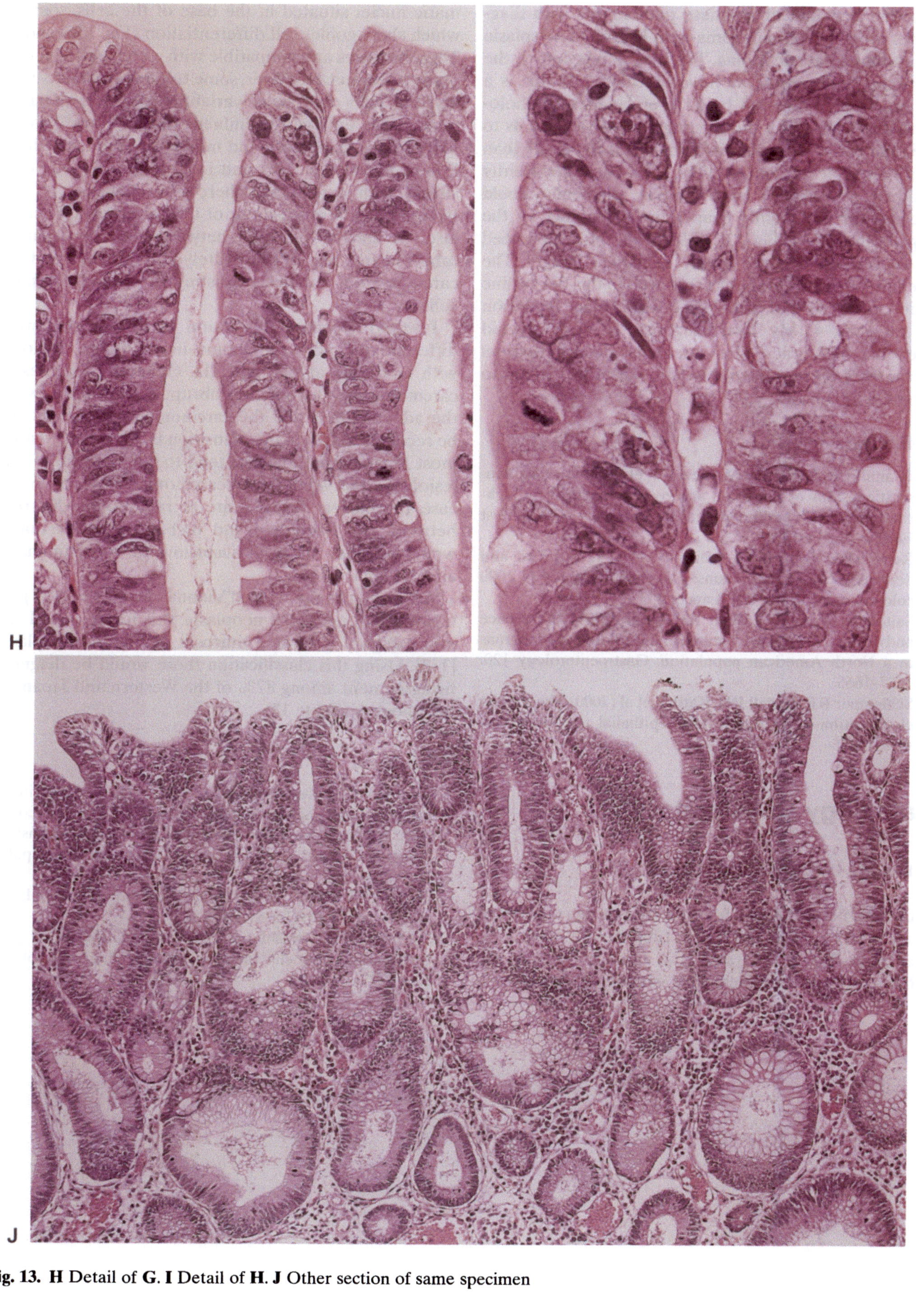

Fig. 13. **H** Detail of **G**. **I** Detail of **H**. **J** Other section of same specimen

broader than that of Japanese pathologists with diagnoses ranging from adenoma with low-grade dysplasia to intramucosal carcinoma. The case is relevant to the controversy regarding *de novo* carcinoma. If this is a carcinoma as suggested by 64% of Japanese pathologists, did it arise in a pre-existing adenoma? Glands to the right of the lesion appear to be of a lower grade than those of the center and left (Fig. 13F). These apparently residual low-grade adenomatous elements could account for the slightly heaped-up appearance of the edge of the lesion (Fig. 13C). However, this would need to be verified in more highly magnified images. The Vienna classification [4] succeeds well in this borderline lesion in that 84% of pathologists would place the lesion in category 4. My own diagnosis is non-polypoid adenoma, high-grade. Most adenomas do not progress to cancer. Left untreated, I would expect this lesion to progress to cancer.

References

1. Jaramillo E, Watanabe M, Slezak P, et al (1995) Flat neoplastic lesions of the colon and rectum detected by high-resolution video endoscopy and chromoscopy. Gastrointest Endosc 42:114–122
2. Rembacken BJ, Fujii T, Cairns A, et al (2000) Flat and depressed colonic neoplasms: a prospective study of 1000 colonoscopies in the UK. Lancet 355:1211–1214
3. Saitoh Y, Waxman I, West AB, et al (2001) Prevalence and distinctive biologic features of flat colorectal adenomas in a North American population. Gastroenterology 120: 1657–1665
4. Schlemper RJ, Riddell RH, Kato Y, et al (2000) The Vienna classification of gastrointestinal epithelial neoplasia. Gut 47:251–255

Pathology Commentary

Akinori Iwashita (Japan)

This superficial elevated lesion is structurally composed of relatively regular and simple tubules with no or little branching (Fig. 13F, G, and J). A large number of the tubules consist of atypical cells with round hyperchromatic nuclei situated in the base of the cells, some of which show goblet cell differentiation (Fig. 13G and J). These features are compatible with a conventional low-grade adenoma. However, some tubules are made up of atypical cells that have variably sized and enlarged nuclei with enlarged prominent nucleoli, and show a loss of nuclear polarity and moderate pseudostratification of nuclei (Fig. 13H and I). Such features are consistent with carcinoma. There is no invasion of the lamina propria mucosae or of the submucosa. There is also no abrupt transition between the adenomatous tubules consisting of moderately atypical cells and the carcinomatous tubules consisting of severely atypical cells.

I would diagnose this lesion as a suspected well-differentiated adenocarcinoma in a tubular adenoma with moderate atypia, type IIa. Generally, in cases of carcinoma in adenoma, an abrupt transition between the adenomatous and the carcinomatous portions can be recognized. When this transition is not clearly visible, most Japanese pathologists tend to diagnose the whole lesion as either adenoma or carcinoma. However, in this case, the nuclear features are so remarkably different between the low-grade and high-grade areas that I would consider this to be suspicious for a carcinoma in an adenoma.

According to the revised Vienna classification of gastrointestinal epithelial neoplasia, this lesion would fall into category 4, termed mucosal high-grade neoplasia [1–3]. Using this classification there would be diagnostic agreement among 87% of the Western and Japanese pathologists (Table 13).

References

1. Schlemper RJ, Kato Y, Stolte M (2000) Diagnostic criteria for gastrointestinal carcinomas in Japan and Western countries: proposal for a new classification system of gastrointestinal epithelial neoplasia. J Gastroenterol Hepatol 15:G49–G57
2. Dixon MF (2002) Gastrointestinal epithelial neoplasia: Vienna revisited. Gut 51:130–131
3. Schlemper RJ, Iwashita A (2004) Classification of gastrointestinal epithelial neoplasia. Curr Diagn Pathol 10: 128–139

Case 14, IIa

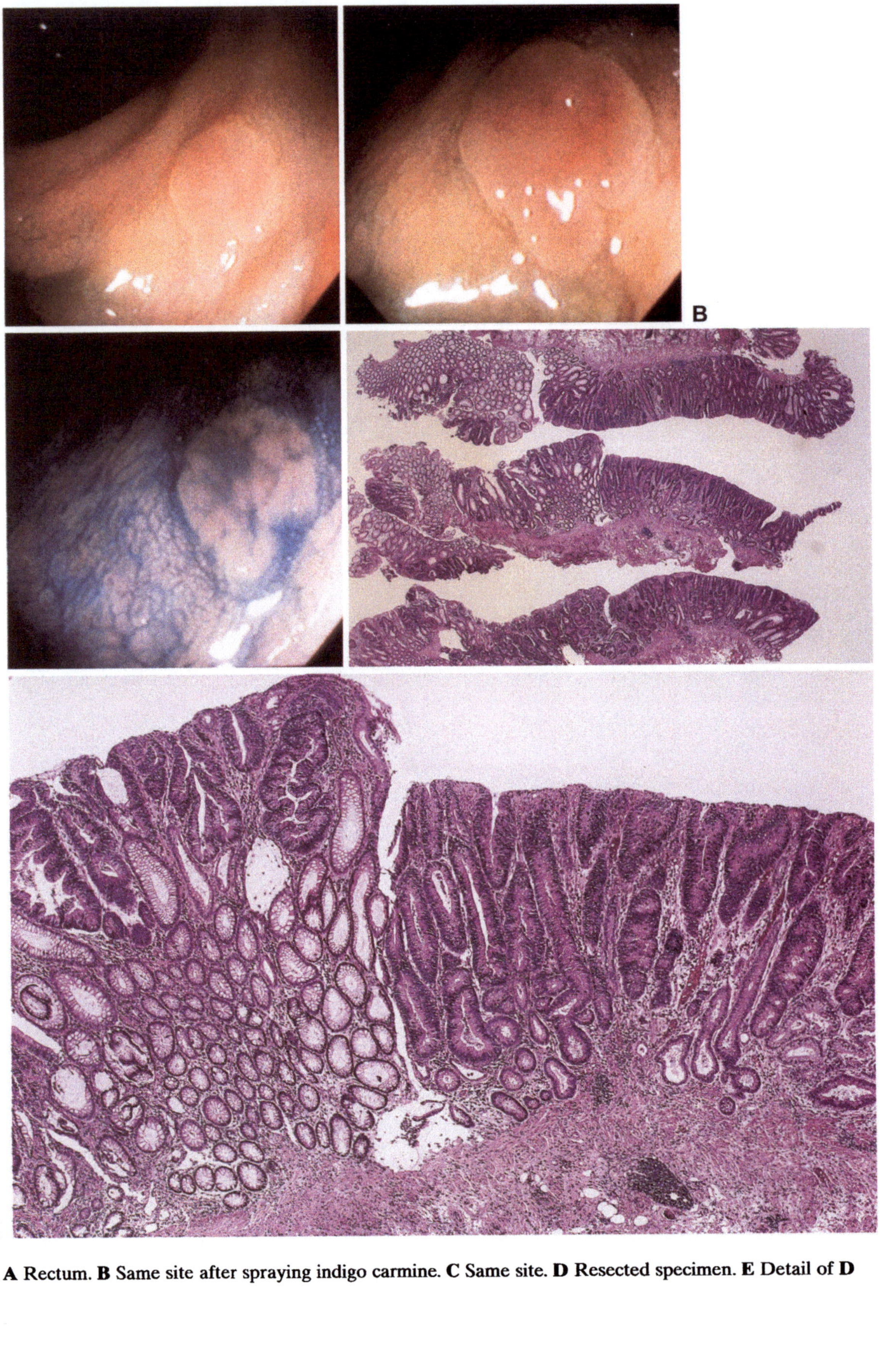

A B C D E

Fig. 14. A Rectum. **B** Same site after spraying indigo carmine. **C** Same site. **D** Resected specimen. **E** Detail of **D**

Case Description

A man, aged 60 years, with a history of lung tuberculosis, was symptom-free and had a screening test for fecal occult blood. Because this was positive, he underwent radiologic and subsequently endoscopic examination of the lower gastrointestinal tract. A lesion of about 5 mm in diameter was found in the rectum. Endoscopic resection was performed. The resection margins were free of tumor. On follow-up endoscopic examinations no local recurrence was found.

Endoscopy Commentary

Christopher B. Williams (UK)

This type of 5-mm lesion would require a minor management decision by the endoscopist—whether to manage by "hot biopsy" (probably unwise over 4 mm diameter), by simple snaring, or by EMR. The lesion has a configuration that most endoscopists would call "sessile" but that a few might categorize as "slightly elevated." Although image resolution is suboptimal, visually its morphological features at first sight give mixed messages. The scalloped margins of the lower part of the lesion and its pale shiny surface (sculptured on dye spray) suggest a hyperplastic nature, but the matt surface and relative protuberance of the upper part show that of an adenoma.

"If in doubt take it out;" I would palpate the lesion with the closed (mini-) snare tube to check soft consistency and mobility over the underlying surface (benign and noninfiltrating), then remove it by simple electrosurgical snaring. Submucosal injection would be easy, but probably an unnecessary waste of time. Such lesions may be accompanied by several others around the colon, so it would be desirable to save time in removal in order to have time to obtain an accurate examination of the colon overall. The snared specimen would be small enough to aspirate down the instrumentation/suction channel into a polyp suction trap, or into a gauze inserted into the suction line.

Endoscopy Commentary

Masaki Kawahara (Japan)

The endoscopic pictures (Fig. 14A and B) demonstrate a roundish-shaped small, superficial elevation (type IIa). The color of this lesion is almost normal compared with the surrounding colonic mucosa. This lesion shows no stiffness, expansiveness, fold convergence, or coexisting white spots. The surface of the lesion is rather smooth, with no erosion or granular pattern. The dye-scattering picture (Fig. 14C) clarifies the margin of the lesion, which is demonstrated by a mild elevation around the lesion from the adjacent colonic mucosa. The surface of the lesion has a slight unevenness, but there are no obvious signs that this lesion is malignant. This IIa lesion was considered to be an adenoma.

Pathology Commentary

Jeremy R. Jass (Canada)

The rectal lesion is slightly elevated and only 5 mm in diameter. As compared with Case 13, the nuclear:cytoplasmic ratio is relatively low, nuclei are elongated and pseudostratified, and the chromatin is condensed. Although some nucleoli are prominent, they remain small and there is only focal loss of nuclear polarity

Table 14. Colorectal lesion 14

Resection: ○	WW WW WW WW WJ	W W WWW WWW WJJ	J J J	J J J J J	W W
Adenoma/dysplasia					
low-grade	○				
high-grade		○			
Carcinoma					
suspected			○		
non-invasive				○	
intramucosal					○

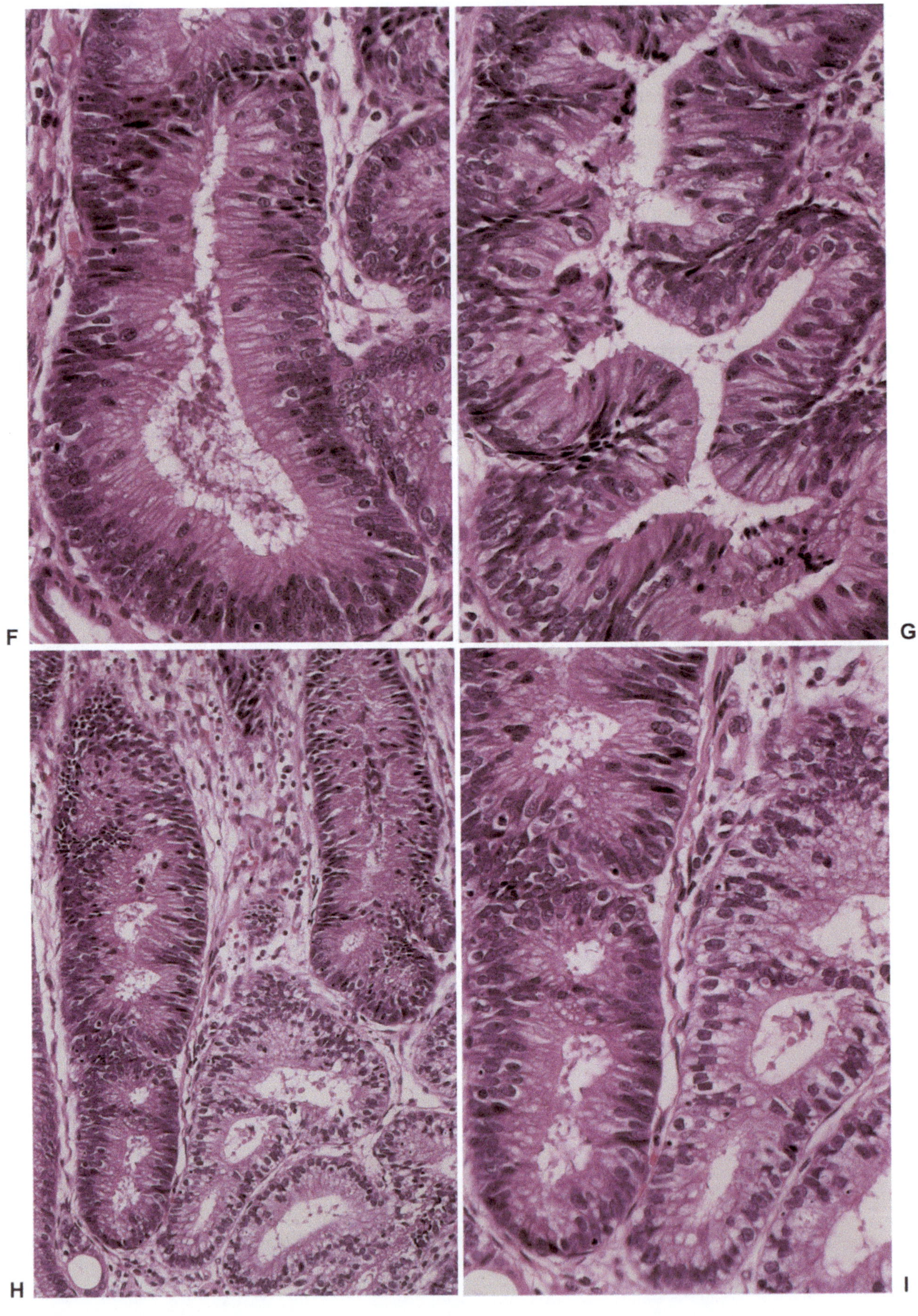

Fig. 14. F Detail of **E**. **G** Detail of **E**. **H** Detail of **E**. **I** Detail of **H**

(Fig. 14F). Architecturally, the lesion shows some glandular complexity as evidenced by infolding, branching, and budding (Fig. 14G and H).

The cytological and architectural appearances fit with adenoma rather than carcinoma, and I would classify the lesion as low-grade. In a three-grade system, I would diagnose this as a nonpolypoid adenoma with moderate dysplasia (intraepithelial neoplasia), and acknowledge that the cytological and architectural changes were unusually advanced for such a small lesion. The Vienna classification is less successful for this lesion than in Case 13, with 32%, 61%, and 6% of diagnoses being placed within categories 3, 4, and 5, respectively [1]. Western pathologists were more likely than Japanese pathologists to perceive Case 14 as being a lower grade lesion than Case 13. The distributions of opinion amongst Japanese pathologists are similar for cases 13 and 14. Amongst the Japanese pathologists it is possible that the more pronounced architectural complexity in Case 14 as compared with Case 13 has compensated for the reduced cytological atypia. The architectural complexity may also account for the suspected or definite diagnosis of noninvasive carcinoma by 73% of Japanese pathologists.

Reference

1. Schlemper RJ, Riddell RH, Kato Y, et al (2000) The Vienna classification of gastrointestinal epithelial neoplasia. Gut 47:251–255

Pathology Commentary

Akinori Iwashita (Japan)

This superficial elevated lesion is architecturally made up of atypical glands, some of which show complex infolding, budding and branching (Fig. 14E, G, and H). The neoplastic cells have rounded, markedly hyperchromatic nuclei and thick nuclear membranes (Fig. 14F, G, and I) and show a loss of nuclear polarity and moderate nuclear pseudostratification (Fig. 14F and G). These nuclear features are not compatible any more with a conventional adenoma, although the artificial distortion of the tissue makes a proper assessment of the cytological features somewhat difficult (Fig. 14D and E). There are no findings suggestive of invasion into the lamina propria mucosae or the submucosa.

From these structural and cellular appearances, I would diagnose this lesion as suspicious for well-differentiated adenocarcinoma, type IIa. Using the revised Vienna classification [1–3], the diagnostic opinions of Western pathologists are divided between mucosal low-grade and mucosal high-grade neoplasia, whereas almost all Japanese pathologists would agree this to be a mucosal high-grade neoplastic lesion, i.e., category 4, for which endoscopic resection is definitely indicated (Table 14). Not only the architectural structures but also the cytological features would be regarded as high-grade by most Japanese pathologists.

References

1. Schlemper RJ, Kato Y, Stolte M (2000) Diagnostic criteria for gastrointestinal carcinomas in Japan and Western countries: proposal for a new classification system of gastrointestinal epithelial neoplasia. J Gastroenterol Hepatol 15:G49–G57
2. Dixon MF (2002) Gastrointestinal epithelial neoplasia: Vienna revisited. Gut 51:130–131
3. Schlemper RJ, Iwashita A (2004) Classification of gastrointestinal epithelial neoplasia. Curr Diagn Pathol 10: 128–139

Case 15, IIa

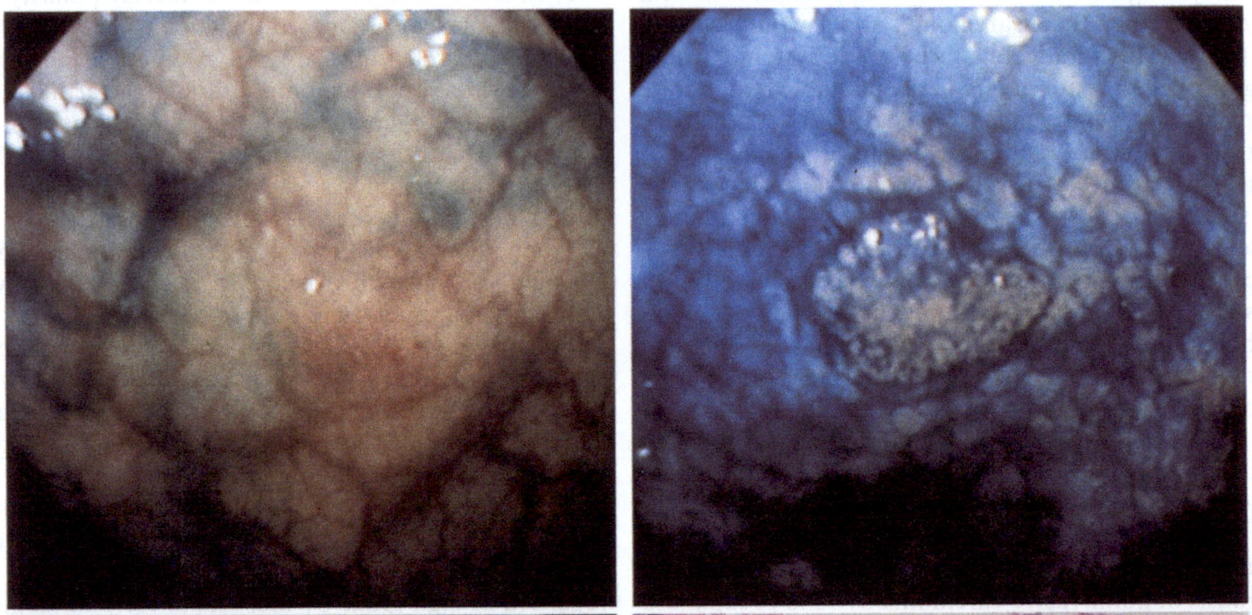

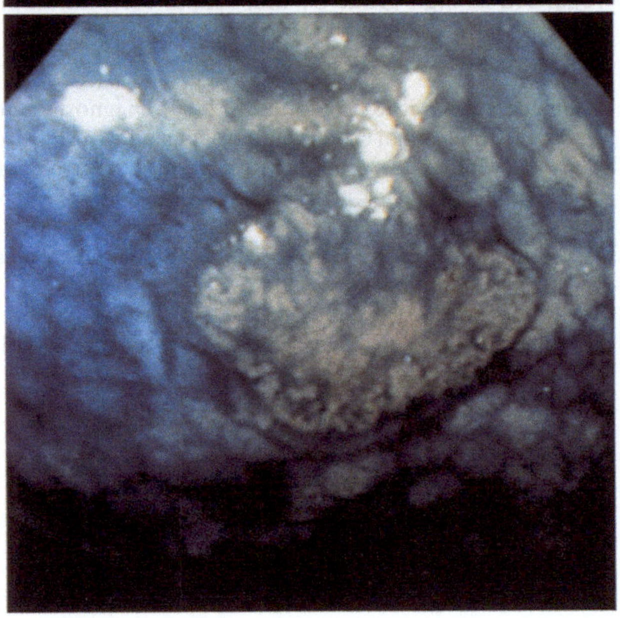

Table 15. Colorectal lesion 15

Resection: ○	W W	W J		
	W W J	W W		
	W W J	W W		
	W W J	W J		
	W W J	W J		
	W J J	W J	J	W
Adenoma/dysplasia				
low-grade	○			
high-grade		○		
Carcinoma				
suspected			○	
intramucosal				○

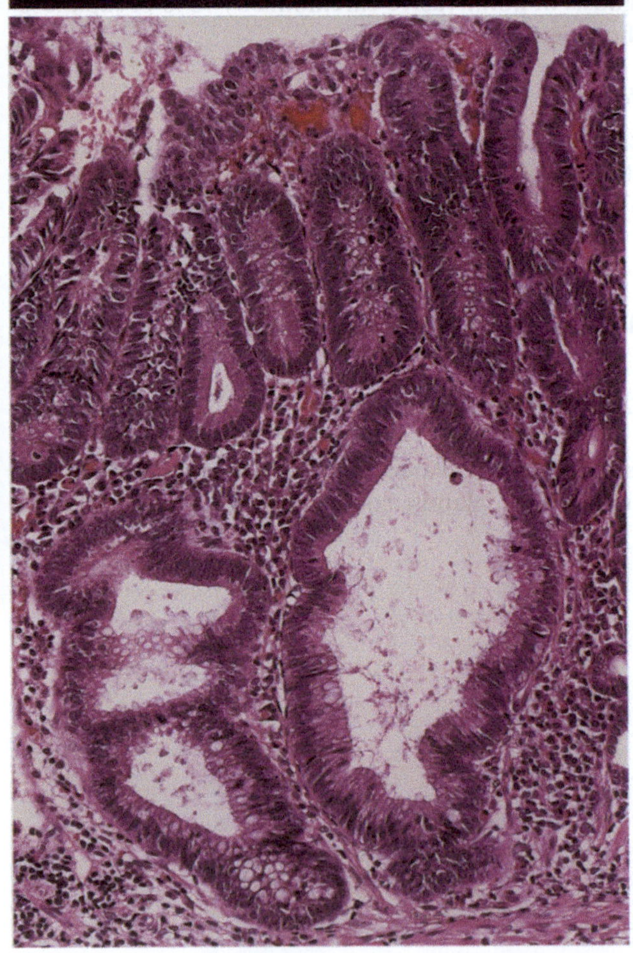

Fig. 15. **A** Sigmoid colon. **B** Same site after spraying indigo carmine. **C** Same site. **D** Detail of resected specimen

Case Description

A man, aged 70 years, complaining of chronic diarrhea underwent a colonoscopic examination. A lesion of about 5 mm in diameter was found in the sigmoid colon. Endoscopic resection was performed.

Endoscopy Commentary

Christopher B. Williams (UK)

The slightly reddened and rough/matt surface of this 5-mm slightly elevated lesion mark it out as an adenoma. Lesions of this size and shape are easily missed by endoscopists, especially if bowel preparation is poor or examination technique is not scrupulous—with patient position change, irrigation or aspiration, and hand skills needed to obtain a good view. Visually the small size, even coloration, and surface symmetry (enhanced on dye spray) all suggest a benign nature.

For certainty of removal and ideal histology, injection polypectomy (EMR) would be ideal, but many Western endoscopists might manage with conventional snare polypectomy. "Cold snaring" without electrocoagulation would be an alternative option at this small size, providing that deflation of the colon and puckering-up of the mucosal surface allowed sufficient snare entrapment. The specimen would be retrieved by aspiration.

Endoscopy Commentary

Masaki Kawahara (Japan)

The endoscopic picture (Fig. 15A) shows a very small, reddish-colored lesion with a superficial elevation (type IIa) or without an elevation (type IIb). The vascular network pattern is disturbed in the lesion, enabling the small lesion to be recognized. The dye-scattering pictures (Fig. 15B and C) show that the lesion has an irregular shape with a clear sphere and an amorphous surface. No signs of deep invasion into the submucosal layer, such as ulceration, stiffness, or expansiveness, are present. Therefore, this lesion is thought to be a mucosal lesion and may be a mucosal cancer because of its irregular surface. Endoscopic removal of this lesion is recommended.

Pathology Commentary

Jeremy R. Jass (Canada)

This sigmoid colon lesion is a small (5 mm), superficial elevated adenoma. The nuclei are small and basal, but tend to be ovoid with some nucleolar prominence and hyperchromatism (Fig. 15G). The glands are simple tubular structures (Fig. 15D and F). The lack of architectural complexity may explain why most Japanese and Western pathologists agree on the diagnosis of adenoma as opposed to carcinoma in this case but not in Case 14.

The main disagreement is on the grade of the lesion. This means that the distribution of diagnoses according to the Vienna classification is 55%, 42%, and 3% for categories 3, 4, and 5, respectively [1]. This is a surprisingly poor agreement and illustrates the subjectivity of grading benign lesions on morphological grounds. The split on grade is similar for Japanese and Western pathologists. This indicates that the different diagnostic approaches by the Japanese and the Western pathologists relate more to labeling lesions as cancer and noncancer and less to the grading of adenoma. Better systems for grading are now required, though the benefits will be more for research than clinical management. In the future, grading on the basis of cytology, architecture, and differentiation needs to be correlated with genetic alterations and related to different tumorigenic pathways. Cytological grade is likely to vary according to whether neoplasms develop in a background of DNA or chromosomal instability [2]. A grading system that assesses only a single pathway of tumorigenesis is not realistic.

It is notable that a few diagnoses of intramucosal carcinoma have been attached to cases 13, 14, and 15. In each case, this diagnosis was by one or more Western pathologists and not Japanese pathologists. This diagnosis is clearly at variance with both Western and Japanese consensus and shows that more aggressive diagnoses are not necessarily limited to Japanese pathologists.

References

1. Schlemper RJ, Riddell RH, Kato Y, et al (2000) The Vienna classification of gastrointestinal epithelial neoplasia. Gut 47:251–255
2. Jass JR (1999) Towards a molecular classification of colorectal cancer. Int J Colorect Dis 14:194–200

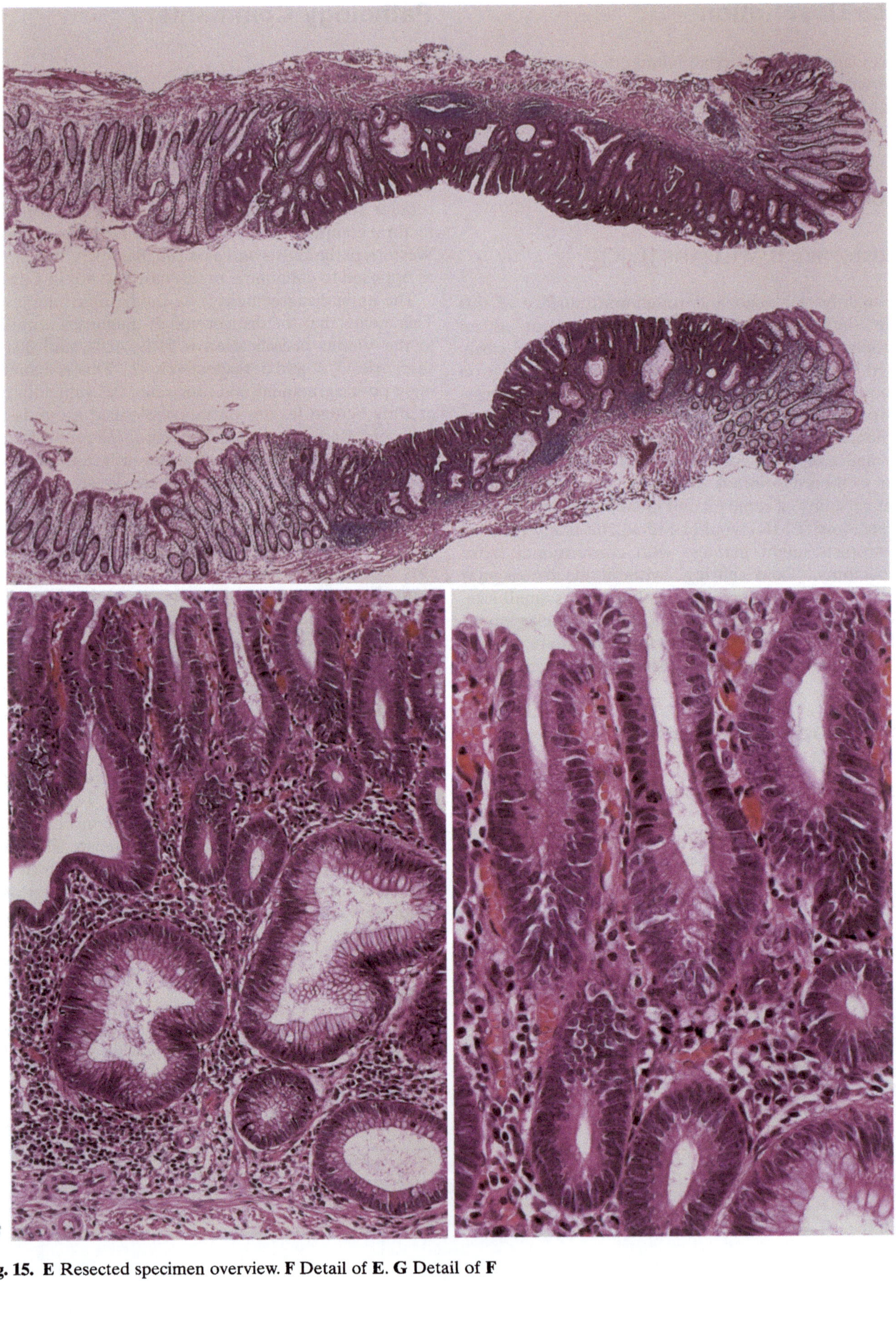

E F G

Fig. 15. **E** Resected specimen overview. **F** Detail of **E**. **G** Detail of **F**

Pathology Commentary

Akinori Iwashita (Japan)

This superficial elevated lesion is architecturally composed of slightly crowded and regularly arranged simple tubular glands. Cytologically, the neoplastic cells have basally oriented spindle shaped nuclei, and show very mild or no pseudostratification of the nuclei (Fig. 15D, F, and G). However, the cells in the proliferative zones have ovoid nuclei with some nucleolar prominence and hyperchromatism (see the cells in the center of the upper half of Fig. 15G). In general, one should not diagnose high-grade neoplasia on the basis of the nuclear features of cells in the proliferative zones. No evidence of invasion of the lamina propria mucosae is found in this lesion.

My diagnosis is tubular adenoma with mild to moderate atypia, i.e., low-grade adenoma, type IIa, or mucosal low-grade neoplasia according to the revised Vienna classification [1–3].

References

1. Schlemper RJ, Kato Y, Stolte M (2000) Diagnostic criteria for gastrointestinal carcinomas in Japan and Western countries: proposal for a new classification system of gastrointestinal epithelial neoplasia. J Gastroenterol Hepatol 15:G49–G57
2. Dixon MF (2002) Gastrointestinal epithelial neoplasia: Vienna revisited. Gut 51:130–131
3. Schlemper RJ, Iwashita A (2004) Classification of gastrointestinal epithelial neoplasia. Curr Diagn Pathol 10: 128–139

Case 16, IIc+IIa

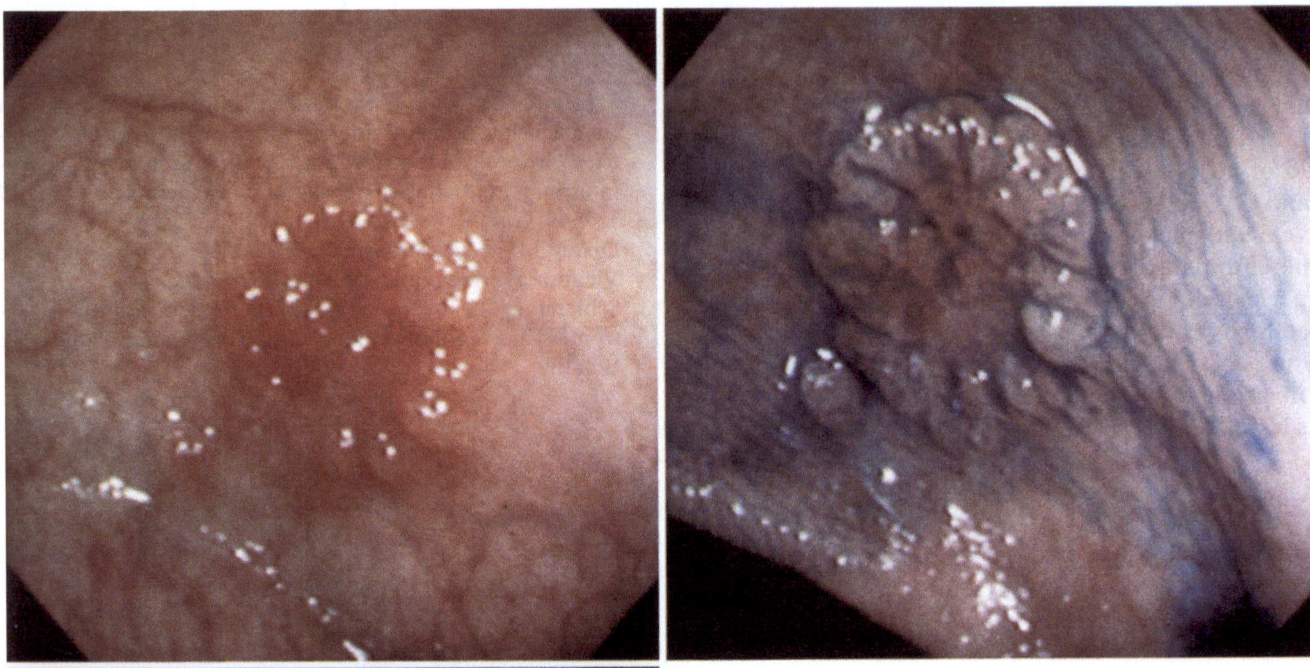

A B

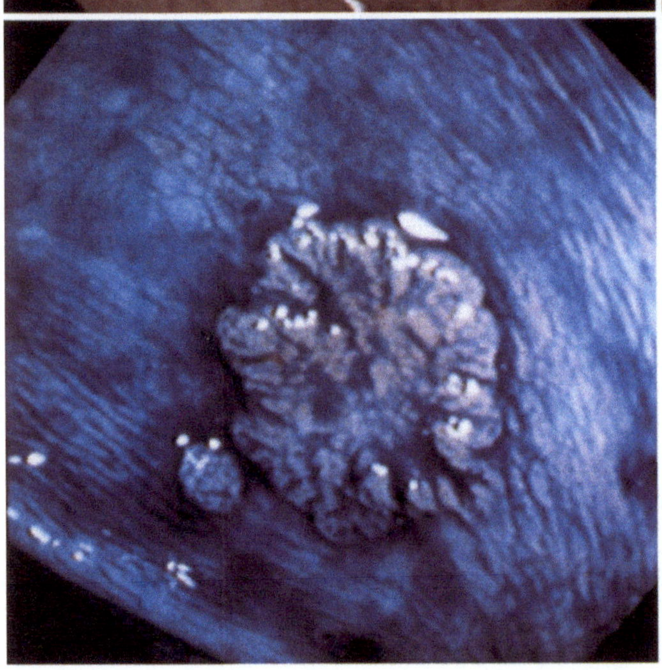

C

Fig. 16. **A** Ascending colon. **B** Same site after spraying indigo carmine. **C** Same site

Table 16. Colorectal lesion 16

Resection: ○	W W W W	W	W	W W W	W J W J W J J W J J W W J W W J W W J W J J
Adenoma/dysplasia					
high-grade	○				
Carcinoma					
suspected		○			
intramucosal			○		
intra- or submucosal				○	
submucosal					○

Case Description

A woman, aged 65 years, had undergone a curative left-sided colectomy for an early carcinoma in the descending colon without lymph node metastases. Since then she had been symptom-free. On follow-up colonoscopic examination three years later, a lesion of about 11 mm in diameter was found in the ascending colon. Endoscopic resection was performed. The resection margins were free of tumor. Several months later, a partial colectomy with lymph node dissection was performed.

Endoscopy Commentary

Christopher B. Williams (UK)

The reddened color and slightly depressed center of this 11-mm lesion suggest an aggressive nature; however, the apparently even surface on dye spray make it relatively unlikely that invasive malignancy will be found. If endoscopic ultrasound facilities were available the endoscopist could prove the point with an ultrasound miniprobe; most would simply ensure complete removal by submucosal injection (watch for "no-lifting sign" during injection) before conventional snaring—also destroying the adjoining 1-mm satellite lesion. If there was doubt about adequate snaring, the snare tip could be used (gently) for additional basal or marginal electrocoagulation, but argon plasma coagulation would be preferable in view of the hazards of full-thickness damage in the thin proximal colon.

For certainty of location on subsequent follow-up, especially as the lesion is in the proximal colon, it would be desirable to leave one or more adjacent 1-cc India ink tattoos. In the (unlikely) event of histological evidence of malignancy the endoscopist would have nothing further to contribute, so localization for the surgeon or laparoscopist has relevance and tattooing takes only 2–3 minutes to achieve.

Endoscopy Commentary

Masaki Kawahara (Japan)

The endoscopic picture (Fig. 16A) reveals an irregular depression with a marginal slight elevation (type IIc+IIa). The depressed part of the lesion is reddish in color. Moreover, the marginal elevation has the same color as the surrounding colonic mucosa. The dye-scattering pictures (Fig. 16B and C) show that the margin of the depression exhibits so-called dendritic changes or a zig-zag pattern. These dendritic changes in the margin consist of an intricate pattern of normal glands and neoplastic glands. The horizontal progression of early superficial colon cancer is considered to show heterogeneity in expansion during the initial stage of development, leading to an asteroid pattern at the tumor front and an elevated margin.

The central depression (IIc) has an irregular granular surface but does not exhibit erosion or ulceration. The lesion as a whole is superficial and does not exhibit fold convergence or stiffness. The bowel wall shows no rigidity either. The marginal dendritic pattern indicates that the development of this lesion was basically expansive. Although such IIc+IIa lesions may have some areas of submucosal invasive cancer, the greater part of this lesion is probably a mucosal cancer. Another small lesion is located adjacent to the main lesion.

Pathology Commentary

Jeremy R. Jass (Canada)

The ascending colon lesion measuring 11 mm in diameter is a superficial mucosal neoplasm with raised edges and a depressed center. At the point of central depression, the mucosa is thin with glandular atrophy and possible focal erosion of surface epithelium (Fig. 16D–F). Nuclei are enlarged, elongated, and hyperchromatic, and show loss of polarity (Fig. 16G). Lower grade appearances are retained in some glands (Fig. 16H). Overall, the cytological and architectural changes are indicative of a high-grade nonpolypoid mucosal neoplasm. At one point, however, neoplastic glands are present within the submucosa, but confined to mucosa-associated lymphoid tissue (MALT).

The main issue raised by this case centers on the significance of the finding of neoplastic epithelium in MALT. The muscularis mucosae is normally breached at the site of MALT. The latter straddles this breach and occupies both mucosa and superficial submucosa. This means that the epithelium can project through the defect in the muscularis mucosae and come to lie within submucosal lymphoid tissue without having to invade the muscularis mucosae. The glands within the MALT appear no different from those within the mucosa and have not excited a desmoplastic reaction. Therefore, although there is neoplastic epithelium within the submucosal compartment, nine of the Western pathologists have indicated that the lesion does not show definite submucosal spread as opposed to 11 who are prepared

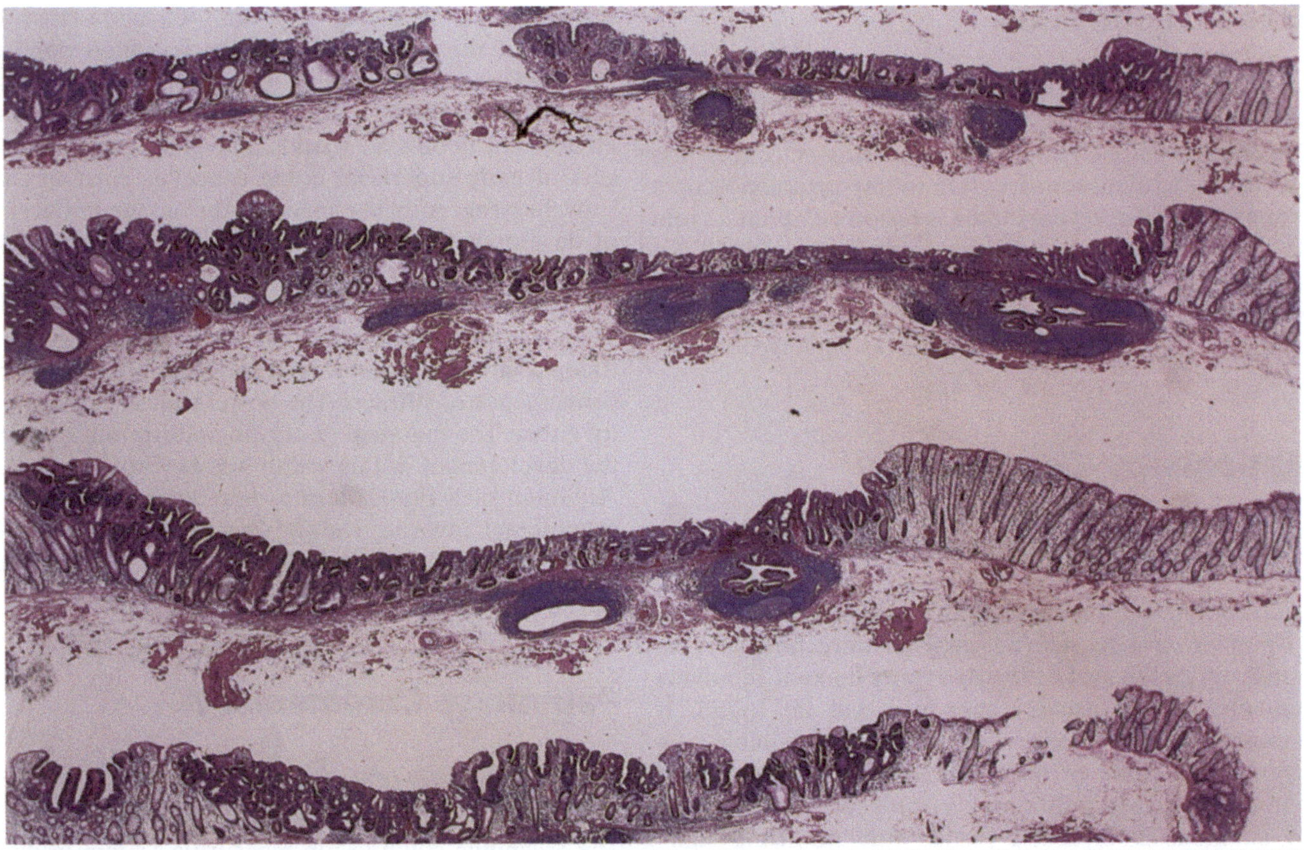

D

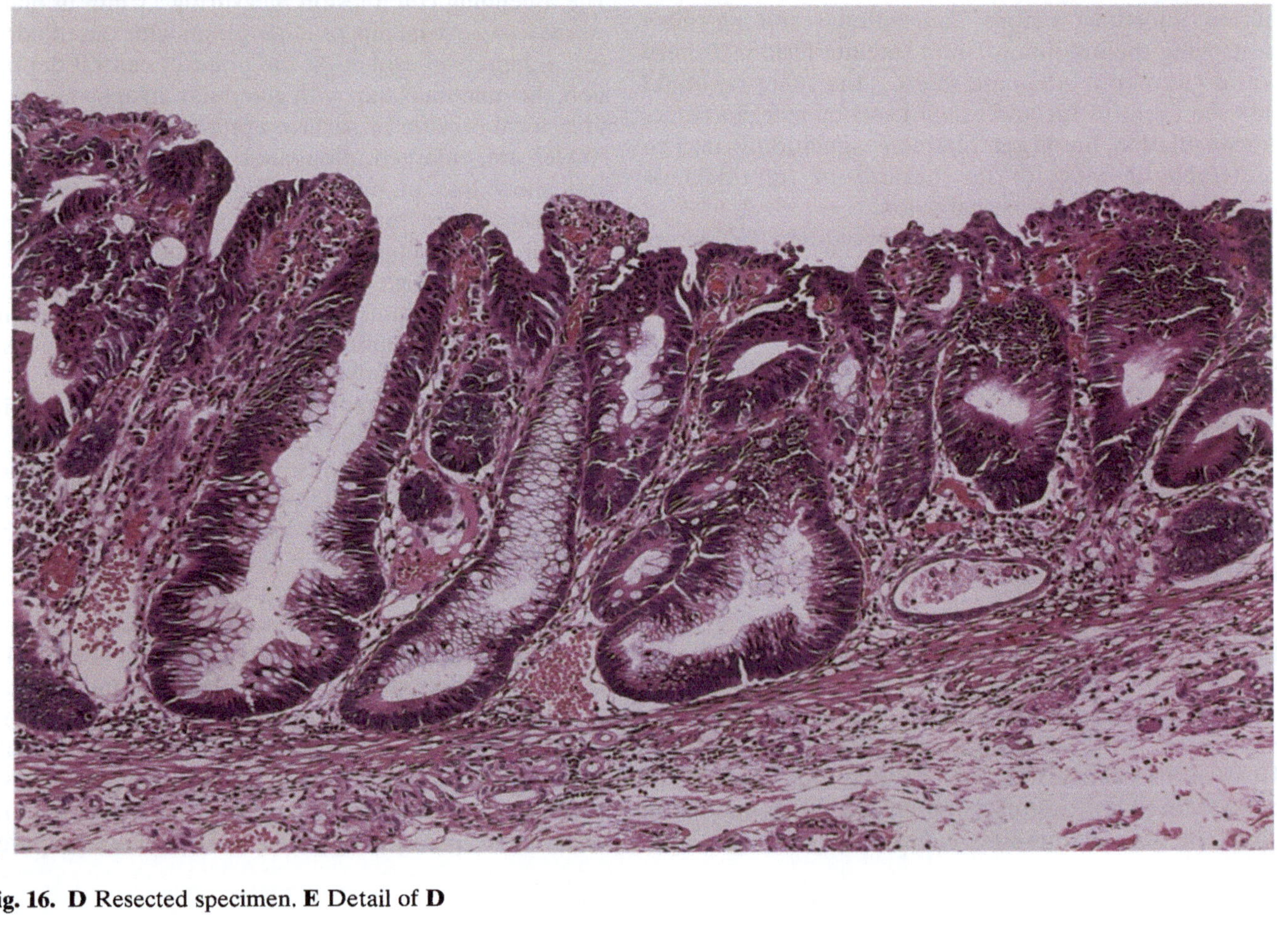

E

Fig. 16. **D** Resected specimen. **E** Detail of **D**

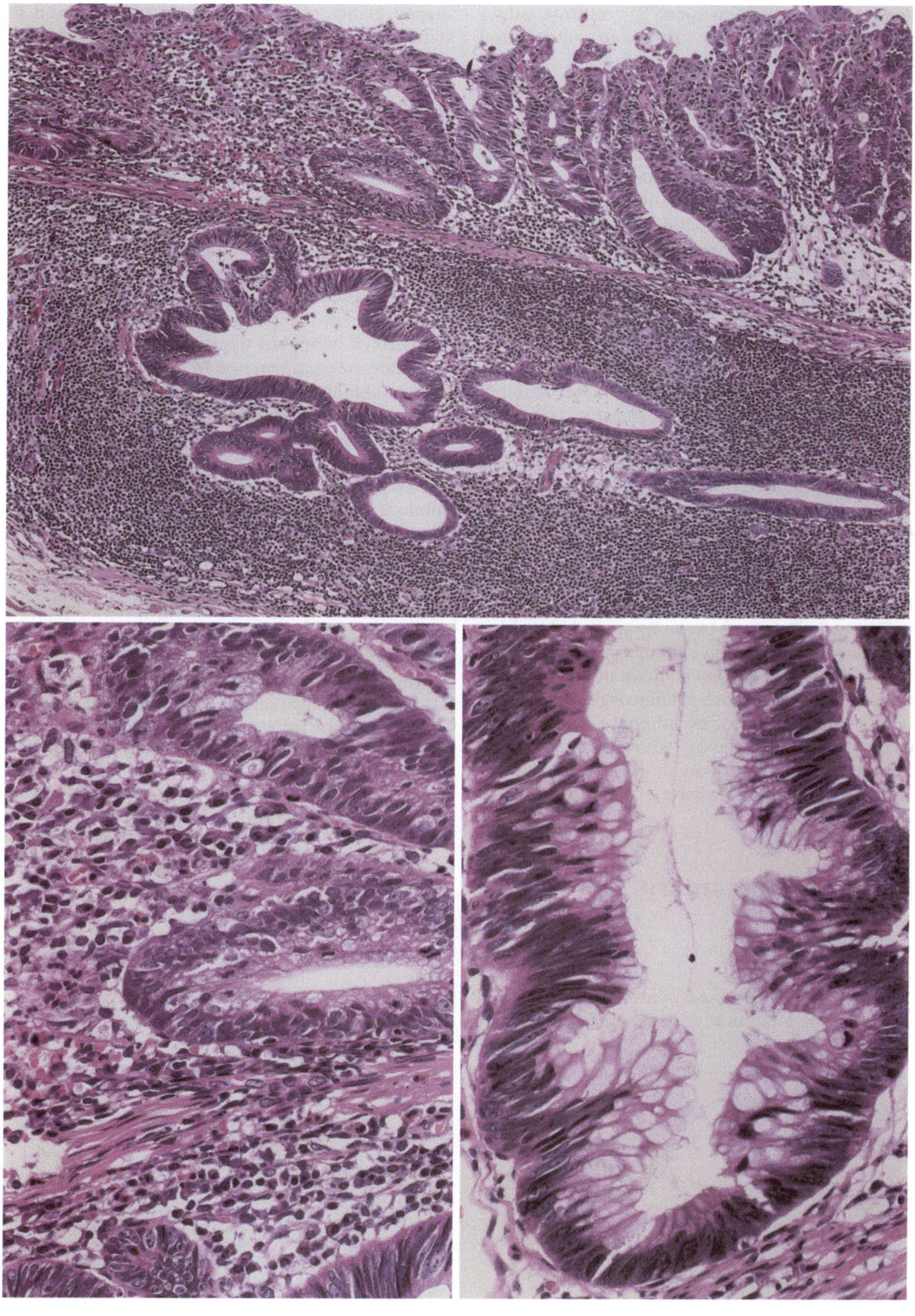
F
G
H

Fig. 16. **F** Detail of **D**. **G** Detail of **F**. **H** Detail of **E**

to diagnose submucosal invasion. By contrast, all 11 Japanese pathologists have diagnosed submucosal invasion.

Currently there is no specific evidence on the clinical significance of submucosal involvement that is limited to MALT. Since the neoplastic glands have not necessarily acquired active invasive properties in order to invade the muscularis mucosae and gain access to MALT, it is reasonable to speculate that the finding does not provide evidence for the acquisition of invasive and metastatic potential but represents a form of pseudoinvasion. On the other hand, it could be argued that the neoplastic glands in MALT may be able to spread easily via lymphatic channels to regional lymph nodes. In practice, it would be most surprising to find lymph node involvement in such an early neoplastic lesion. In other words it will be difficult to correlate the observation of MALT involvement with more extensive lymphatic spread.

Low-power scans of the lesion (lowest section in Fig. 16D) indicate that some of the mucosal glands have a complex or cribriform architecture. On this basis, the diagnosis of carcinoma-in-situ or intramucosal carcinoma might be considered. In the absence of poor differentiation, there are few objective criteria for establishing the existence of invasion of the lamina propria. Nevertheless, some of the Western pathologists who are unconvinced by the submucosal invasion are prepared to countenance the diagnosis of intramucosal carcinoma. I would diagnose submucosal invasion but qualify this with the caveats noted above. The mucosal component includes glands showing high-grade dysplasia (amounting to carcinoma-in-situ) and residual adenomatous glands, suggestive of a pre-existing nonpolypoid adenoma.

Pathology Commentary

Akinori Iwashita (Japan)

This lesion with a depressed center and superficial elevated edges is structurally made up of irregularly shaped glands showing features such as gland within gland (Fig. 16F), bridging (Fig. 16E and F), and a cribriform pattern (Fig. 16D, bottom left). The nuclei of the neoplastic cells are markedly hyperchromatic with thick nuclear membranes, and show a loss of polarity and moderate to marked pseudostratification (Fig. 16G and H). These glandular and cellular features alone would be sufficient for a diagnosis of carcinoma from the Japanese point of view. In addition, there is convincing evidence of submucosal invasion of severely atypical glands. The fact that the longitudinal axis of the glands in the submucosa is parallel to the muscularis mucosae, i.e., perpendicular to the axis of normal mucosal glands, is an argument for invasive carcinomatous growth. The presence of lymphoid tissue is another argument. It is sometimes seen in reaction to invasive growth, not only in the colon and rectum but also in the esophagus.

From these microscopic findings, I would diagnose this lesion as a well-differentiated adenocarcinoma with submucosal invasion, type IIc+IIa. According to the revised Vienna classification [1–3], the diagnostic opinions of Western pathologists are divided between mucosal high-grade neoplasia and submucosal invasion by carcinoma, whereas all Japanese pathologists would agree this to be a category 5 lesion, i.e., a carcinoma invading the submucosa (Table 16).

References

1. Schlemper RJ, Kato Y, Stolte M (2000) Diagnostic criteria for gastrointestinal carcinomas in Japan and Western countries: proposal for a new classification system of gastrointestinal epithelial neoplasia. J Gastroenterol Hepatol 15:G49–G57
2. Dixon MF (2002) Gastrointestinal epithelial neoplasia: Vienna revisited. Gut 51:130–131
3. Schlemper RJ, Iwashita A (2004) Classification of gastrointestinal epithelial neoplasia. Curr Diagn Pathol 10: 128–139

Case 17, IIa+IIc-like

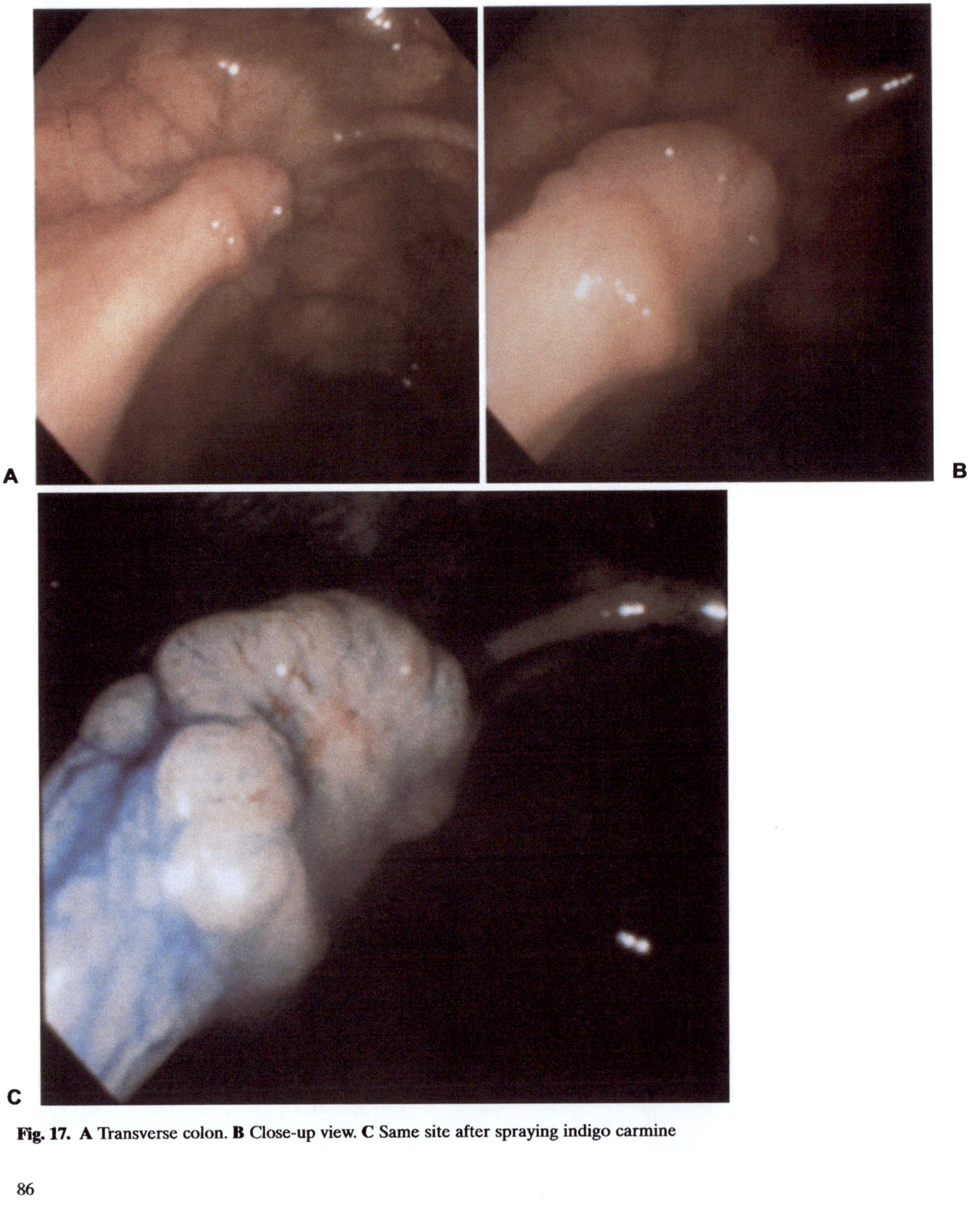

Fig. 17. A Transverse colon. **B** Close-up view. **C** Same site after spraying indigo carmine

Case Description

A woman, aged 68 years, had a past history of appendectomy and had no recent abdominal symptoms. Because a screening test showed that her feces were positive for occult blood, she underwent a colonoscopic examination. A lesion of about 10 mm in diameter was found in the transverse colon and biopsied. One week later a partial colectomy was performed. In the surgical specimen, none of the 9 resected lymph nodes was positive for tumor, but blood vessel invasion could be observed. Four years later, she died of pulmonary metastases.

Endoscopy Commentary

Christopher B. Williams (UK)

This lesion has the highly sinister characteristic appearance of a "malignant polyp." The saddle-shaped (slightly excavated) shape, with "rolled" or everted margins combine to suggest endoscopically that invasion is certain. Most endoscopists, on the basis of this visual assessment, would do no more—apart from palpating with the biopsy forceps to confirm the firm and immobile nature of the lesion and taking several biopsies from the margin to confirm dysplastic tissue.

Any attempt at submucosal injection would be highly likely to show the typical "no-lift" sign, with the injection bleb speading around the fixed lesion, but failing to elevate it for safe snaring. Surgical management is indicated and any attempt at endoscopic management absolutely contraindicated. The endoscopist can, however, aid surgical or laparoscopic localization by placing 3–4 India ink tattoos around the circumference, making it easy for the surgeon to find.

Endoscopy Commentary

Masaki Kawahara (Japan)

The endoscopic pictures show a small, elevated lesion with an irregular central depression (type IIa+IIc). Although the shape of this lesion is similar to that in Case 16, it is a totally different type of lesion. Stiffness, fold convergence, and a rigid deformity of the bowel wall are visible. In addition, the converging fold is very thick. These endoscopic findings suggest that this lesion is a submucosally massively invasive cancer (sm-massive cancer) or advanced cancer.

In this case, the rigidity of the bowel wall is obvious. However, in some cases without an obvious rigid deformity, the lack of air-induced deformation, or wall deformity as air is insufflated, may be informative. Air-induced deformation is indicated by three findings: a straight rigidity of the bowel lumen, a stand-like (trapezoid) lifting of the lesion, and multiple convergence folds. These findings indicate a difference in the expansibility of tissues between the part with submucosal invasion and the part without invasion. Therefore, these findings are not observed in mucosal lesions or submucosal cancer with slight invasion (sm-slight cancer).

Table 17. Colorectal lesion 17

Biopsy: × Resection: ○	W	W W J	WW WW WW WW WWJ	W W	W W J J	J J J J J	W W W J J
Regenerative changes	×						
Indefinite for neoplasia		×					
Adenoma/dysplasia							
low-grade			×				
high-grade				×			
Carcinoma							
suspected					×		
non-invasive						×	
intramucosal							×
> submucosal	○	○	○	○	○	○	○

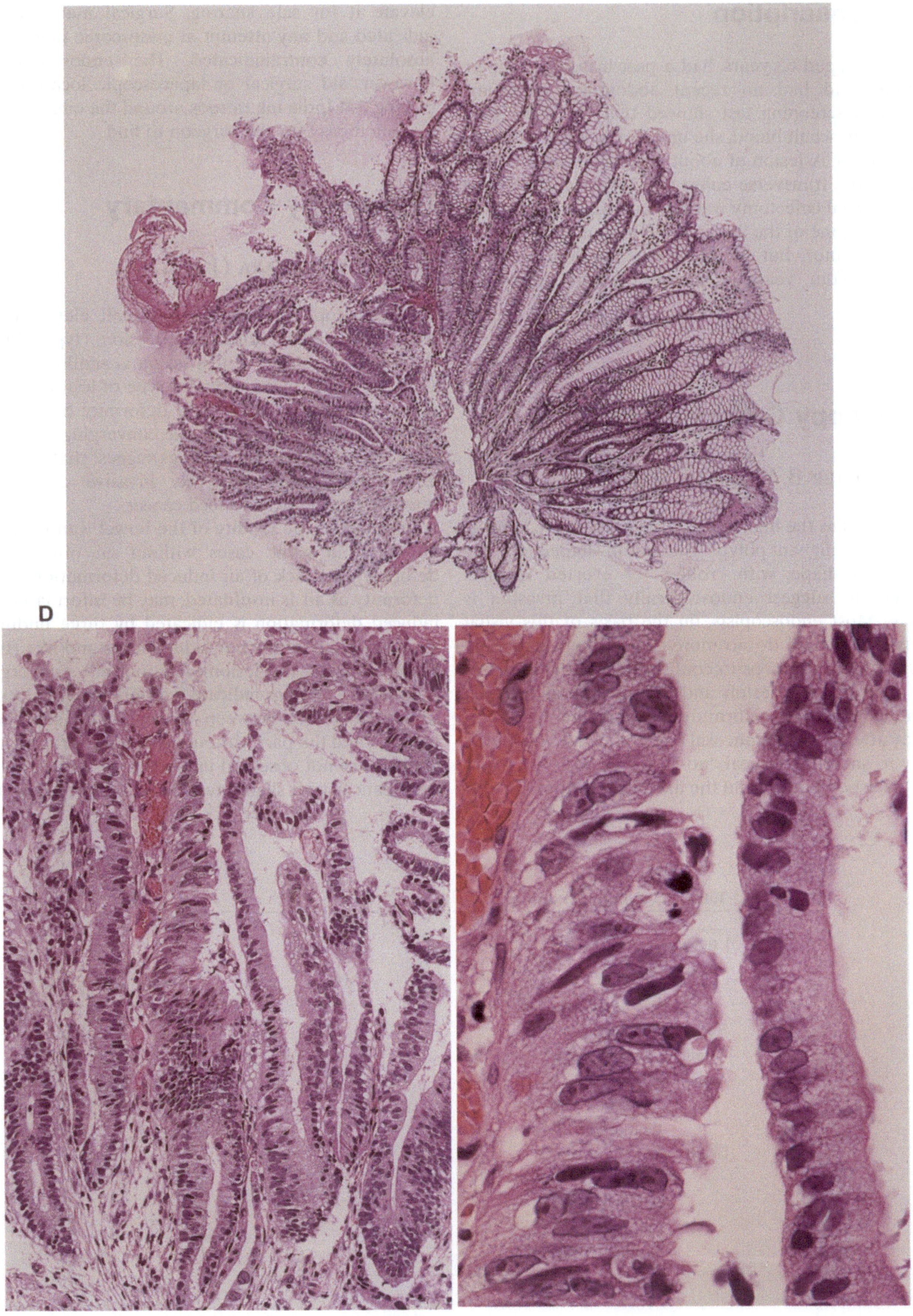

D E F

Fig. 17. **D** Biopsy specimen. **E** Detail of **D**. **F** Detail of **E**

The central depression of this lesion lacks ruggedness or a granular pattern, indicating that the depressed surface is a cancerous erosion with the loss of glandular structure. The marginal elevation is covered with normal mucosa similar to a submucosal tumor, suggesting that the growth of the lesion occurred mainly in the submucosal layer. This finding also designates the histological depth of the lesion as deeper than the mucosal layer. Such lesions should be treated surgically, not endoscopically.

Pathology Commentary

Jeremy R. Jass (Canada)

The tumor is a nonpolypoid lesion 10 mm in diameter with a raised rolled edge and a depressed center. In its endoscopic appearance highlighted by dye spray (Fig. 17C) the lesion resembles a minute ulcerated cancer. The diagnosis amongst Western pathologists ranges from regenerative change to intramucosal carcinoma, but most favor a diagnosis of low-grade adenoma. The diagnostic range amongst Japanese pathologists is less wide; most favor a diagnosis of noninvasive carcinoma. The discrepancy is therefore very wide and is not resolved by the use of the Vienna classification [1]. Resection of the entire lesion showed an adenocarcinoma extending through the submucosa to involve the superficial muscularis propria. This was a unanimous diagnosis amongst both Western and Japanese pathologists.

This is an important case that appears to highlight a major deficiency in Western reporting practices. The original biopsy is unlike an adenoma. The nuclei are ovoid to round, vary in size and shape, and several contain one or more prominent nucleoli. Chromatin is finely dispersed and glassy (Fig. 17F). There is focal loss of polarity. Apoptotic activity is apparent (Fig. 17F). The cells are cuboidal to columnar with eosinophilic and undifferentiated cytoplasm (Fig. 17F). No intracellular mucin droplets are apparent. The subepithelial tissues are not desmoplastic but show proliferation of myofibroblasts and a paucity of normal lamina propria cellular constituents (Fig. 17E). The latter is seen in solitary rectal ulcer syndrome and may account for the diagnosis of regenerative change by one Western pathologist. Although definite evidence of invasion is lacking, the overall features are suspicious of well-differentiated adenocarcinoma.

In the resected specimen (Fig. 17G), the detail of the mucosal portion (Fig. 17H) shows adenomatous glands with pseudostratified elongated nuclei and apical mucin droplets. This probably represents residual adenoma from the edge of the lesion. The appearances are unlike the original biopsy which (in retrospect) probably includes malignant epithelium abutting against normal colorectal mucosa.

The lesson to be drawn from this case is that malignant epithelium can occur within colorectal mucosa. It is often present in specimens of advanced cancer and may represent lateral and/or upward spread with gradual replacement of normal (or adenomatous) epithelium by malignant epithelium. This pattern of carcinoma-in-situ may also precede the development of invasive malignancy but be too transient or unstable to be diagnosed with any frequency. The same pattern may be observed in metastases from one part of the gut to another. Metastatic malignant epithelium may infiltrate and grow within the pre-existing cryptal sheath of normal mucosa and mimic adenoma [2]. In the present case, the subtle cytological changes have led to an erroneous diagnosis of low-grade adenoma by several pathologists. Cancers showing such subtle cytological changes may be characterized by a near-normal chromosomal content.

References

1. Schlemper RJ, Riddell RH, Kato Y, et al (2000) The Vienna classification of gastrointestinal epithelial neoplasia. Gut 47:251–255
2. Shepherd NA, Hall PA (1990) Epithelial-mesenchymal interactions can influence the phenotype of carcinoma metastases in the mucosa of the intestine. J Pathol 160:103–109

Pathology Commentary

Akinori Iwashita (Japan)

The biopsy specimen of this IIa+IIc-like lesion shows proliferation of irregularly shaped and relatively small tubules in association with a slight stromal proliferation compatible with a desmoplastic reaction in the colonic mucosa (Fig. 17E, left side of Fig. 17D). The atypical tubules are comprised of cells having a monotonous appearance without goblet cell differentiation (Fig. 17E) and showing rounded and vesicular nuclei of variable size and shape with a thick nuclear membrane (Fig. 17F). Several nuclei contain one or more prominent eosinophilic nucleoli (Fig. 17F). A focal loss of nuclear polarity can be recognized. From the biopsy findings mentioned above, I would diagnose this biopsy specimen as a well-differentiated adenocarcinoma with suspected invasion of the lamina propria mucosae.

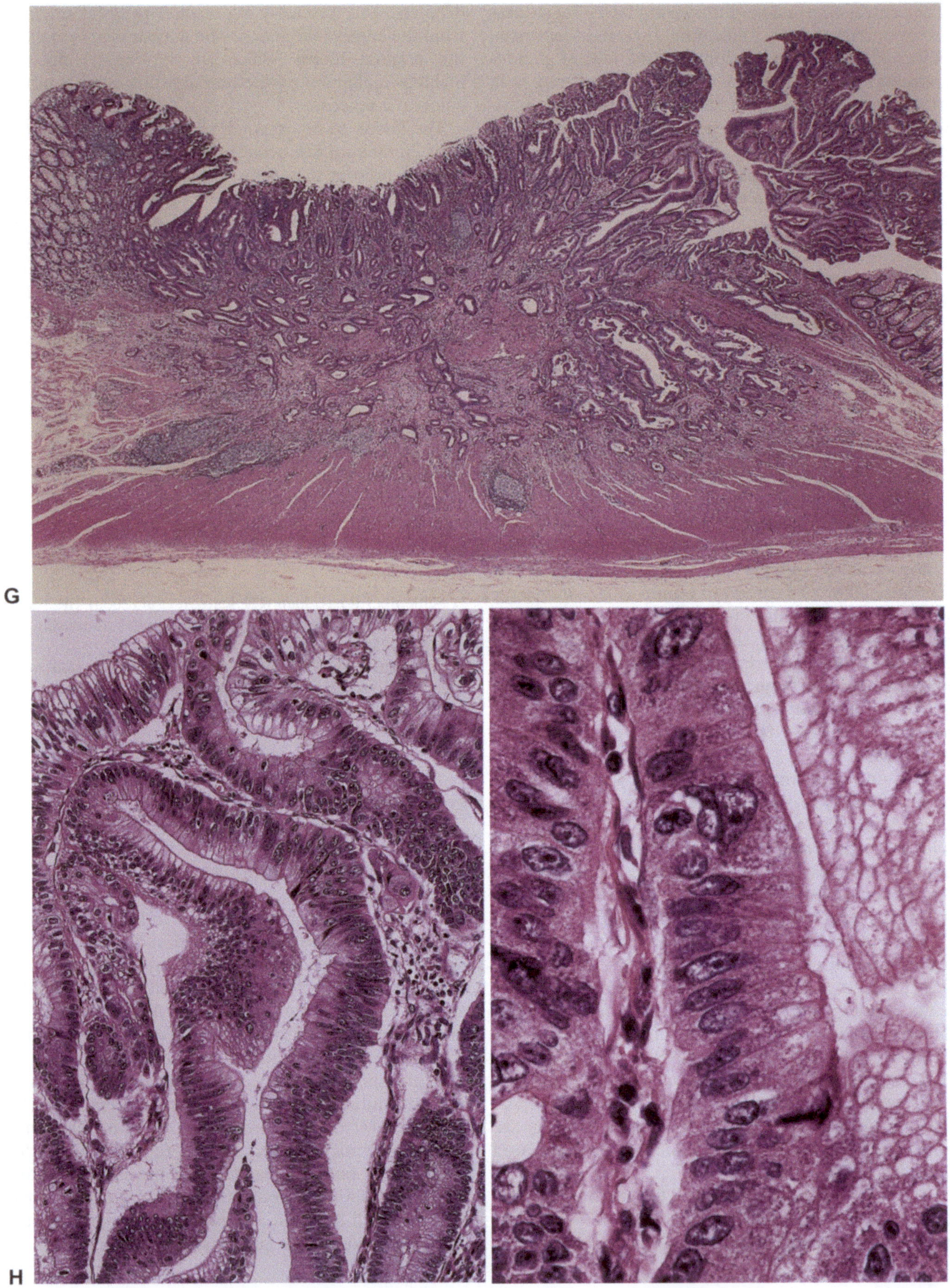

Fig. 17. **G** Resected specimen. **H** Detail of **G** (mucosal portion). **I** Detail of **G** (mucosal portion)

In the resected specimen neoplastic glands are observed in the mucosa, submucosa and muscularis propria (Fig. 17G). Details of the mucosal portion show architectural and cytological features of well-differentiated adenocarcinoma, as indicated by irregularly shaped glands, nuclear enlargement and pleomorphism, loss of nuclear polarity, and nucleolar prominence (Fig. 17H and I). My diagnosis is well-differentiated adenocarcinoma invading down into the muscularis propria, without an adenomatous component.

Using the terminology of the revised Vienna classification [1–3], the most common Western diagnosis of the biopsy specimen was mucosal low-grade neoplasia, i.e., category 3, whereas almost all Japanese pathologists diagnosed mucosal high-grade neoplasia, i.e., category 4 (Table 17). The lack of recognition by many Western pathologists of the high-grade cytological features of the biopsy specimen could have major clinical implications. Such an underdiagnosis could erroneously lead to endoscopic follow-up of this patient instead of nondelayed complete resection of the lesion. This case demonstrates that Western clinicians should not merely rely on the pathological diagnosis of biopsy specimens but also on their endoscopic assessment of malignant features and their estimation of the depth of invasion of suspicious lesions. Good communication between clinicians and pathologists is essential.

References

1. Schlemper RJ, Kato Y, Stolte M (2000) Diagnostic criteria for gastrointestinal carcinomas in Japan and Western countries: proposal for a new classification system of gastrointestinal epithelial neoplasia. J Gastroenterol Hepatol 15:G49–G57
2. Dixon MF (2002) Gastrointestinal epithelial neoplasia: Vienna revisited. Gut 51:130–131
3. Schlemper RJ, Iwashita A (2004) Classification of gastrointestinal epithelial neoplasia. Curr Diagn Pathol 10:128–139

Case 18, Is

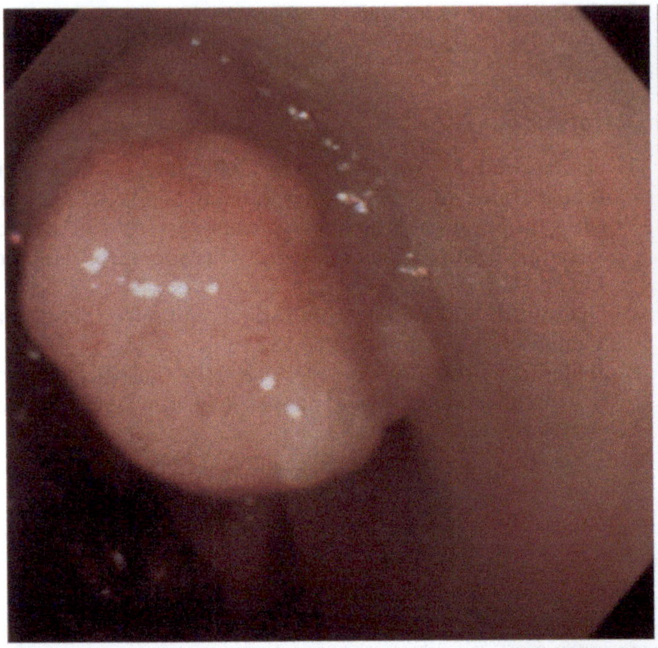

A

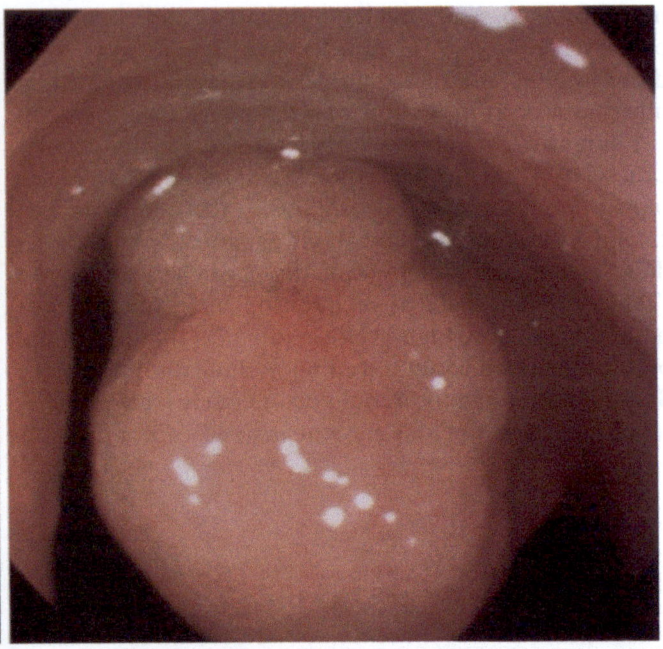

B

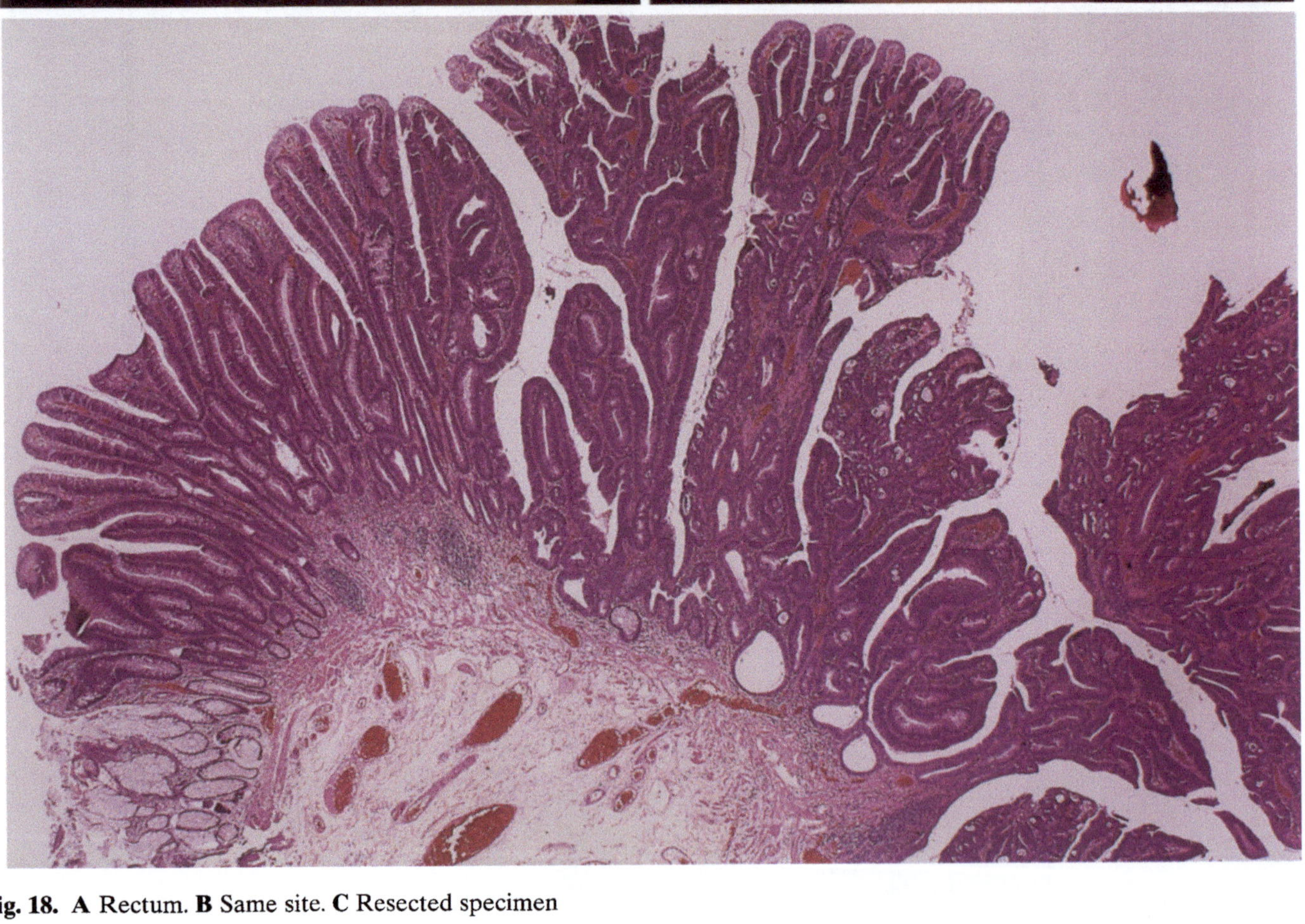

C

Fig. 18. A Rectum. **B** Same site. **C** Resected specimen

Case Description

A man, aged 70 years, was symptom-free and requested a colonoscopic examination for the purpose of cancer screening. A polyp of about 13mm in diameter was found in the rectum. Endoscopic resection was performed. The resection margins were free of tumor. On follow-up endoscopic examinations no local recurrence was found.

Endoscopy Commentary

Christopher B. Williams (UK)

At first sight this is a typical medium-sized protuberant adenomatous polyp, with a visibly "gyral" or "sulcal" surface pattern. The view is, however, limited and gives no clue as to whether it is broad-based or stalked, fixed, or mobile. There is on both images (centrally in Fig. 18A, to the right side in Fig. 18B) a small, reddened, slightly depressed area which could represent focal more severe abnormality.

Palpation with the snare tube would check for soft overall texture and some mobility, before snare polypectomy—preferably in a single portion or several large bits, to facilitate histological interpretation. Finding "invasion at the margin of the specimen" is a drawback of piecemeal polypectomy, so careful orientation of the resected specimen(s) is an important contribution by the endoscopic team. The endoscopist can sometimes obtain a better assessment of "completeness of resection" from overall judgment than the pathologist looking at disorganized partial portions of polyp.

This particular polyp was in the rectum, so retrieval and localization would not have been a problem.

Endoscopy Commentary

Masaki Kawahara (Japan)

The endoscopic pictures reveal a protruded lesion with a broad base (type Is). Macroscopically this lesion has a rough nodular or lobular surface with some luster. The color of the lesion is almost normal, with a faint redness. No ulcerative changes or erosion is seen on the surface of the lesion. Fold convergence, rigidity of the wall, coexisting white spots, and submucosal bulging (like a submucosal tumor) are not visible around the lesion. No apparent signs of malignancy or submucosal invasion are present. However, this lesion is rather large (about 20mm in diameter), so there is some possibility that the lesion may contain a focal cancer histologically (cancer in adenoma), although this possibility cannot be confirmed by the endoscopic findings. Endoscopic resection is the treatment of choice for such lesions.

Pathology Commentary

Jeremy R. Jass (Canada)

The rectal lesion is a sessile polypoid mass 13mm in diameter. The low-power view shown in Fig. 18C includes tubulovillous adenoma with areas of a suggestive serrated architecture. The overall diagnosis is based on a high-grade focus characterized by a gland-within-gland architecture (Fig. 18D and F). The complex pattern falls short of true cribriforming. Cytologically the high-grade focus shows nuclear elongation, enlargement, and marked stratification. Nuclei are vesicular with a prominent nucleolus (Fig. 18F). Some mucus secretion is retained by goblet-like cells.

Table 18. Colorectal lesion 18

Resection: ○	W WW WW WW WW	W W	J J JJ JJ JJ	W WW WWJ WWJ WWJ
Adenoma/dysplasia				
high-grade	○			
Carcinoma				
suspected		○		
non-invasive			○	
intramucosal				○

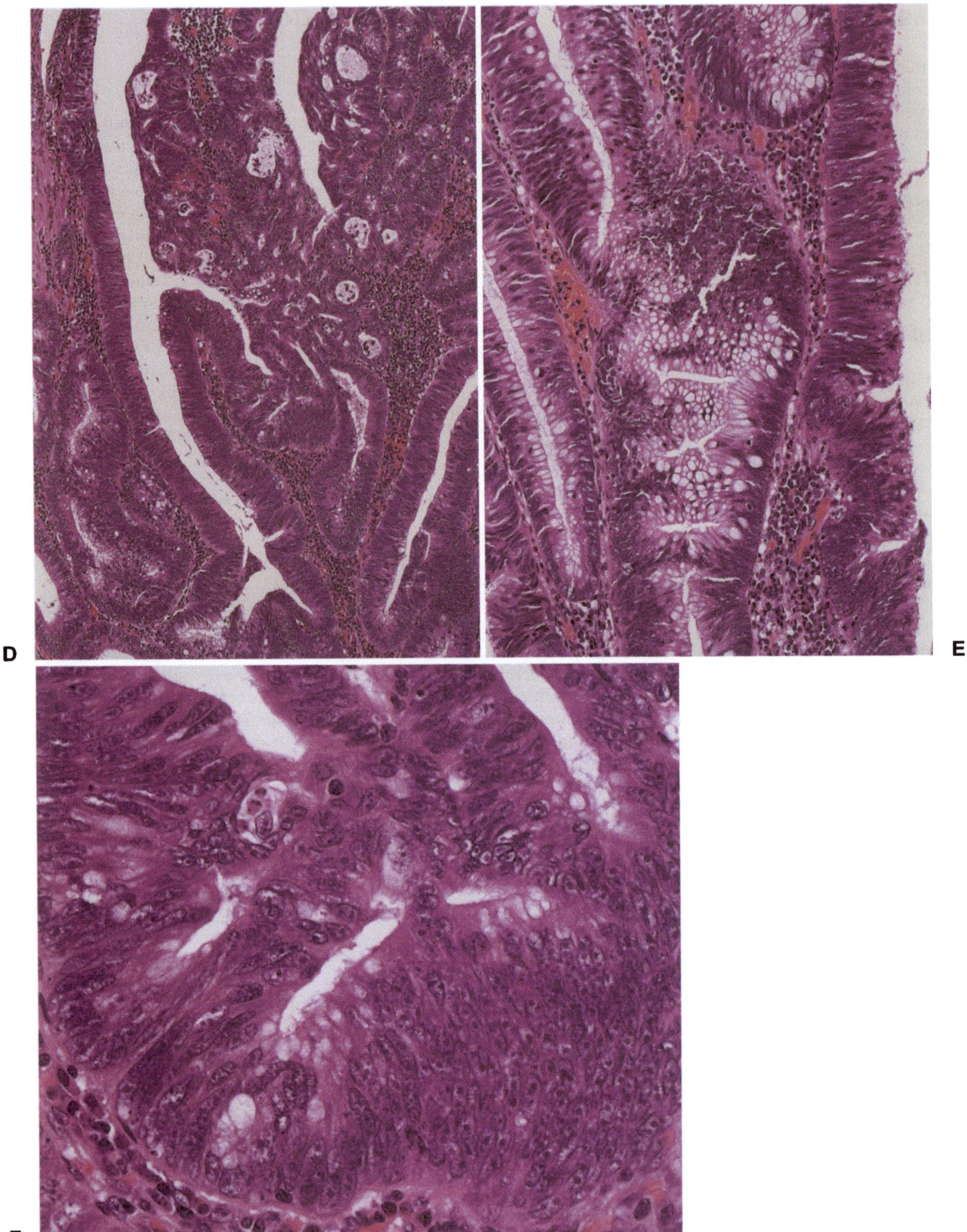

Fig. 18. **D** Detail of **C**. **E** Detail of **C**. **F** Detail of **D**

The Western pathologists fall mainly into two equally matched groups favoring either high-grade adenoma or intramucosal carcinoma. Most Japanese pathologists favor a diagnosis of noninvasive carcinoma. The Vienna classification has failed in this instance, with 61% and 39% of diagnoses within Categories 4 and 5 [1]. It is unclear why so many Western pathologists have rather uncharacteristically preferred the relatively "aggressive" diagnosis of intramucosal carcinoma. There is no definite evidence of invasion of the lamina propria and the gland-within-gland pattern fits with Western descriptions of high-grade intraepithelial neoplasia or carcinoma-in-situ. It could be argued that the extensive glandular budding shown in Fig. 18D must equate with invasion of the lamina propria. Nevertheless, intramucosal carcinoma is generally not a frequent diagnosis in the West. It may be an appropriate diagnosis in rare instances such as poorly differentiated or signet-ring cell carcinoma complicating ulcerative colitis. My diagnosis is focal high-grade intraepithelial neoplasia (amounting to carcinoma-in-situ) within a tubulovillous adenoma with areas of architectural serration.

Reference

1. Schlemper RJ, Riddell RH, Kato Y, et al (2000) The Vienna classification of gastrointestinal epithelial neoplasia. Gut 47:251–255

Pathology Commentary

Akinori Iwashita (Japan)

This polypoid lesion is architecturally composed of relatively large, regular and simple tubules with a small focus characterized by a cribriform and gland within gland structure (Fig. 18C, D, and F). The regular and simple tubules are lined by cells that have basally oriented spindle shaped nuclei, show goblet cell differentiation and little or no pseudostratification of the nuclei (Fig. 18E, and the left side and bottom right of Fig. 18D). On the other hand, the cells in the focus with severe architectural changes have enlarged, vesicular nuclei with a prominent nucleolus, and show marked pseudostratification of the nuclei and little or no goblet cell differentiation (Fig. 18F). There is no definite evidence of intramucosal invasion and no submucosal invasion.

From the microscopic appearances mentioned above, I would diagnose this lesion as a well- to moderately differentiated adenocarcinoma in a tubulovillous adenoma with moderate atypia, restricted to the mucosa, type Is. According to the revised Vienna classification there is complete agreement among both Western and Japanese pathologists that this is a mucosal high-grade neoplastic lesion, i.e., category 4 (Table 18), requiring local resection [1–3]. If the (unrevised) Vienna classification were used, the diagnostic opinions of the pathologists would be divided between noninvasive high-grade neoplasia and (intramucosally) invasive neoplasia. The extent of disagreement would be remarkable (Table 18). Pathologists have different ideas as to which histologic features should be regarded as invasion into the lamina propria mucosae. This case demonstrates that the use of the revised Vienna classification in which high-grade adenoma and intramucosal carcinoma are grouped together in one category, would avoid problems with defining intramucosal invasion and would be clinically more useful, as patients with such mucosal high-grade neoplastic lesions would require the same local treatment.

References

1. Schlemper RJ, Kato Y, Stolte M (2000) Diagnostic criteria for gastrointestinal carcinomas in Japan and Western countries: proposal for a new classification system of gastrointestinal epithelial neoplasia. J Gastroenterol Hepatol 15:G49–G57
2. Dixon MF (2002) Gastrointestinal epithelial neoplasia: Vienna revisited. Gut 51:130–131
3. Schlemper RJ, Iwashita A (2004) Classification of gastrointestinal epithelial neoplasia. Curr Diagn Pathol 10:128–139

Case 19, Ip

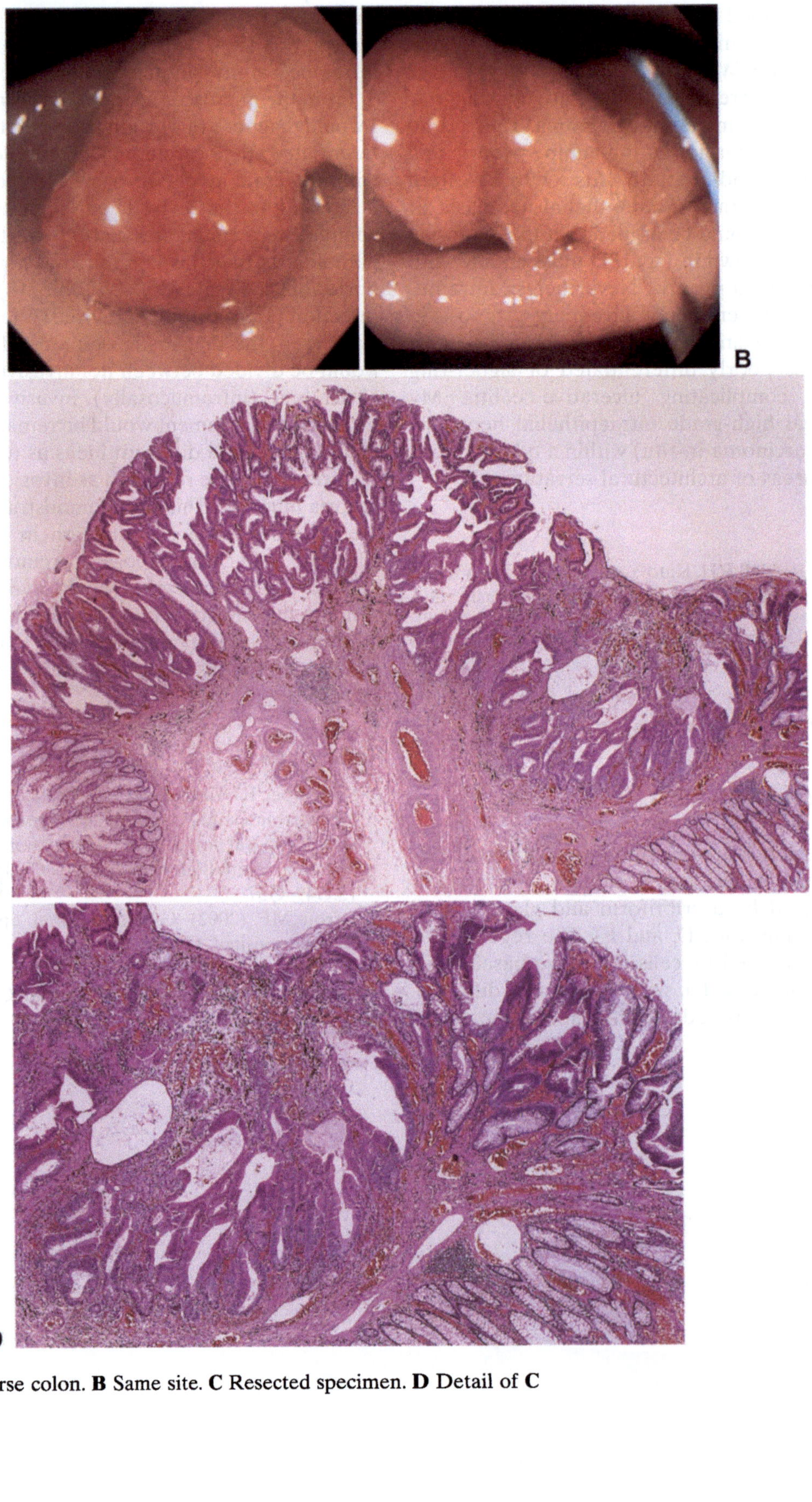
A B C D

Fig. 19. **A** Transverse colon. **B** Same site. **C** Resected specimen. **D** Detail of **C**

Case Description

A woman, aged 57 years, underwent a colonoscopic examination, because a screening test had shown that her feces were positive for occult blood. A polyp of about 15 mm in diameter was found in the transverse colon (Fig. 19A and B) and polypectomy was performed. The histology of this polypectomy specimen is shown in Fig. 19C–G. During the same colonoscopic examination also an ulcerative tumor compatible with an advanced colon carcinoma was found in the transverse colon. This diagnosis was confirmed by a biopsy and two months later a partial colectomy was performed.

Endoscopy Commentary

Christopher B. Williams (UK)

Although this polyp is described as 15 mm in size, endoscopically the main "give-away" in its appearance is the disproportion between head size (perhaps 7–8 mm wide and 4–5 mm long) and the substantial stalk (6–7 mm wide and around 1 cm long). The stalk size is that of a polyp head of 15–20 mm diameter. The inference is that the head has partially infarcted off—probably from malignancy invading and occluding the vascular plexus. Although mechanical trauma *can* cause polyps to infarct, this normally occurs at stalk level, so a small or asymmetric head should be considered suggestive of malignancy. The close-up view (Fig. 19B) may suggest local deformity and induration, which would be further evidence of invasive malignancy.

These warning signs are an indication to the endoscopist to snare the stalk as low down as possible, flush with the colon wall. This gives the best chance of including all invasive malignancy, and also helps the histologist to make the fullest assessment. Local India ink tattoo is also indicated for follow-up purposes, although it is extremely rare to find any recurrence locally. For this polyp, providing histological criteria are favorable, and both the histologist and endoscopist consider removal to be complete, it is highly likely that endoscopic removal alone would be sufficient. Only when invasion reaches too close to the resection line or in the 1% of malignancies which are poorly differentiated is surgery mandatory (because of the increased likelihood of metastasis to local nodes—potentially curable by surgical resection).

Table 19. Colorectal lesion 19

Resection: ○	W	W W W W W W W J	W W W J	W W J	J J J J J	W W W W W W J	W	J J
Regenerative changes	○							
Adenoma/dysplasia								
low-grade		○						
high-grade			○					
Carcinoma								
suspected				○				
non-invasive					○			
intramucosal						○		
intra- or submucosal							○	
submucosal								○

Endoscopy Commentary

Masaki Kawahara (Japan)

The endoscopic pictures show a rather small, pedunculated lesion (type Ip). The color of the protruding tip (head) of the lesion is reddish. The stalk of this lesion is thick and exhibits expansiveness (Fig. 19A); this feature (known as a "snowman" deformity) suggests that the cancer may have invaded the stalk. The head is rigid and shows an irregular unevenness. The lesion has a clear depression in the head (Fig. 19B), giving the lesion a rugged, stiff appearance. These endoscopic findings suggest that this lesion is malignant, and there is a possibility that submucosal invasion of the cancer has occurred in the depressed part. Endoscopic resection could be attempted, but the resected specimen should be carefully examined for histological risk factors of lymph node metastasis, especially in the depressed part of the lesion.

Pathology Commentary

Jeremy R. Jass (Canada)

The transverse colon lesion is a lobulated, polypoid mass measuring 15 mm in diameter. The low-power overview (Fig. 19C) shows a tubulovillous adenoma and a smaller, circumscribed subclone with a higher grade appearance. The tubulovillous adenoma may show some glandular serration.

The diagnosis is based upon the higher grade subclone illustrated in Fig. 19D–G. This subclone shows superficial ulceration, and appears to expand and push against the muscularis mucosae but not to penetrate this structure and invade the submucosa. The neoplastic glands range in size and many are back-to-back. The surrounding stroma is not desmoplastic but includes

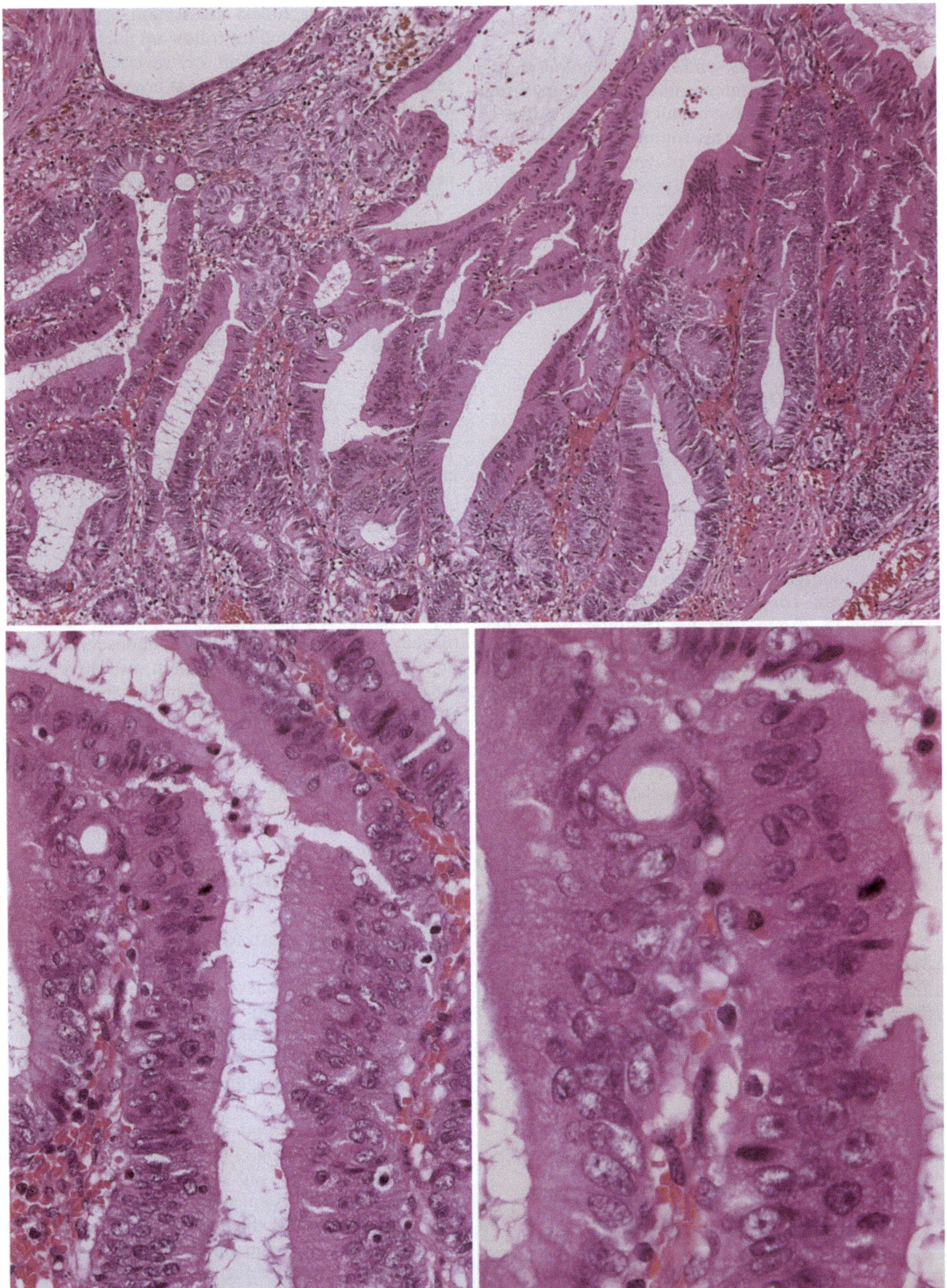

E F G

Fig. 19. **E** Detail of **D**. **F** Detail of **E**. **G** Detail of **F**

granulation tissue adjacent to the ulcerated surface. The glands are lined by eosinophilic columnar cells. Luminal secretory mucin is present (Fig. 19E). The nuclear:cytoplasmic ratio is relatively low. Nuclei are ovoid to round with little variation of size or shape. The nuclei are vesicular with a prominent nucleolus. There is loss of nuclear polarity (Fig. 19F and G). Intraepithelial lymphocytes may be present (Fig. 19F). Although the appearances could be described as "low-grade" they are unlike those of a conventional adenoma. The "low-grade" cytological appearance of the lesion may be explained by its origin within a serrated adenoma and a pathway of tumorigenesis that is associated with DNA microsatellite instability, rather than chromosomal instability and aneuploidy [1].

The diagnostic opinion is wide. Using the Vienna classification, the diagnostic distribution is 3%, 26%, 39%, and 32% within Categories 1, 3, 4, and 5, respectively [2]. Western pathologists fall into two main groups, one group diagnosing low-grade adenoma/dysplasia and the second preferring the diagnosis of intramucosal carcinoma. By contrast, most Japanese pathologists favor noninvasive carcinoma. This difference in opinion reflects the lack of guidelines for correlating morphological appearances with different pathways of molecular evolution. As evidence accumulates on the molecular profiles characterizing different pathways of tumorigenesis, appropriate guidelines will need to be developed for grading cytology, architecture, and differentiation according to premises that provide meaningful correlation with each pathway. Our current approach is to grade features as though there was a single pathway to cancer requiring a single set of rules. Such an approach cannot be correct. My "biological" interpretation is focal mucosal carcinoma within a tubulovillous adenoma (possibly serrated), but I would report the lesion as high-grade intraepithelial neoplasia as there is no unequivocal evidence of invasion into the lamina propria.

References

1. Jass JR (2001) Serrated route to colorectal cancer: back street or super highway? J Pathol 193:283–285
2. Schlemper RJ, Riddell RH, Kato Y, et al (2000) The Vienna classification of gastrointestinal epithelial neoplasia. Gut 47:251–255

Pathology Commentary

Akinori Iwashita (Japan)

This pedunculated polyp consists of a large tubulovillous low-grade adenomatous area showing slightly crowded and regularly arranged tubules with branching, and a small high-grade focus showing variably shaped and variably sized glands with downward extension (Fig. 19C). These high-grade neoplastic glands are probably invading the superficial portion of the submucosa, as in the bottom left corner of Fig. 19D a relatively large artery can be seen in the vicinity of a neoplastic gland; the artery and the gland are not separated by smooth muscle bundles of the muscularis mucosae. In general, arteries of this size are not present in the mucosa but only in the submucosa or beyond. The cells in the high-grade neoplastic glands have a monotonous appearance, show no goblet cell differentiation (Fig. 19E), and have rounded vesicular nuclei with a thick nuclear membrane and a prominent nucleolus (Fig. 19F and G). There is loss of nuclear polarity and also marked pseudostratification of the nuclei (Fig. 19F and G).

From the structural and cytological features mentioned above, I diagnose this lesion as a well-differentiated adenocarcinoma in a tubulovillous adenoma, with probable superficial submucosal invasion. Using the revised Vienna classification [1–3], the diagnostic opinions of most Western pathologists are divided between mucosal low-grade and mucosal high-grade neoplasia (category 3 versus 4), whereas most Japanese pathologists diagnose either mucosal high-grade neoplasia or submucosal invasion by carcinoma (category 4 versus 5) (Table 19). For polypoid colorectal carcinomas with submucosal invasion but without lymphatic or blood vessel invasion, local resection is considered adequate treatment [1–3]. Thus, in this patient a diagnosis of category 4 or 5 would have the same clinical implication.

From the diversity of diagnoses shown in Table 19, it is clear that the use of conventional terminology without classification into clinically meaningful categories may confuse clinicians. It is hoped that the use of the revised Vienna classification may not only contribute to a better understanding between Western and Japanese pathologists but also to a better communication between pathologists and clinicians, resulting in a reduction of undertreatment and overtreatment.

References

1. Schlemper RJ, Kato Y, Stolte M (2000) Diagnostic criteria for gastrointestinal carcinomas in Japan and Western countries: proposal for a new classification system of gastrointestinal epithelial neoplasia. J Gastroenterol Hepatol 15: G49–G57
2. Dixon MF (2002) Gastrointestinal epithelial neoplasia: Vienna revisited. Gut 51:130–131
3. Schlemper RJ, Iwashita A (2004) Classification of gastrointestinal epithelial neoplasia. Curr Diagn Pathol 10: 128–139

4. Superficial Carcinoma of the Esophagus (Cases 20–24)

Case 20, IIc

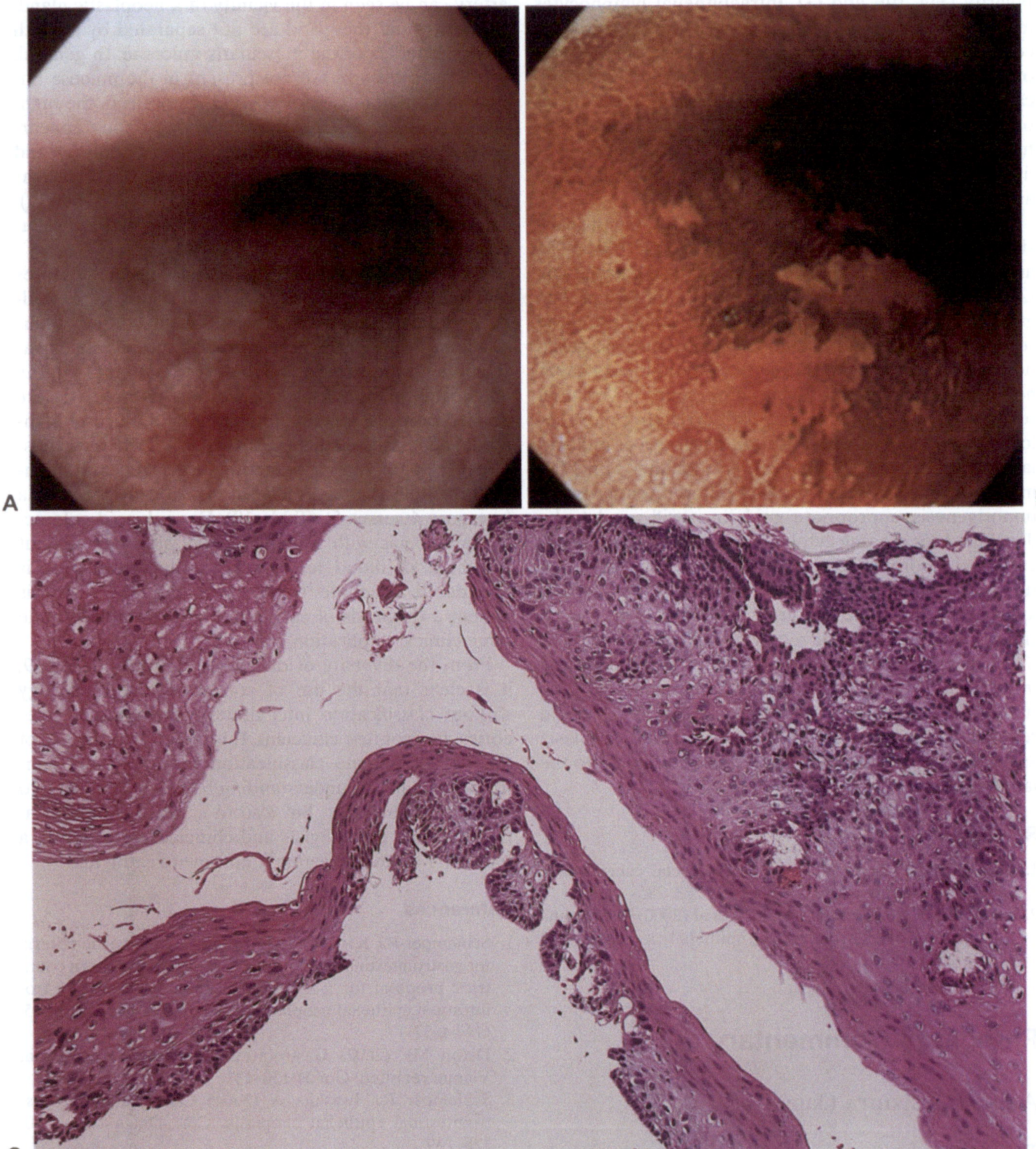

Fig. 20. A Distal esophagus. B Same site after spraying Lugol's iodine. C First biopsy specimen

Case Description

A man, aged 59 years, complaining of occasional epigastric pain, underwent an upper GI endoscopic examination. At 33 cm from the teeth a lesion was found and biopsied. Three weeks thereafter endoscopic resection was performed. Histological examination of the two resected pieces revealed that not all resection margins were free of neoplastic change. However, on follow-up endoscopy 2 weeks later, no unstained area could be seen around the postresection ulcer; also, no neoplastic changes could be observed in 16 biopsies taken from the ulcer margin.

Endoscopy Commentary

Massimo Crespi (Italy)

The lesion located at the lower third of the esophagus is slightly depressed, and well differentiated from the surrounding apparently normal mucosa only by the Lugol staining. The location, just above the gastroesophageal junction, and the endoscopic patterns suggest a Barrett's type epithelium with possible dysplastic changes, as confirmed by the first and second biopsy as interpreted by most of the Western pathologists and by the examination of the resected specimen. The Lugol staining, easy to perform, has to be considered in our opinion as a mandatory step in any endoscopic examination when irregularities of the mucosa are detected: in our experience in high-risk populations for esophageal cancer in Iran and China, it was of great help in aiming the bioptic samplings and in detecting dysplasia, even in the absence of intestinalized mucosa [1]. The endoscopic mucosal resection (EMR) procedure performed seems appropriate and a strict follow-up is highly advisable.

Reference

1. Crespi M, Grassi A, Munoz N, et al (1984) Endoscopic features of suspected precancerous lesions in high-risk areas for oesophageal cancer. Endoscopy 16(3):85–91

Endoscopy Commentary

Kimiya Takeshita (Japan)

A red lesion, about 2 cm long (in the vertical dimension), is endoscopically visible on the posterior wall of the middle esophagus (Fig. 20A). On iodine staining (Lugol's staining), the lesion is observed as a two-chained islet-like unstained area with an irregular shape (Fig. 20B). Its margin has a map-like form. It is gently protrusive laterally (a sign specific to cancer). The mucosal surface of the lesion, however, shows few irregularities and the cancer is confined to a narrow area, suggesting very shallow cancer invasion (m1 or m2).

Pathology Commentary

Sanford M. Dawsey (USA)

Both biopsies show squamous epithelium, without lamina propria. Portions of both biopsies are well oriented, with papillae extending upward from the base of the epithelium in the plane of the section, but other portions are less well oriented, so the papillae are cut across tangentially. Both biopsies contain atypical cells with enlarged, hyperchromatic, dyspolaric nuclei which vary

Table 20. Esophageal lesion 20

Biopsy 1: $\times^1$
Biopsy 2: $\times^2$
Resection: ○

	W	W W W W	W	W W J	W W J	W	W W W W W W	W W	W	J	J J J	J J J J J
Indefinite for neoplasia	○		$\times^1$									
Dysplasia												
low-grade	$\times$	$\otimes$	$\times^2$	$\times$	$\times^1$	$\times^2$		$\times$				
high-grade			○	○	$\otimes^2$	$\otimes^1$	$\otimes$		○			
Carcinoma												
suspected								○	$\times^2$	$\times$	$\times^1$	
non-invasive										○	$\otimes^2$	$\otimes$
intramucosal									$\times^1$			

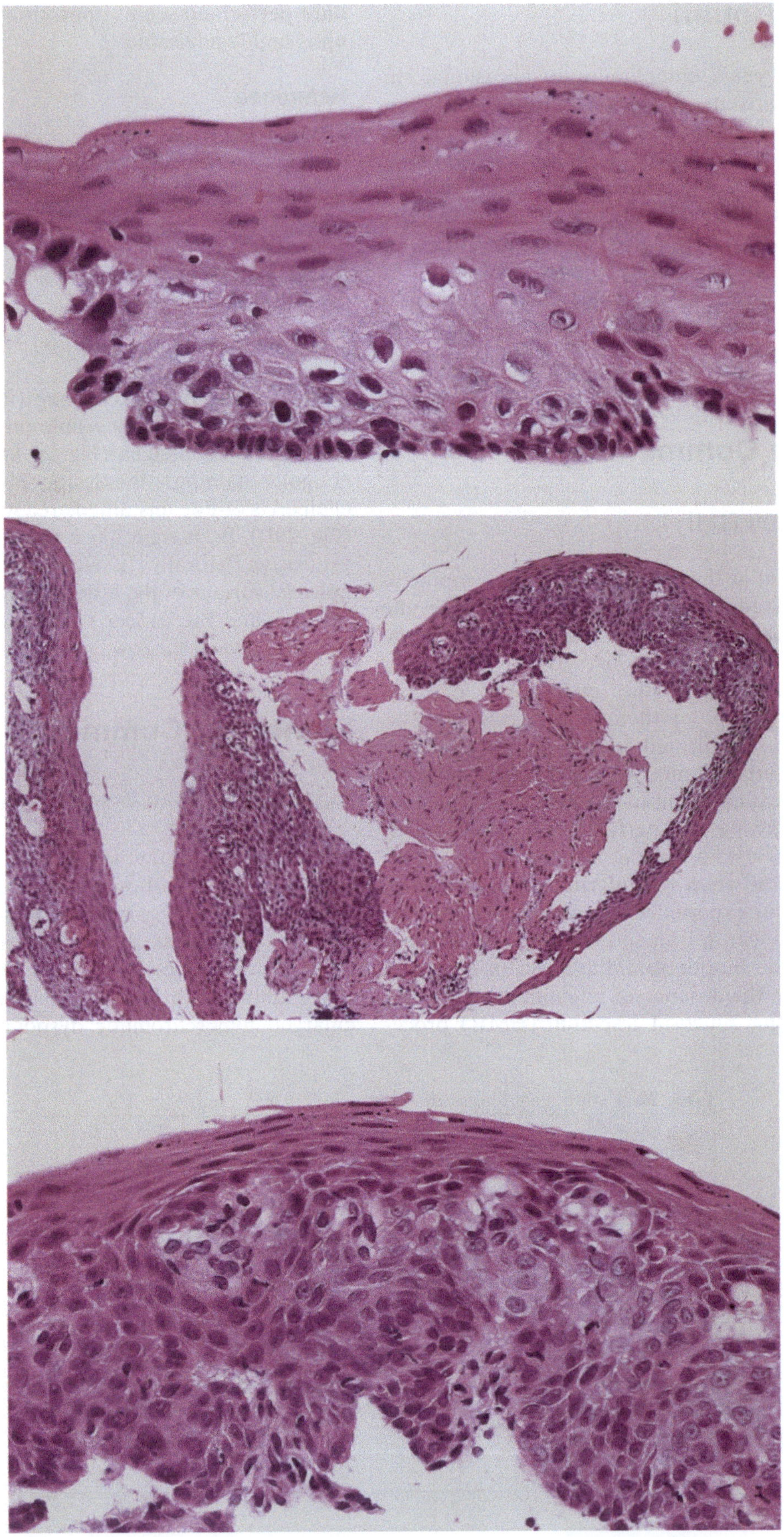

D

E

F

Fig. 20. **D** Detail of **C**. **E** Second biopsy specimen. **F** Detail of **E**

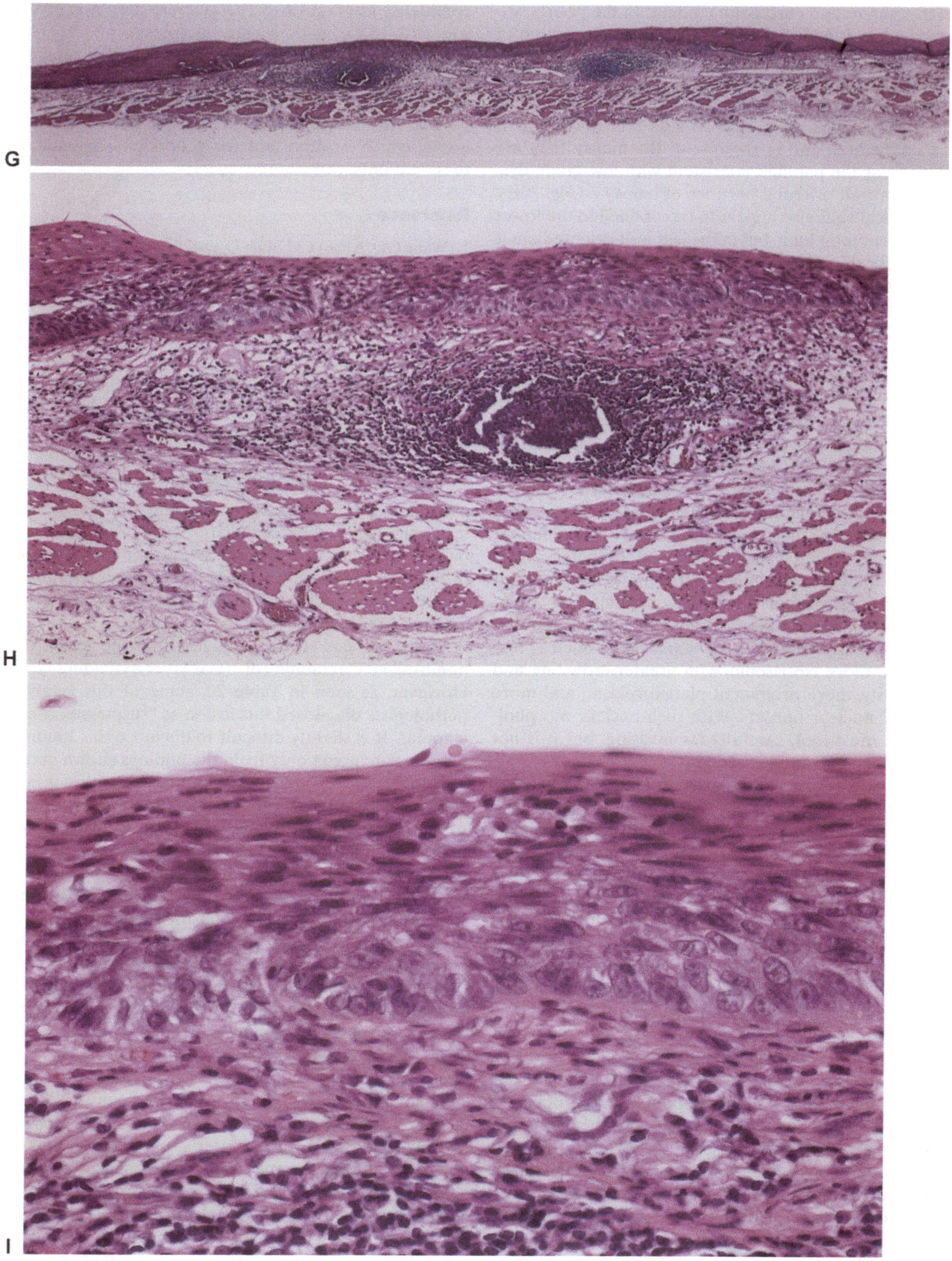

Fig. 20. **G** Resected specimen. **H** Detail of **G**. **I** Detail of **H**

in size, shape, and chromatin content. In the poorly oriented areas, it is difficult to evaluate the proportion of the epithelial thickness that is involved by these atypical cells, which is important for the grading of squamous dysplasia. In well-oriented portions of biopsy 1 (Fig. 20D), the atypical cells are confined to the lower half of the epithelium, and in the rest of the biopsy they are found near the papillae, consistent with low-grade dysplasia. In well-oriented portions of biopsy 2 (Fig. 20E), the atypical cells also appear to be confined to the lower half of the epithelium, but in the less well-oriented areas (Fig. 20F), they appear to be more widely distributed, filling the spaces between papillae and extending into the upper half of the epithelium, consistent with high-grade dysplasia. There is no evidence of invasion in either biopsy.

The resection specimen contains the full thickness of the mucosa, including the epithelium, lamina propria, and muscularis mucosae, and a superficial portion of the submucosa. At low power (Fig. 20G), one can see that the epithelium is of variable thickness and cellularity and that the lamina propria contains lymphoid aggregates and inflammatory cells. Higher power views (Fig. 20H,I) show that the thinner central part of the epithelium is filled with crowded atypical dyspolaric cells which extend into the upper half of the epithelium but show no evidence of invasion, consistent with high-grade squamous dysplasia. While the distribution of cells is similar to that seen in biopsy 2, the nuclear features are more worrisome, with greater crowding and dyspolarity, more prominent pleomorphism, and more irregular nuclear borders. With such nuclear morphology, one must look carefully for invasion, but it is not present in the examined sections.

Among Western pathologists, grading of squamous dysplasia is largely based on the proportion of the epithelial thickness that is involved by the dysplastic cells. In three-grade systems, the dysplasia is graded as mild if the atypical cells are confined to the lower third, moderate if they are confined to the lower two thirds, and severe if they are present in all three thirds of the epithelium. In two-grade systems, the dysplasia is graded as low grade if the atypical cells are confined to the lower half, and high grade if they are present in both halves of the epithelium. The usefulness of such grading is shown by follow-up studies in which patients with a range of biopsy findings are followed for the development of invasive squamous cell carcinoma. In one such study, performed in a high-risk population in northern China, 682 adults were endoscoped and then followed for 13.5 years [1]. Categorizing the patients by their worst initial biopsy diagnosis, the cumulative incidences and relative risks for developing invasive squamous cell carcinoma during this follow-up period were: normal 8.3%, 1.0 (reference); mild dysplasia 23.7%, 2.9 (95% confidence interval 1.6–5.2); moderate dysplasia 50.0%, 9.8 (5.3–18.3); and severe dysplasia 73.9%, 28.3 (15.3–52.3). It is clear from such studies that morphologic grading of squamous dysplasia, as defined above, can identify patients with dramatically different levels of risk for developing invasive squamous cell carcinoma, which is important for proper management of these patients.

Reference

1. Wang GQ, Abnet CC, Shen Q, et al (2005) Histological precursors of oesophageal squamous cell carcinoma: results from a 13 year prospective follow up study in a high risk population. Gut 54:187–192

Pathology Commentary

Masayuki Itabashi (Japan)

In low magnification of the first biopsy from the distal esophagus (Fig. 20A), squamous epithelium shows atypical cells with hyperchromatic nuclei in basal and parabasal layers (Fig. 20C). High-power magnification of Fig. 20C shows more clearly the basal and parabasal atypical cells with hyperchromatic nuclei, which vary in size and are irregular in shape (Fig. 20D).

These findings strongly suggest that the lesion is a noninvasive carcinoma (of basal layer-extending type). However, as seen in Table 20, some of the Japanese pathologists diagnosed this lesion as "suspicious of carcinoma." It is slightly difficult to diagnose this lesion as definite carcinoma only from the findings shown above.

Another biopsy specimen from the same lesion also shows growth of atypical cells in the deeper two-thirds of the squamous epithelium (Fig. 20E). A higher power magnified picture of Fig. 20E shows multilayered growth of atypical cells with enlarged nuclei in the deeper two thirds of the epithelium (Fig. 20F). The findings of Fig. 20C–F are sufficient for a diagnosis of noninvasive (intraepithelial) carcinoma (or at least "highly suspicious of carcinoma") to be made.

A scanning power view of an endoscopic mucosal resection (EMR) specimen reveals a slightly depressed lesion and mild inflammation beneath the epithelium (Fig. 20G). Higher magnification of Fig. 20G shows multilayered growth of neoplastic cells with marked nuclear atypism, which is enough to provide a diagnosis of noninvasive carcinoma (carcinoma in situ) (Fig. 20H,I).

According to Japanese criteria, pathologists make a diagnosis of carcinoma only with marked nuclear atypism and/or disorganized arrangement of atypical cells regardless of the presence of definite invasion to the stroma.

Case 21, IIc

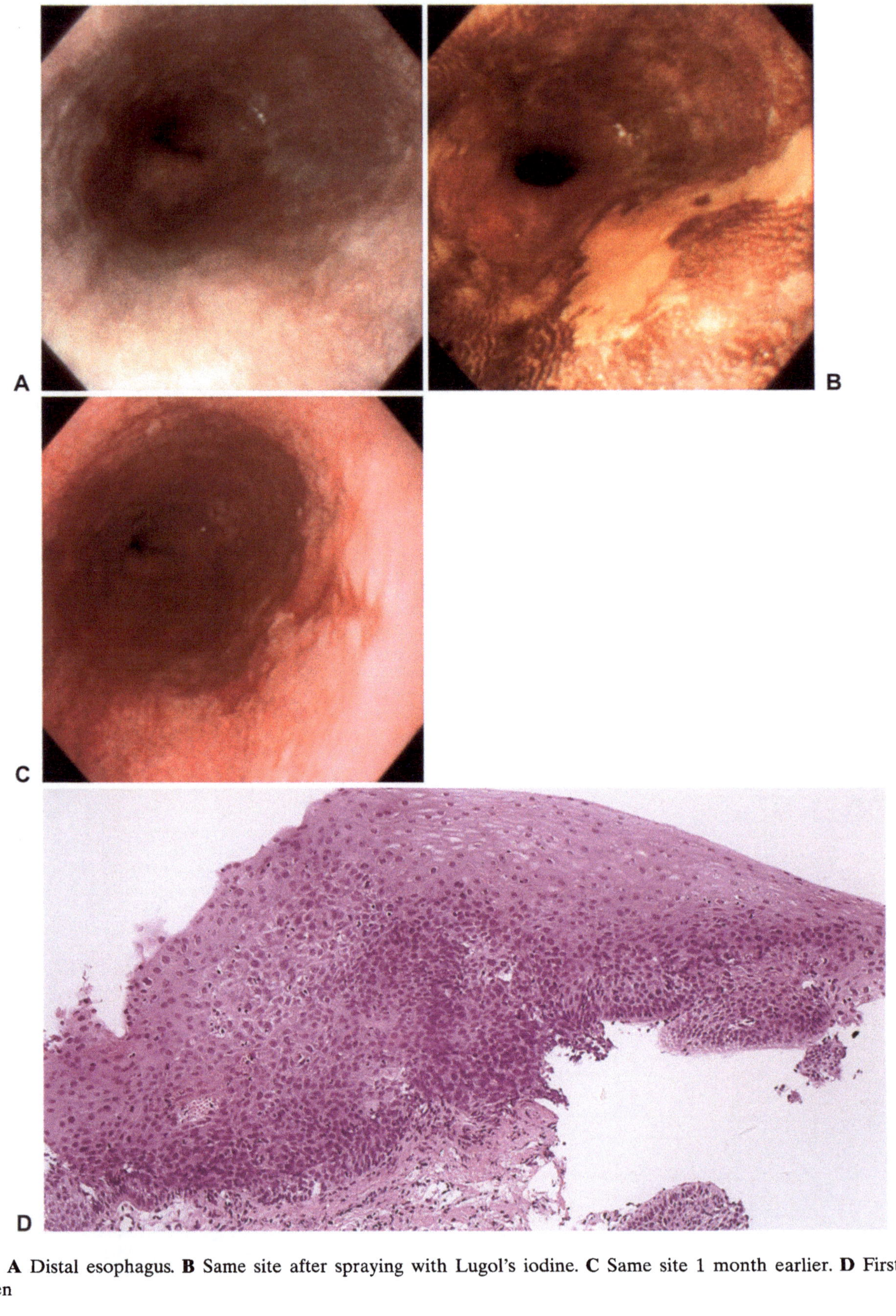

Fig. 21. **A** Distal esophagus. **B** Same site after spraying with Lugol's iodine. **C** Same site 1 month earlier. **D** First biopsy specimen

Case Description

A man, aged 71 years, with a history of heavy smoking, chronic obstructive pulmonary disease, and gastroduodenal ulcers, had no recent dyspeptic symptoms but underwent yearly upper GI screening by endoscopy. At 38 cm from the teeth a lesion was found and biopsied. About 1 month later endoscopic ultrasonographic examination was performed and 2 months thereafter the lesion was endoscopically resected in two pieces. On follow-up endoscopic and histological examinations, no neoplastic changes could be observed.

Endoscopy Commentary

Massimo Crespi (Italy)

The decision to prescribe an upper gastrointestinal endoscopic examination was a wise one, because age (71 years) and the long history of heavy smoking could well suggest the possibility of esophageal lesions. The endoscopic appearance is rather disturbing because the whole area of the lower esophagus is characterized by an irregular mucosal surface with redness and edema. The Lugol spray revealed a large, irregular, unstained area but also smaller areas of discolored mucosa. One question that arises is the result and reliability of the endoscopic ultrasonography, because the histology of the resected specimen is mostly in agreement with intramucosal carcinoma. In any case, the decision to perform an EMR was the only option considering the age and general condition of the patient.

The finding of "intramucosal carcinoma" or "noninvasive cancer" at the follow-up biopsies was limited mostly to the interpretation by Japanese pathologists, and the possibility of an overdiagnosis based on different criteria has to be taken into account.

Endoscopy Commentary

Kimiya Takeshita (Japan)

A red lesion, longer in its vertical dimension, appearing partially erosive, is visible in the posterior wall of the lower esophagus (Fig. 21C). Routine endoscopy revealed no sign of reflux esophagitis in the surrounding areas, although the view was not very clear. The presence of a hiatal hernia seems to be very likely. On iodine staining, the lesion is observed as a broad V-shaped unstained area (Fig. 21B). Although areas affected by esophagitis are also observed as unstained areas on iodine staining, an essential feature of esophageal lesions which distinguishes them from tumorous lesions is the presence of a healed area of a certain width at the border with intact tissue, which shows a fuzzy skin-like chromatic response to iodine staining. The lesion shows only minimal irregularities, suggesting that the tumor is confined to the intramucosal region.

Pathology Commentary

Sanford M. Dawsey (USA)

Both biopsies contain squamous epithelium and lamina propria. Biopsy 1 (Fig. 21D–F) is poorly oriented, with all papillae cut tangentially. The cells near the base of the epithelium and around the papillae are crowded, disorganized, and overlapping, with prominent loss of

Table 21. Esophageal lesion 21

Biopsy 1: $\times^1$
Biopsy 2: $\times^2$
Resection: $\bigcirc$

	W	J	W	J	W	W	W	W	W	WW WW WW WW W	W	J	W	WW	JJ	JJ	JJ	JJ
Regenerative changes	$\times$ $\times^1$ $\times^1$ $\times$ $\times^1$ $\times^1$																	
Indefinite for neoplasia	$\times^2$ $\times^1$																	
Dysplasia																		
low-grade	$\bigcirc$ $\times^2$ $\times^2$ $\times$ $\times^1$ $\times^1$ $\times^1$ $\times^1$																	
high-grade	$\otimes^2$ $\times^2$ $\times^2$ $\times^2$ $\times^1$ $\times^1$ $\times^1$																	
Carcinoma																		
suspected	$\bigcirc$ $\bigcirc$ $\bigcirc$ $\times^2$ $\times^2$ $\times^1$ $\times^1$																	
non-invasive	$\times^2$ $\times^2$ $\times^2$ $\times$																	
intramucosal	$\bigcirc$ $\bigcirc$ $\bigcirc$ $\bigcirc$ $\bigcirc$ $\bigcirc$ $\bigcirc$ $\bigcirc$ $\otimes^2$ $\bigcirc$ $\bigcirc$ $\otimes^2$ $\bigcirc$																	

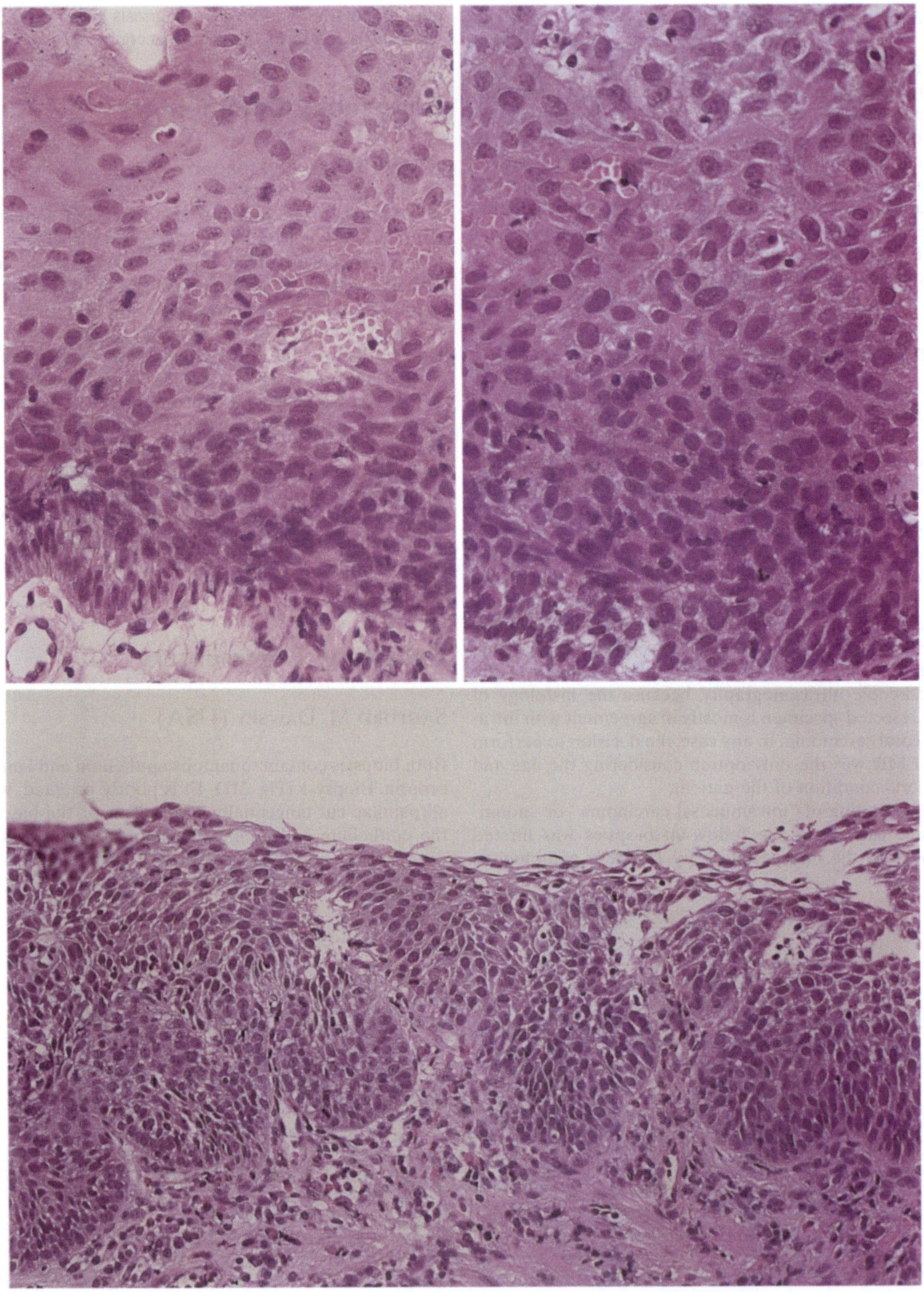

E F G

Fig. 21. **E** Detail of **D**. **F** Detail of **D**. **G** Second biopsy specimen normal polarity. The nuclei are hyperchromatic, but are only mildly enlarged and show only mild variation in size and shape. Because of the suboptimal orientation of the biopsy, it is unclear what portion of the epithelial thickness is involved by the atypical cells, but most of them appear to be confined to the lower half, consistent with low-grade dysplasia.

Biopsy 2 (Fig. 21G), in contrast, is well oriented and contains atypical cells throughout the full thickness of the epithelium. The nuclei are hyperchromatic and are more pleomorphic than those seen in biopsy 1. This biopsy certainly represents high-grade dysplasia; the question in this sample is whether it represents invasive carcinoma. Although the epithelial tongues have rounded "pushing" lower borders, consistent with enclosure by a basement membrane, and the inflammatory reaction in the lamina propria is only moderate, the epithelial tongues appear disorganized, and growing in different directions, as though they are unaware of each others' presence. This pattern is not diagnostic of invasion, but it is certainly very worrisome for it in the limited view we have of this lesion, and the communication to the clinician should reflect this concern. Thus I would call this biopsy suspicious for invasive carcinoma, with a comment that further sampling of the lesion is warranted to rule out definite invasion. A diagnosis of high-grade dysplasia with a comment suggesting further sampling to rule out invasive carcinoma would also be appropriate. In either case, the clinician should be called and alerted to the seriousness of the lesion and the possibility that the biopsies may not have sampled the worst part of the lesion.

The resection specimen contains mucosa and submucosa, and shows a squamous cell carcinoma invading into the lamina propria. The low-power views (Fig. 21H,I) show multiple tumor nests, lymphoid aggregates with germinal centers, and a moderate inflammatory infiltrate. The tumor nests have rounded, pushing borders, and do not appear to invade the muscularis mucosae. In Fig. 21H, the surface of the tumor appears depressed below the adjacent normal epithelium, consistent with the endoscopic finding of a IIc lesion, and the tumor focally undermines the adjacent epithelium. In the high-power view, the nuclear features of the tumor are similar to those seen in biopsy 2.

This case illustrates the variability of histologic patterns that can be seen in single endoscopic lesions, and the resulting need to take multiple biopsies of worrisome endoscopic findings. Biopsy 1 and biopsy 2 have very different morphologic patterns, and the pathologist's concern would be much less if only biopsy 1 had been sent for examination.

This case also illustrates the limits of endoscopic biopsy diagnosis as well as the need for good communication between pathologist and clinician. Although the epithelial cellular morphology is quite similar in biopsy 2 and in the invasive tumor nests of the resection specimen, definite evidence of invasion is not present in the biopsy, and a similar cellular morphology can be seen in cases that are not invasive. Because of the biopsy's size and the tissue that was sampled, it cannot document or rule out invasion, and the clinician needs to know this.

The presence or absence of invasion is the most important single finding that the pathologist can tell the clinician in cases where tissue is removed to evaluate neoplasia, and this finding should be stated explicitly in every pathology report of such cases. Without invasion, neoplasia rarely spreads widely, metastasizes, or kills the host, so the clinician must know the invasion status of each case.

Pathology Commentary

Masayuki Itabashi (Japan)

A first biopsy specimen from the distal esophagus shows high cellularity mainly in the deep one-third layer of thick squamous epithelium (Fig. 21D). A detailed picture of Fig. 21D shows nuclei of a high cellular zone, which are not so hyperchromatic and show even distribution of heterochromatin (Fig. 21E). Furthermore, a high cellular zone (in the deeper layer) gradually transits to a low cellular zone (upper layer of the epithelium). These findings lead the Japanese pathologists to a diagnosis of dysplasia.

Another detailed picture of Fig. 21D shows more multilayered nuclei in an irregular arrangement (Fig. 21F). The nuclear chromatin is evenly distributed. There is also a gradual transition from the deeper layer of high cellularity toward the upper layer of low cellularity. These findings lead to a diagnosis of "suspicion of carcinoma (cis)" but lack enough information to be called "definite noninvasive carcinoma" according to the Japanese criteria.

A second biopsy specimen shows dense growth of atypical cells with hyperchromatic nuclei in the whole layer of the epithelium and elongation of its thickened rete ridge toward the lamina propria mucosae (Fig. 21G). Most of the Japanese pathologists call this lesion "definite carcinoma" either with or without stromal invasion (cf. Table 21).

A resected specimen under EMR shows growth of neoplastic cells in the surface squamous epithelium as well as in the lamina propria mucosae (Fig. 21H). A high-power view of another section of the same

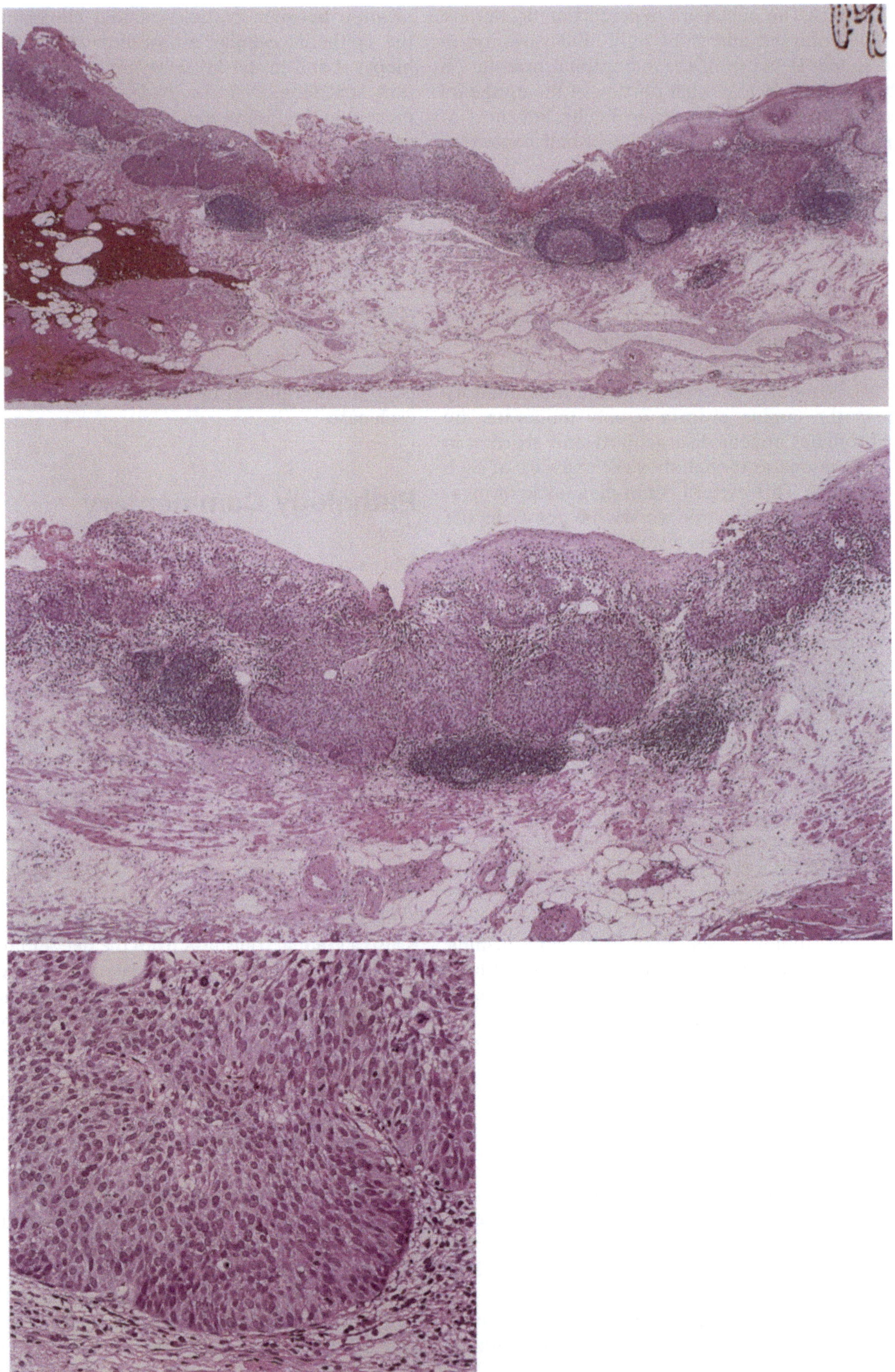

H

I

J

Fig. 21. **H** Resected specimen. **I** Other section of same specimen. **J** Detail of **I**

specimen as Fig. 21H shows definite bulky invasion of neoplastic cells into the lamina propria mucosae (Fig. 21I). A higher power magnification of Fig. 21I shows bulky invasion of neoplastic cells into the lamina propria mucosae almost reaching the muscularis mucosae at the bottom of the picture (Fig. 21J). With these findings (Fig. 21H–J), all of the Japanese pathologists made a diagnosis of intramucosal invasive carcinoma (cf. Table 21).

Case 22, IIc

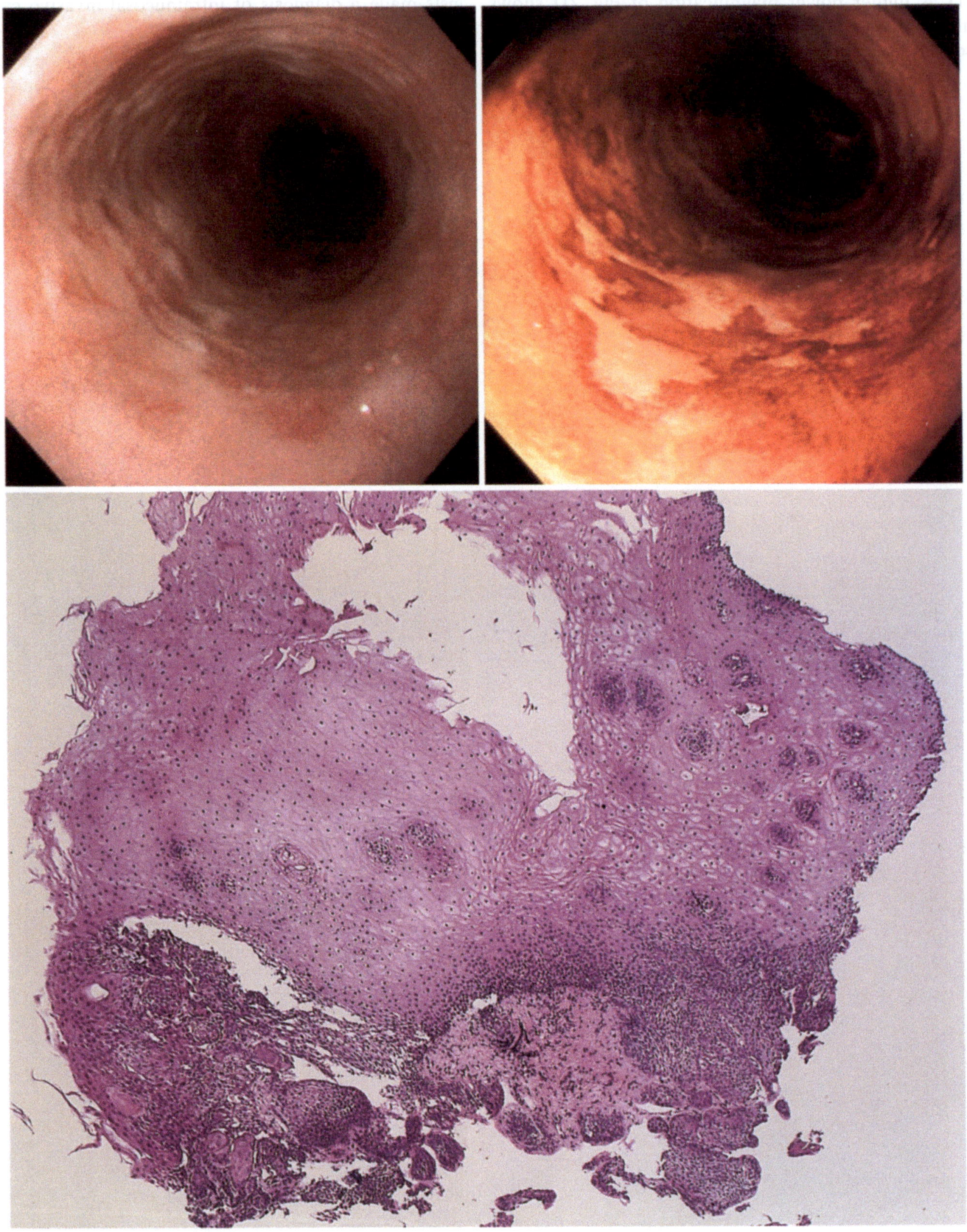

Fig. 22. **A** Distal esophagus. **B** Same site after spraying Lugol's iodine. **C** Biopsy specimen

Case Description

A man, aged 54 years, had undergone total gastrectomy for stage IIIA gastric carcinoma. On follow-up upper GI endoscopic examination 3 months later, a lesion was found at 32 cm from the teeth and biopsied. Two months thereafter endoscopic resection was performed. The resection margins (one piece) were free of neoplastic change.

Endoscopy Commentary

Massimo Crespi (Italy)

From the scanty clinical information about the extension of EMR, it is difficult to assess whether the patient may be considered healed from the esophageal lesion. In fact, the endoscopic pictures show a diffused area of unstained mucosa not only at the bottom but also on the right side of the picture, together with diffuse irregularities of the mucosal surface. Considering the previous gastric surgery, EMR was in any case the only possible approach. The histology is again perplexing, with interpretations scattered from normal to intra- and submucosal cancer. Who may be trusted?

Endoscopy Commentary

Kimiya Takeshita (Japan)

A case after total gastrectomy for stomach cancer. The lesion is discolored in the region extending from the posterior to the anterior wall of the middle esophagus. The capillary network cannot be seen. A lesion affecting about one quarter of the circumference, mostly depressed, is visible. Iodine staining revealed an unstained area corresponding almost exactly to the lesion (Fig. 22B). However, regenerative changes, possibly secondary to biopsy, are visible in the surrounding area. These features seem to represent those of a typical mucosal cancer.

Pathology Commentary

Sanford M. Dawsey (USA)

The biopsy contains both squamous epithelium and lamina propria, but it is quite poorly oriented, with all papillae cut across, so the relationship of the epithelium and the lamina propria is difficult to evaluate. In the higher power view (Fig. 22D), nests of epithelial cells appear closely associated with the lamina propria, possibly consistent with invasion, but the orientation is so problematic that no definite statement concerning invasion can be made. Additionally, the magnification in Fig. 22D does not allow full evaluation of the nuclear features of the epithelial cells. The technical difficulties associated with this biopsy are reflected in the wide range of diagnoses rendered by the pathologists who reviewed these pictures. In a clinical setting, I would examine this slide at higher power to look more closely at the nuclear features, and I would examine more tissue sections from deeper levels in the block to evaluate further the possibility of invasion. With only the current information, I would call this biopsy suspicious for invasive carcinoma, and I would communicate to the clinician, both verbally and in my report, that my view of the biopsy was technically suboptimal. I would mention

Table 22. Esophageal lesion 22

Biopsy: ×
Resection: ○

	W	W	W J	W	W W	W W	W	W J	W	W	W	W W	W	W W	J	J J J J	J	W J J J	W
Regenerative changes	×																		
Indefinite for neoplasia		×	×	×															
Dysplasia																			
low-grade	○	○			⊗	×	○	×		○									
high-grade			○			○			⊗		○	×							
Carcinoma																			
suspected				○			×	○					⊗	○	×				
non-invasive															○	⊗	×		
intramucosal										×	×	○		×			○	⊗	○
submucosal																			×

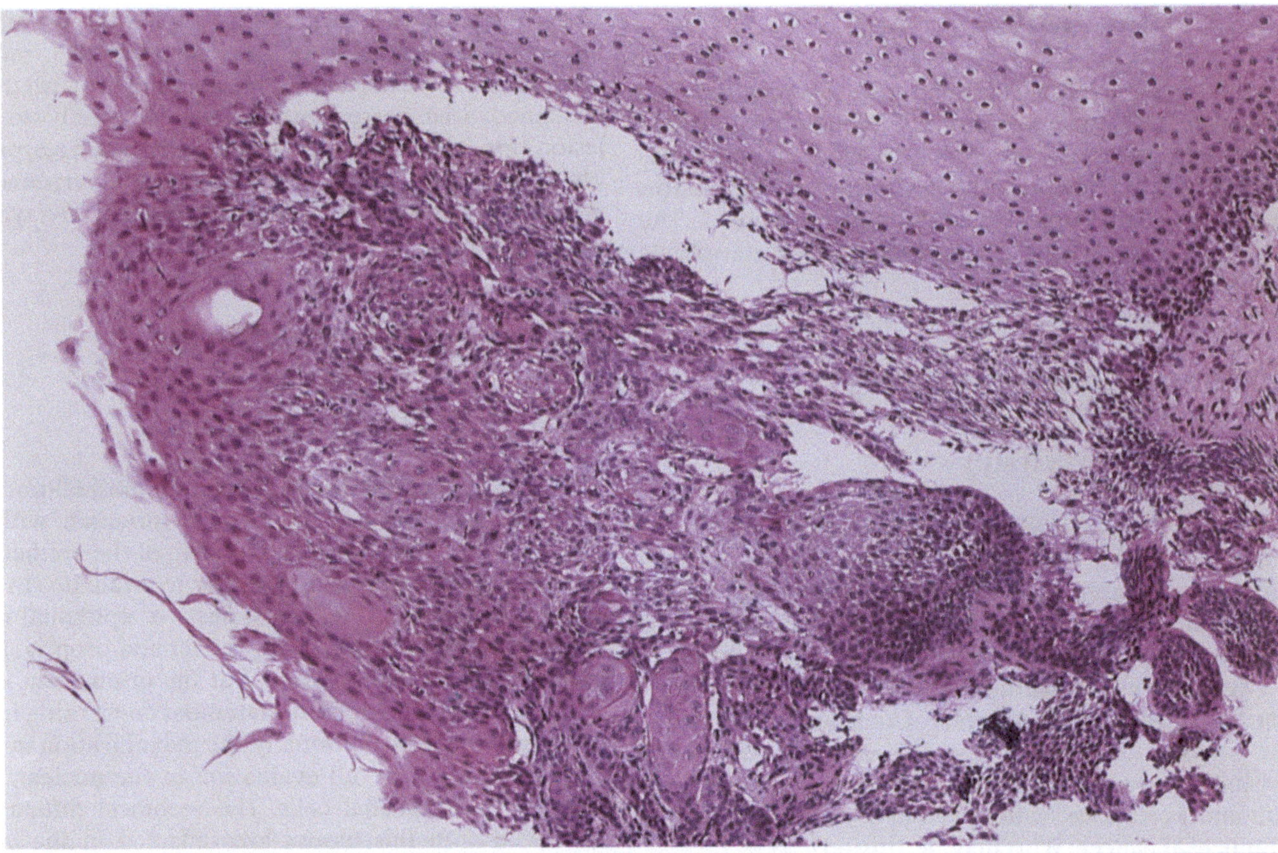

D

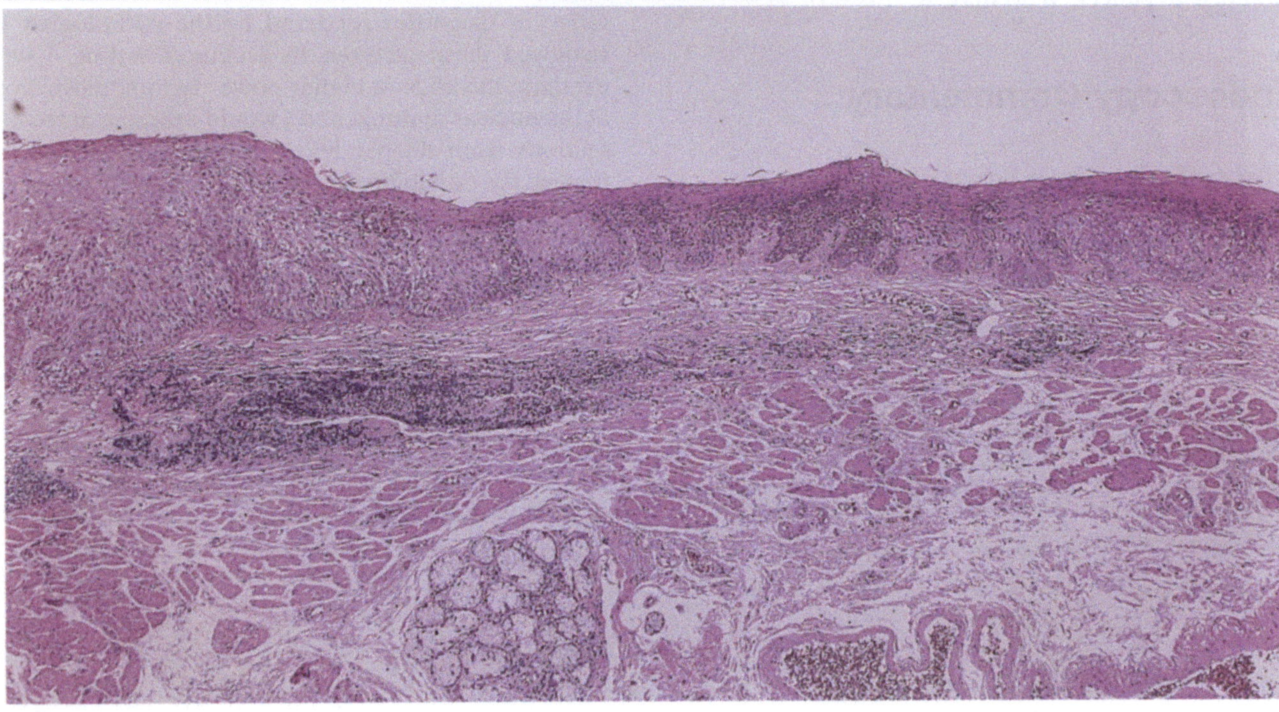

E

Fig. 22. **D** Detail of **C**. **E** Resected specimen

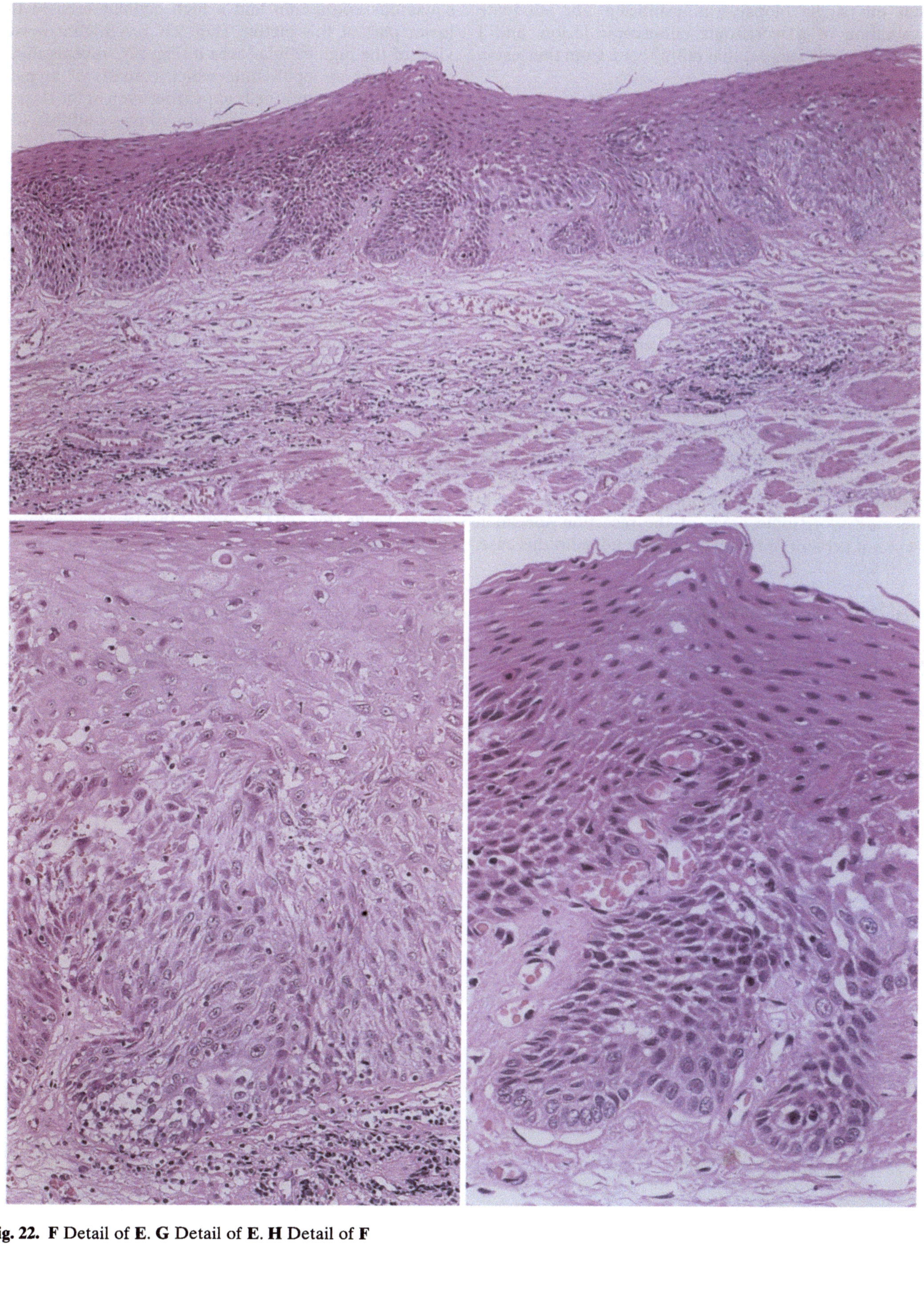

F

G

H

Fig. 22. **F** Detail of **E**. **G** Detail of **E**. **H** Detail of **F**

that this single biopsy was insufficient for adequate evaluation of a worrisome endoscopic lesion, and I would strongly suggest that more tissue from this lesion be examined.

The resection specimen contains both mucosa and submucosa. The epithelium shows variable morphologic features. In the right half of the low-power view, some epithelial tongues show atypical cells only in the lowest cell layers, with orderly maturation from base to surface (Fig. 22H). In contrast, in the left half of the low-power view the epithelium is thickened and contains atypical cells with enlarged, pleomorphic nuclei and distinct nucleoli throughout much of its thickness (Fig. 22G). Although invasion is not definite, the left side of the lesion is highly suspicious for early invasion of the lamina propria. Such a lesion certainly needs to be removed fully, so it is reassuring to know that the resection margins were free of neoplastic change.

This case illustrates again the importance of biopsy orientation for proper evaluation of neoplastic invasion, and the need for multiple biopsies to capture the variable histologic patterns that can be seen in a single endoscopic lesion. The pleomorphic morphology seen in the most worrisome areas of the resection specimen were not present in the single biopsy taken in this case.

Pathology Commentary

MASAYUKI ITABASHI (Japan)

A low-power view of an endoscopic biopsy from the distal esophagus shows a tangentially cut section of squamous epithelium and a high cellular area in the lower part of this picture (Fig. 22C). A higher power view of the high cellular area in Fig. 22C reveals thickened squamous epithelium which consists of atypical cells and dyskeratotic cells appearing even in the deeper layer of the epithelium, and also shows budding–like growth toward the lamina propria mucosae (Fig. 22D). Most of the Japanese pathologists diagnosed the lesion as "definite carcinoma". However, one gave a diagnosis of suspicion of carcinoma.

A scanning power view of the EMR specimen shows a slightly depressed lesion with rete ridge-like downward growth toward the lamina propria mucosae (Fig. 22E). A low-power view of Fig. 22E shows growth of atypical neoplastic cells in the deeper half of the epithelium and a thickened rete ridge-like extension toward the lamina propria mucosae (Fig. 22F). A higher power view of Fig. 22E shows atypical spindle-shaped cell growth in the deeper half of the epithelium and their irregular arrangement (Fig. 22G). A higher power picture of Fig. 22F shows atypical cell growth in the deeper third of the epithelium and a downward, thickened rete ridge-like extension of variable-sized atypical cells (Fig. 22H). Some of the Japanese pathologists diagnosed the lesion of as noninvasive carcinoma, while the others diagnosed intramucosal invasive carcinoma (cf. Table 22). It is sometimes difficult to judge whether a lesion is truly invasive or noninvasive, as seen in Table 22.

Case 23, IIc

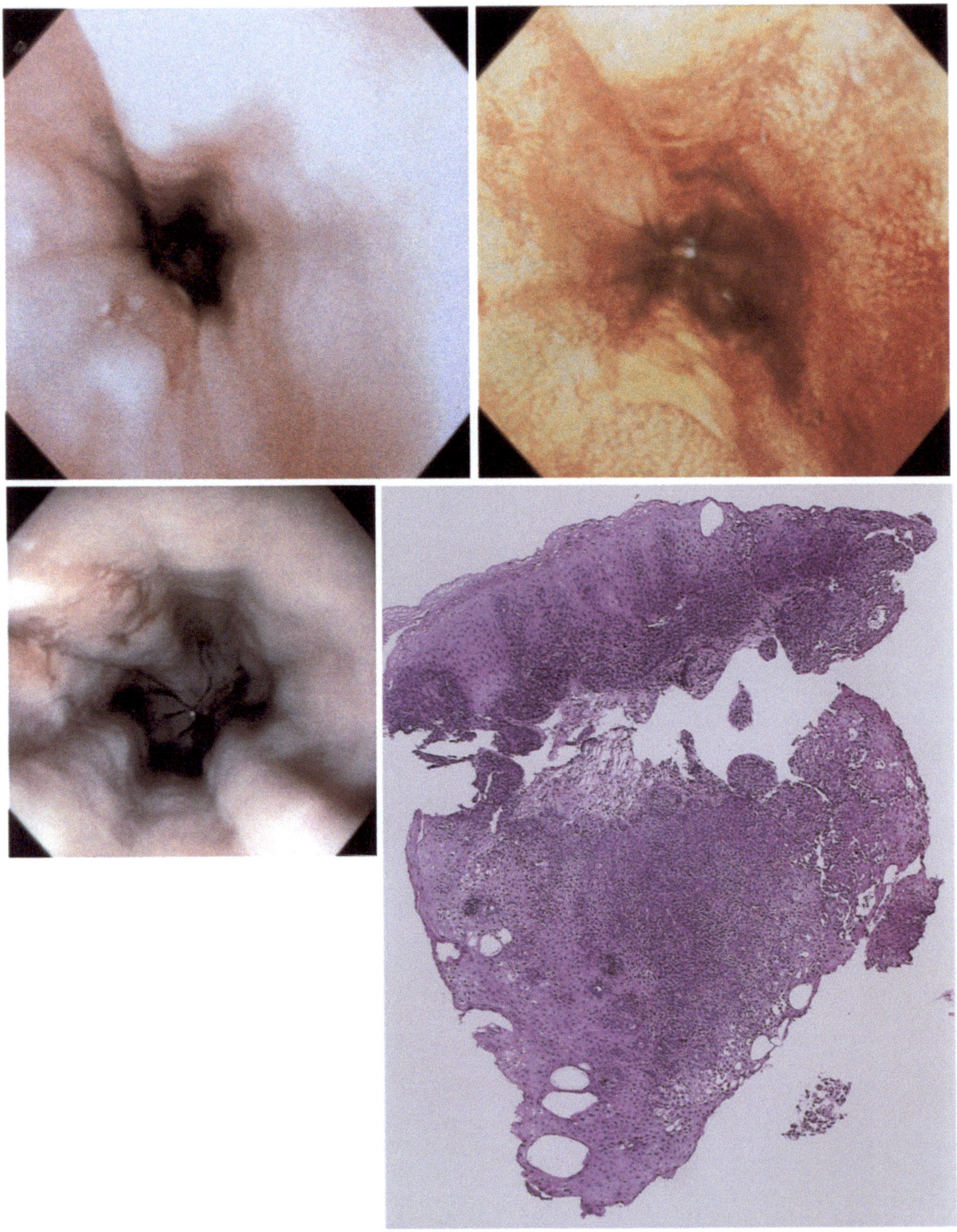

A B C D

Fig. 23. **A** Distal esophagus (after esophageal varices ligation). **B** Same site after spraying with Lugol's iodine. **C** Same site 2 months earlier (before esophageal varices ligation). **D** Biopsy specimen

Case Description

A man, aged 55 years, with a history of heavy drinking and smoking, chronic hepatitis C, liver cirrhosis, cerebral infarction, and pulmonary hypertension, complained of chest pain and underwent upper GI endoscopy. From 25 to 40 cm from the teeth, esophageal varices were seen; moreover, at 35 cm an esophageal lesion and at the angulus a small, discolored, shallow, depressed lesion were found and biopsied. Five months later endoscopic ultrasonographic examination and esophageal varices ligation were performed, and shortly thereafter the esophageal lesion was endoscopically resected in three pieces and the gastric lesion, a minute signet-ring cell carcinoma, in one piece. On follow-up endoscopic and histological examinations no neoplastic changes could be detected.

Endoscopy Commentary

Massimo Crespi (Italy)

Considering the underlying pathological conditions (cirrhosis, cerebral infarction, etc.), both EMRs seem to fall into an "overtreatment" attitude: in any case EMR was the only possible therapy. The endoscopic pictures (Fig. 23A and B), taken after variceal ligation, clearly show the esophageal lesion, which previously was overshadowed by the large varices shown in Fig. 23C. This fact is of interest because it teaches us the importance of a second-look endoscopy, completed with Lugol staining, after cure of the varices, especially in high-risk subjects (heavy drinkers and smokers) as in this case. Again we have to remark on the very perplexing variability of histological interpretations.

Endoscopy Commentary

Kimiya Takeshita (Japan)

A case with concomitant liver cirrhosis, esophageal varices, and early gastric cancer. The varices were almost full-circumferential along the segment of the esophagus extending between 25 and 40 cm from the incisors. A small lesion, which was red and erosive and about 1 cm in diameter, was visible endoscopically in the lower segment of the esophagus after variceal ligation. Iodine staining revealed a small unstained zone corresponding to this lesion (Fig. 23B). In this case, an immediate endoscopic diagnosis of cancer was difficult to make based only on the size and superficial features of the lesion. Considering the possibility of bleeding from the varices after endoscopic mucosal resection, piecemeal resection was performed, by which resection of small portions of the lesion was repeated. We believe that this operative procedure was the most appropriate option for this patient.

Pathology Commentary

Sanford M. Dawsey (USA)

The biopsy includes squamous epithelium and lamina propria. The orientation is fairly good in half of the biopsy but is poor in the other half. In the well-oriented portion of the biopsy (Fig. 23D,E), the nuclei in the lower two thirds of the epithelium are markedly hyperchromatic and show moderate variation in size and shape. The upper epithelium shows orderly maturation, with only a few scattered atypical cells. The poorly ori-

Table 23. Esophageal lesion 23

Biopsy: × Resection: ○	W	W	W	W W J	W W W	WW WW WW WW WW	W	J	J	J J JJ JJ JJ	W
Regenerative changes	○		×								
Indefinite for neoplasia				×							
Dysplasia											
low-grade		⊗			×			×			
high-grade	×		○	○	○	⊗	○				
Carcinoma											
suspected							×		○		
non-invasive								○		⊗	
intramucosal									×		⊗

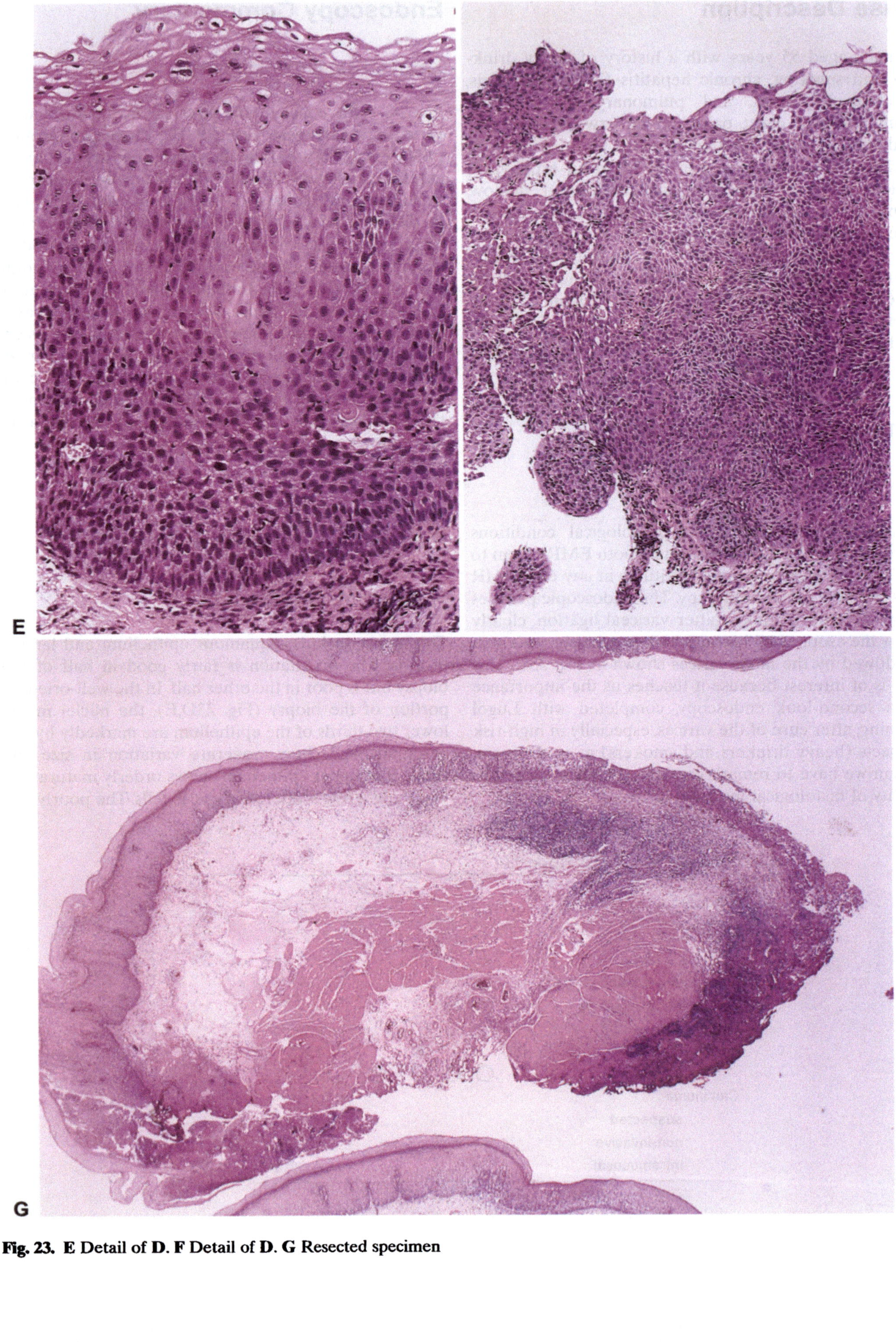

Fig. 23. E Detail of **D**. **F** Detail of **D**. **G** Resected specimen

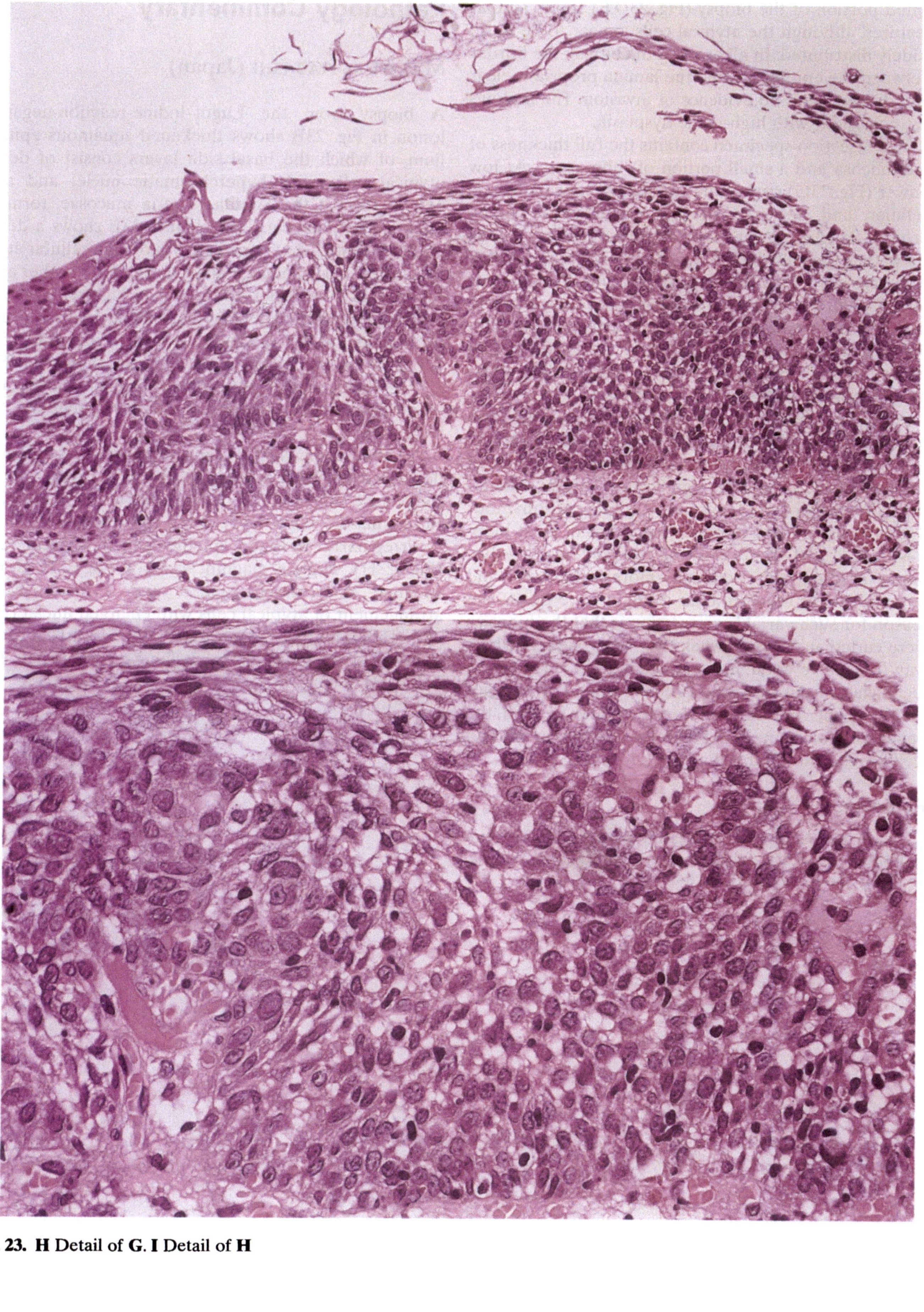

H

I

Fig. 23. **H** Detail of **G**. **I** Detail of **H**

ented portion of the biopsy (Fig. 23D,F) shows similar features, although the atypical cells appear to be more widely distributed. In all areas of the biopsy, the border between the epithelium and the lamina propria is clear and distinct, with no evidence of invasion. The findings are consistent with high-grade dysplasia.

The resection specimen contains the full thickness of the mucosa and a small portion of submucosa. At low power (Fig. 23G) part of the epithelium appears hypercellular, and this part overlies an inflamed lamina propria. Higher power views of this area (Fig. 23H,I) show that the full thickness of the epithelium is filled with atypical cells with enlarged, pleomorphic vesicular nuclei, small nucleoli, and relatively scant cytoplasm. As in the biopsy, however, the border between the epithelium and the lamina propria is clear and distinct, with no evidence of invasion. Thus the findings are again most consistent with high-grade dysplasia.

As discussed in Case 20, grading of squamous dysplasia based on the proportion of the epithelial thickness that is involved by the dysplastic cells has been shown to have prognostic significance. Biopsy orientation is very important for accurate grading of squamous dysplasia using these criteria. Most areas of most biopsies in Cases 20–24 are not well oriented, making dysplasia grading more difficult, more subjective, and potentially less accurate than it might have been. The reason for such variable orientation is that the biopsies were curled and twisted when they were fixed. The best way to achieve good, uniform orientation is to have a technician in the endoscopy room spread the biopsies on filter paper before they are fixed. After fixation, the paper can be removed and the biopsies remain flat and well oriented for embedding and sectioning [1].

Reference

1. Lewin KJ, Riddell RH, Weinstein WM (1992) Gastrointestinal pathology and its clinical implications, 1st edn. Igaku-Shoin, New York, pp 8–11

Pathology Commentary

Masayuki Itabashi (Japan)

A biopsy from the Lugol–iodine-reaction-negative lesion in Fig. 23B shows thickened squamous epithelium, of which the basal side layers consist of dense atypical cells with hyperchromatic nuclei and also extend toward the lamina propria mucosae, forming thick trabeculae (Fig. 23D). Figure 23E shows a detail of Fig. 23D, with downward growth of high cellular atypical cells of varied nuclear sizes. A detail of another area of Fig. 23D shows thick epithelium of high cellularity of atypical cells, with hyperchromatic nuclei and a bud-like protrusion toward the lamina propria mucosae (Fig. 23F). From the histological findings shown in Fig. 23D–F, the Japanese pathologists diagnosed the lesion as noninvasive carcinoma or invasive carcinoma (cf. Table 23).

An endoscopically resected specimen shows a slightly depressed but high cellular lesion on the right side of the picture (Fig. 23G). A detail of the lesion in Fig. 23G shows that the whole layer of the epithelium is replaced by irregularly arranged spindle-shaped atypical cells (Fig. 23H). Higher magnification of Fig. 23H shows widened intercellular spaces and a disorganized arrangement of atypical cells with enlarged nuclei (Fig. 23I). This lesion was diagnosed as intraepithelial carcinoma (cis) by most of the Japanese pathologists (cf. Table 23).

Case 24, IIb

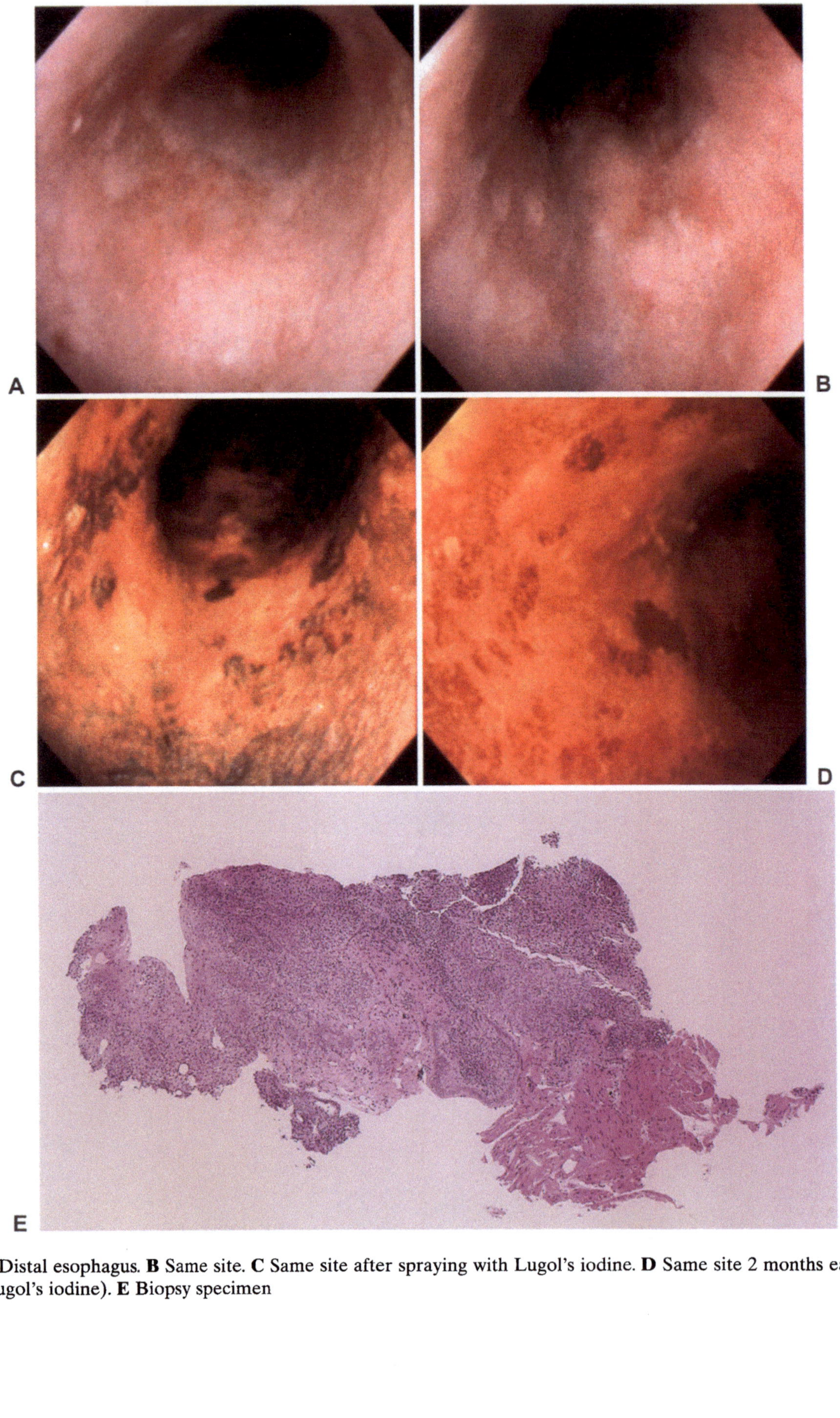

Fig. 24. **A** Distal esophagus. **B** Same site. **C** Same site after spraying with Lugol's iodine. **D** Same site 2 months earlier (after spraying Lugol's iodine). **E** Biopsy specimen

Case Description

A man, aged 70 years, with diabetes mellitus, had no recent dyspeptic symptoms but underwent upper GI screening by endoscopy. At 30 cm from the teeth a lesion was found and biopsied. Two months later endoscopic ultrasonographic examination was performed and 1 week thereafter the lesion was endoscopically resected in four pieces. On follow-up endoscopic and histological examinations, no neoplastic changes could be observed.

Endoscopy Commentary

Massimo Crespi (Italy)

This is a very interesting case, where EMR demonstrated its crucial value as treatment of early lesions in subjects at high risk for surgery. The endoscopic pictures, both the ones obtained before and after Lugol staining, clearly show a flat, mucosal lesion with irregular margins. It is not clear why 2 months elapsed between the first endoscopy and EMR: in fact Fig. 24D shows the lesion already well enhanced by the Lugol stain. The small area on the left, mimicking elevated, convergent folds, is obviously the primary target for multiple biopsies and EMR.

In this case the histology is more uniform, pointing mostly to an intramucosal carcinoma.

Endoscopy Commentary

Kimiya Takeshita (Japan)

The posterior wall of the middle esophagus shows discolored mucosa and an extensive area lacking in capillary networks. Iodine staining revealed the lesion as a semi-circumferential, unstained area (Fig. 24C). At some points, the extent of the lesion was greater than that usually observed by routine endoscopy. This case seems to be a type of superficial carcinoma that is poorly demarcated and difficult to diagnose, and emphasizes the importance of bearing in mind that a large type IIb-like cancer with little superficial irregularity can show deep invasion into the lamina propria in some parts of the lesion.

Pathology Commentary

Sanford M. Dawsey (USA)

The biopsy is another example of poor orientation limiting the information that can be obtained from a biopsy specimen. The biopsy contains squamous epithelium, a small amount of lamina propria, and a portion of muscularis mucosae. The epithelium is filled with atypical cells with enlarged dyspolaric nuclei and distinct to prominent nucleoli. The cytologic features are clearly dysplastic and are worrisome for invasive carcinoma, but they are not more atypical than the abnormal cells seen in Case 20 (Fig. 20I), which were not invasive. Cells with these morphologic features represent invasive carcinoma only when they are shown to invade the lamina propria or deeper structures.

Focally, nests of the atypical cells are present near the muscularis mucosae, making them highly suspicious for invasive nests, but the orientation is so poor that the exact relationship of the various tissue components is not certain. I have previously seen biopsies of noninvasive lesions where poor orientation caused the epithelium and the muscularis mucosae to appear as closely related as in this case. With better orientation, the biopsy could have looked similar to the upper portion

Table 24. Esophageal lesion 24

Biopsy: ×
Resection: ○

	W	W	W W	W W W	W W	W W W J	J	J	J J	J J J W J W J	W	W W W	W W J
Indefinite for neoplasia	×												
Dysplasia													
high-grade		⊗	×	×	×								
Carcinoma													
suspected			○			×							
non-invasive							⊗	○	×				
intramucosal	○			○		○		×	○	⊗	○	×	
submucosal					○						×	○	⊗

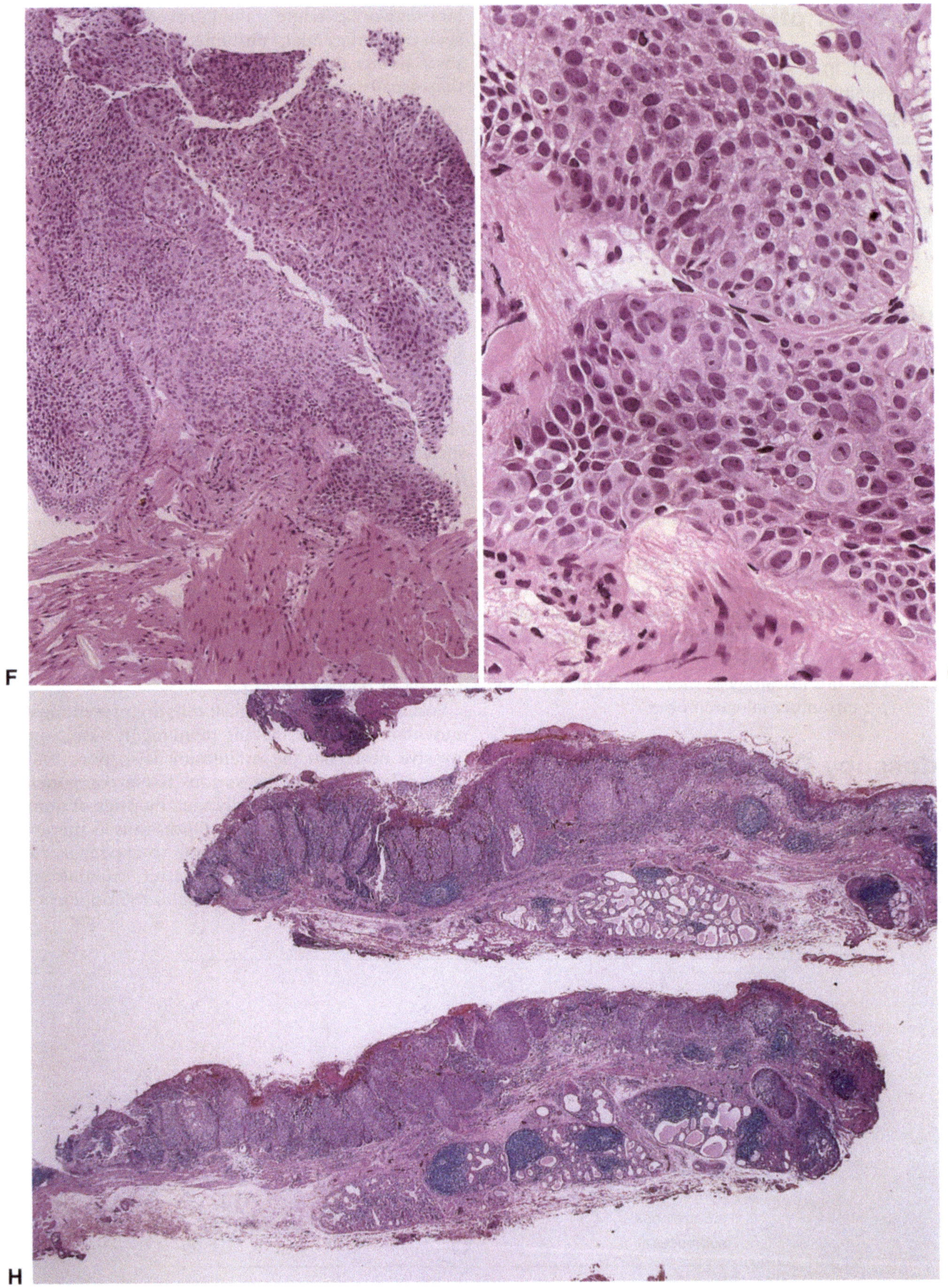

Fig. 24. **F** Detail of **E**. **G** Detail of **F**. **H** Resected specimen

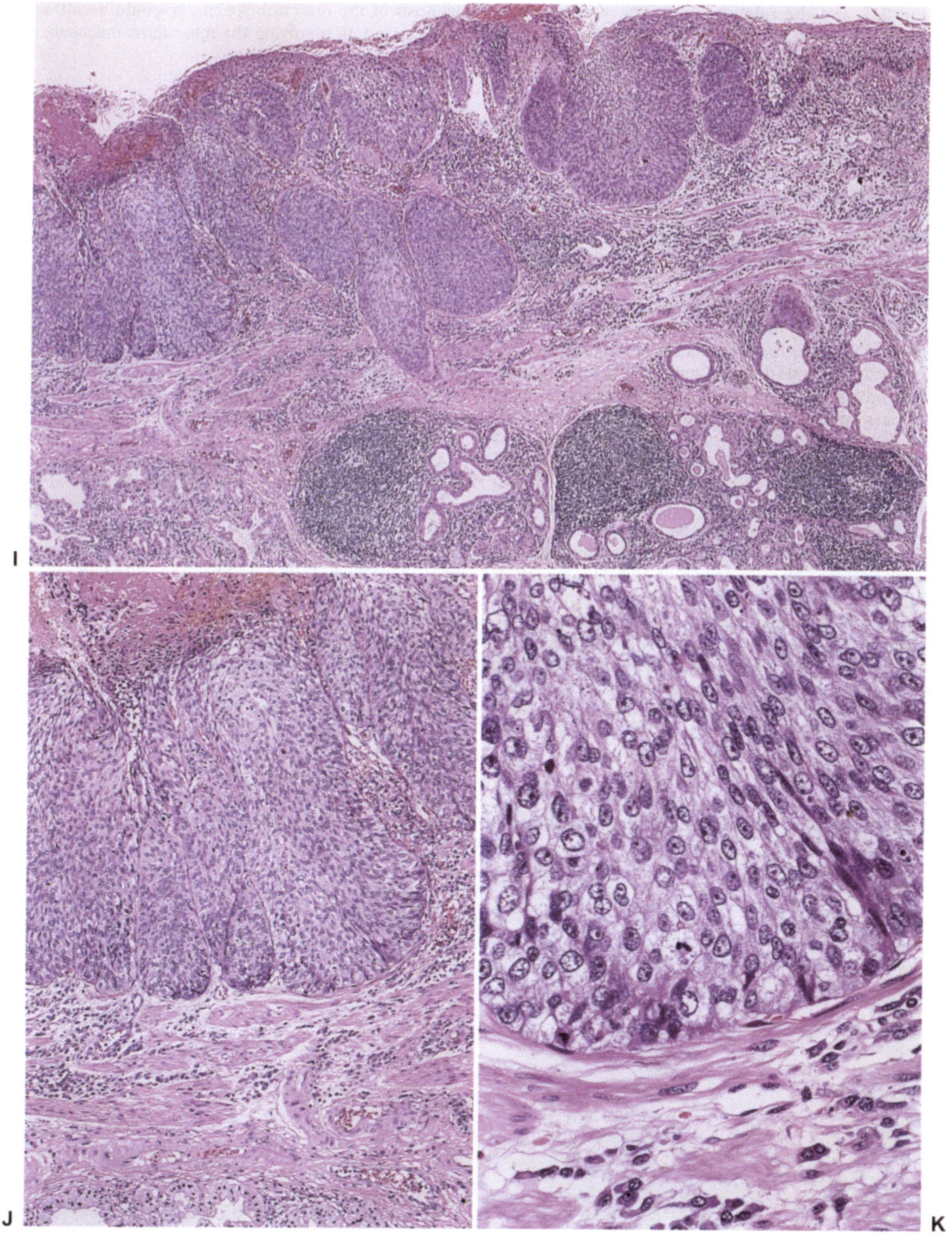

Fig. 24. **I** Detail of **H**. **J** Detail of **I**. **K** Detail of **J**

of Fig. 24I, and the relationship of the various tissue components would be clear. Thus, this biopsy certainly represents high-grade dysplasia and may well represent intramucosal carcinoma, and I can understand any diagnosis in this spectrum, but I myself cannot be sure of invasion from the section illustrated. If I had this case in a clinical setting, I would cut through the block looking for more definite evidence of invasion. If I found nothing more definitive, my diagnosis would be suspicious for invasive carcinoma, with a written and verbal comment to the clinician that I am highly suspicious of invasion but cannot prove it without examining additional tissue.

As mentioned in Case 21, invasion is the most important single variable that a pathologist must evaluate in a biopsy of a neoplastic lesion, because it is only through invasion that neoplastic cells gain access to lymphatic and blood vessels and the ability to metastasize. When invasion is not clear in the submitted tissue, pathologists should be conservative in their interpretation and discuss their findings with the clinician. In most cases it is not too difficult to rebiopsy the lesion or, if clinical suspicion is high enough, to perform an endoscopic mucosal resection for both diagnosis and treatment.

The resection specimen in this case contains the full mucosa and an ample portion of the submucosa. It shows clear tumor invasion into the muscularis mucosae, and focal involvement of ducts leading to the submucosal glands (Fig. 24I). I do not interpret such duct involvement as submucosal invasion unless I see tumor penetration into the connective tissue surrounding the ducts. True submucosal invasion may be present on the right side of Fig. 24H, but we are not given closer views to further evaluate this possibility. The higher power views (Fig. 24J,K) show nuclear morphology which is similar to that seen in the biopsy (Fig. 24G), taking into account differences in fixation artifact. My diagnosis of the resection specimen would be intramucosal carcinoma involving the muscularis mucosae.

Pathology Commentary

Masayuki Itabashi (Japan)

An endoscopic biopsy from the lesion shows highly cellular and thick epithelium which extends toward the muscularis mucosae, almost reaching it (Fig. 24E). A detail of Fig. 24E shows thick trabeculae of high cellular epithelium almost reaching the muscularis mucosae (Fig. 24F). Higher magnification of Fig. 24F shows a disorganized arrangement of variable-sized neoplastic cells with plump nuclei (Fig. 24G). These findings (Fig. 24E–G) led most of the Japanese pathologists to diagnose the lesion as intramucosal invasive carcinoma (cf. Table 24).

A scanning power view of an EMR specimen shows high cellular epithelium with thick trabecular downward projection of epithelium, and association of inflammatory cell infiltration as well as of lymph follicles (Fig. 24H). A low-power magnification of Fig. 24H shows the thick trabecula-like downward growth of neoplastic epithelium more clearly than Fig. 24H (Fig. 24I). One of the trabeculae reaches the level of the muscularis mucosae, which may be an intraductal extension of the neoplasia. Downward projection of the neoplastic trabeculae reaches the upper layer of the muscularis mucosae (Fig. 24J). Higher magnification of Fig. 24J shows disorganized growth of neoplastic cells with a round nucleus containing a remarkable nucleolus and frequent mitotic figures (Fig. 24K). Carcinoma with invasion to the muscularis mucosae is the diagnosis made by most of the Japanese pathologists.

5. Comments on the Variability of the Diagnoses

Manfred Stolte

At first glance, the variability in the histological differential diagnosis of early epithelial neoplasia of the stomach, first reported by Schlemper et al. [1] and subsequently confirmed in further reports [2–4], is alarming. This variability then gave rise to critical comments [5]. One gastroenterologist was even moved to give his comments the title "Japanese Fairy Tales," [6] and concluded "The high prevalence of early gastric carcinoma in Japan and the successes in combating carcinoma of the stomach are possibly nothing but an artefact." This commentator, however, overlooked the fact that one of the Western pathologists established exactly the same diagnoses, as did the four Japanese pathologists. He also failed to note that, in contrast to this group of four Japanese and one Western pathologist, the diagnoses made by the three other Western pathologists in forceps biopsy material differed considerably from their own diagnoses in the mucosectomy specimens from the same patients. Similar variable results in identical specimens were also revealed by the slide seminar that led to the compromise Vienna classification of gastrointestinal epithelial neoplasia [7], so that we might be justified in claiming that, in this area the term "Western deficiency" might be a more accurate comment than "Japanese fairy tales." [8]

The uncertainty of many Western pathologists in differentiating between dysplasia and well-differentiated carcinoma of the stomach was already known from a number of follow-up studies of high-grade dysplasia of gastric mucosa. In 80% of these cases, a carcinoma was diagnosed within the very short average follow-up time of 6 months [9–16]. This uncertainty is readily understandable since, in comparison, the Japanese pathologists have much greater experience as a result of the much more common endoscopy/biopsy diagnosis of early carcinoma, and the much more frequently practiced endoscopic mucosectomy [17]. Fewer examinations coupled with less training in this area is therefore the likely explanation for the diagnostic uncertainty of many Western pathologists [18].

However, at second glance, the diagnostic discrepancies are not particularly serious in terms of clinical consequences. Only very rarely did a Western pathologist underdiagnose a neoplasm as regenerative change. In almost all cases, neoplasia was correctly diagnosed in the biopsy specimen with the result that, on the basis of the endoscopic findings, the diagnosis would almost always lead to the correct consequence of endoscopic, and not surgical, therapy.

As a subscriber to *Stomach and Intestine* and as a frequent guest in Japan, I learned a great deal from my Japanese colleagues, and early on abandoned the dogma—still upheld by many in the West—that stresses the need to detect isolated invasive tumor cells to establish the diagnosis of invasive carcinoma. I was particularly helped in this respect by the work of Takahashi and Iwama [19–21]. In their three-dimensional reconstructions of the microstructures of well-differentiated tubular adenocarcinomas of the stomach, these authors demonstrated that the carcinomatous tubuli invasively penetrated the lamina propria of the mucosa and anastomosed with the neighboring tubuli to form a network of neoplastic tubuli. The discovery of such a network shows that invasive growth through the lamina propria is present. When these tubuli then infiltrate the muscularis propria and the upper part of the submucosa—without separated tumor cells and with intact basement membrane—Western pathologists also diagnose invasive carcinoma, as in the case of lymph node metastases in well-differentiated adenocarcinomas located elsewhere.

This concept of invasion was also convincingly represented by Borchard [22]: while superficial lateral expansion, luminal extension, and a vertical intratubular extension dominate in adenomas, well-differentiated tubular adenocarcinoma limited to the mucosa has a quite different growth pattern. This "growth pattern of invasion" is characterized by primarily lateral intertubular expansion which is located not in the surface but in the middle part of the mucosa. These abnormally branched carcinomatous glands, without tumor cell dissociation or penetration of atypical epithelial cells through the basement membrane, may lead to secondary changes such as compression and pressure atrophy of neighboring glands, and erosion.

The fact that five of the Western pathologists established their diagnoses in the same manner as their Japanese colleagues shows that this "Japanese viewpoint" has increasingly gained ground outside of Japan too. May the cases discussed in this book help this concept to achieve further international acceptance.

References

1. Schlemper RJ, Itabashi M, Kato Y, et al (1997) Differences and diagnostic criteria for gastric carcinoma between Japanese and Western pathologists. Lancet 349:1725–1729
2. Lauwers GY, Shimizu M, Correa P, et al (1999) Evaluation of gastric biopsies for neoplasia: differences between Japanese and Western pathologists. Am J Surg Pathol 23:511–518
3. Rugge M, Correa P, Dixon MF, et al (2000) Gastric dysplasia: the Padova international classification. Am J Surg Pathol 24:167–176
4. Schlemper J, Borchard F, Dixon MF, et al (2000) International comparability of the pathological diagnosis for early cancer for the digestive tract: Munich meeting. J Gastroenterol 35(suppl 12):102–110
5. Sakamoto J, Yasue M (1997) Do Japanese statistics on gastric carcinoma need to be revised? Lancet 349:1711–1712
6. Anonymous (1997) Magenkarzinom-Früherkennung: Japanische Märchen? Münch Med Wochenschr 139:21
7. Schlemper RJ, Riddell RH, Kato Y, et al (2000) The Vienna classification of gastrointestinal epithelial neoplasia. Gut 47:251–255
8. Stolte M (1999) Diagnosis of gastric carcinoma: Japanese fairy tales of Western deficiency? Virch Arch 334:279–280
9. DiGregorio C, Morandi P, Fante R, et al (1993) Gastric dysplasia. A follow-up study. Am J Gastroenterol 88: 1714–1719
10. Fertitta AM, Comin U, Terruzzi V, et al (1993) Clinical significance of gastric dysplasia. A multicenter follow-up study. Endoscopy 25:265–268
11. Kokkola A, Haapiainen R, Laxen F, et al (1996) Risk of gastric carcinoma in patients with mucosal dysplasia associated with atrophic gastritis: a follow up study. J Clin Pathol 49:979–984
12. Lansdown M, Quirke P, Dixon MF, et al (1990) High grade dysplasia of the gastric mucosa: a marker for gastric carcinoma. Gut 31:977–983
13. Rugge M, Farinati F, Baffa R, et al (1994) Gastric epithelial dysplasia in the natural history of gastric cancer: a multicenter prospective follow-up study. Gastroenterology 107:1288–1296
14. Rugge M, Farinati F, Di Mario F, et al (1991) Gastric epithelial dysplasia: a prospective multicenter follow-up study from the interdisciplinary group on gastric epithelial dysplasia. Hum Pathol 22:1002–1008
15. Saraga EP, Gardiol D, Costa J (1987) Gastric dysplasia: a histological follow-up study. Am J Surg Pathol 11:788–796
16. DeDombal FT, Price AB, Thompson H, et al (1990) The British Society of Gastroenterology early gastric cancer/dysplasia survey: an interim report. Gut 31:115–120
17. Ida K, Okuda J, Katoh T, et al (1996) Recent advances and problems in the endoscopic treatment of early gastric cancer. Dig Endosc 8:46–52
18. Stolte M (2003) The new Vienna classification of epithelial neoplasia of the gastrointestinal tract: advantages and disadvantages. Virchows Arch 442:99–106
19. Takahashi T, Iwama N (1984) Architectural pattern of gastric adenocarcinoma—a 3-dimensional study. Virchows Arch 403:127–134
20. Takahashi T, Iwama N (1984) Atypical glands in gastric adenoma. Three-dimensional architecture compared with carcinomatous and metaplastic glands. Virchows Arch (Pathol Anat) 403:135–148
21. Takahashi T, Iwama N (1985) Three-dimensional microstructure of gastrointestinal tumors. Gland pattern and its diagnostic significance. Path Annu part I: 419–440
22. Borchard F (2000) Formen und Nomenklatur der gastrointestinalen Epithelexpansion: Was ist Invasion? Verh Dtsch Ges Path 84:50–61

II. Vienna Consensus Criteria for Pathological Diagnosis

1. Vienna Consensus Criteria for Pathological Diagnosis

Jeremy R. Jass

1. Introduction

It is generally assumed that the distinction between cancer and noncancer is relatively straightforward and not subject to wide interobserver disagreement. A number of workshops involving the assessment of gastrointestinal lesions by Japanese and Western pathologists have highlighted major discrepancies [1–4]. In general, Japanese pathologists have a lower threshold for the diagnosis of malignancy than Western pathologists. In view of the poor levels of diagnostic agreement, international dialogue and collaboration is impeded, and progress in both clinical and basic research suffers accordingly. The Vienna classification (Table 1) was developed in order to remedy this situation [5]. When the proposed terminology is adopted by Japanese and Western pathologists, the reporting differences are reduced but not eliminated.

2. Basis for Discrepancies

Analysis of discrete criteria used by pathologists in the evaluation of gastrointestinal neoplasms underscores the basis for the discrepancies between Japan and the West [1]. In Japan, emphasis is placed upon cytological features of malignancy, particularly nuclear enlargement, hyperchromatism, pleomorphism, and nucleolar prominence, and architectural features such as complex budding or branching of glands. In the West, emphasis is placed on the demonstration of invasion into the underlying stroma. While these contrasting approaches go some way towards explaining the discrepancies, other less tangible factors are also of importance. These center on definitions of dysplasia, neoplasia, carcinoma-in-situ, invasion, and intramucosal carcinoma, and different attitudes towards clinical utility versus descriptive precision in histopathological reporting.

2.1 Dysplasia, Neoplasia, and Carcinoma-In-Situ

The term "dysplasia" is employed more widely in the West than in Japan [4]. In the West, dysplasia (as applied to the interpretation of gastrointestinal biopsies) is synonymous with intraepithelial neoplasia. Like intraepithelial neoplasia, dysplasia may be graded. Low-grade dysplasia differs slightly from the normal counterpart whereas high-grade dysplasia approximates to carcinoma-in-situ. Other approaches to grading are discussed below. The term "neoplasia" implies autonomous growth and clonal alterations of cancer genes. Malignant potential is not implicit (some neoplasms such as lipomas lack malignant potential) but all gastrointestinal neoplasms are regarded as having increased malignant potential. Within the gastrointestinal tract, neoplasia may present as discrete, protuberant, and well-circumscribed polyps or as superficial elevated, flat, shallow-depressed, and ill-defined lesions. The term "dysplasia," as employed in the West, generally relates to the flat, shallow-depressed, and ill-defined forms of intraepithelial neoplasia. In practice there is no sharp cutoff between polypoid and nonpolypoid dysplasia. For example, adenomas may be flat or depressed whereas dysplasia associated with inflammatory bowel disease may be superficial-elevated or polypoid. In addition, it has been usual in the West to stratify adenomas on the basis of the grade of dysplasia: mild, moderate, and severe, or low- and high-grade. By definition, all adenomas show some degree of dysplasia.

With the exception of the esophagus, many Japanese pathologists have little or no use for the term "dysplasia." Lesions diagnosed as dysplasia in the West may be accommodated by three alternatives in Japan: reactive change, adenoma, or carcinoma. If one looks critically at diagnostic practices in the West, one can certainly sympathize with the Japanese approach. Low-grade dysplasia is problematical in that it is overdiagnosed and subject to considerable interobserver disagreement [6]. Follow-up studies of subjects developing low-grade dysplasia in a background of Barrett's esophagus, chronic gastritis, or ulcerative colitis, and in the absence of an endoscopically visible lesion, show little evidence for malignant progression [7,8]. On the other hand, the diagnosis of high-grade dysplasia frequently implies the presence of an underlying malignancy [9,10].

When a Japanese pathologist diagnoses cancer in a biopsy that would be interpreted as high-grade dysplasia in the West, this is not because the Japanese pathologist has learned that an underlying cancer cannot be

Table 1. Vienna classification of gastrointestinal epithelial neoplasia

Category	Definition
1	Negative for neoplasia/dysplasia
2	Indefinite for neoplasia/dysplasia
3	Noninvasive low-grade neoplasia (low-grade adenoma/ dysplasia)
4	Noninvasive high-grade neoplasia
	4.1 High-grade adenoma/dysplasia
	4.2 Noninvasive carcinoma (carcinoma-in-situ)[a]
	4.3 Suspicion of invasive carcinoma
5	Invasive neoplasia
	5.1 Intramucosal carcinoma[b]
	5.2 Submucosal carcinoma or beyond

[a] Noninvasive indicates absence of evident invasion
[b] Intramucosal indicates invasion into the lamina propria or muscularis mucosae

excluded. Rather, it is a decision based upon cytological and architectural criteria and the premise that cancer must be present within an epithelial layer prior to the onset of invasion. It so happens, however, that when the premise is put to the test Japanese pathologists often turn out to be correct [1–3], i.e., the diagnosis of cancer in a biopsy (interpreted as benign by Western pathologists) is often vindicated when the entire lesion is subsequently resected.

Although dysplasia is frequently overdiagnosed on the one hand and may turn out to be the mucosal component of an invasive carcinoma on the other, lesions do exist that are flat or depressed, neoplastic, noninvasive, and cannot be accommodated by the term "adenoma." These are observed against a background of chronic inflammation in the columnar-lined (Barrett's) esophagus, stomach, and colon (Fig. 1A–D). The latest edition of the World Health Organization classification has recommended that the term "dysplasia" be replaced by "intraepithelial neoplasia" but recognizes the existence of diffuse, non-invasive neoplasia separate from adenoma [11].

2.2 Invasion and Intramucosal Carcinoma

In the West, the presence or absence of invasion has been used as the main discriminant between cancer and noncancer. Superficially this provides an objective and pragmatic approach to the reporting of gastrointestinal neoplasia. An epithelial lesion is either confined to the tissue of origin (intraepithelial) in which case there is no possibility of distant spread, or early invasion has occurred with an associated risk of distant spread. However, the practicalities are not quite so straightforward. In most epithelial surfaces, invasion implies traversion of the basement membrane into the underlying connective tissue stroma. In well-differentiated glandular neoplasia, invasive elements may synthesize a basement membrane and it may be difficult to distinguish between preinvasive and early invasive mucosal neoplasia. The diagnosis is easier in the case of poorly differentiated mucosal carcinoma when cells are grouped into small, irregular clusters or totally discohesive as in the case of signet-ring cell carcinoma. However, many mucosal neoplasms are not poorly differentiated.

In the West, a particular rule has been developed for colorectal but not esophageal or gastric neoplasia. According to this rule, cancer cannot be diagnosed without the demonstration of invasion across the muscularis mucosae into the submucosa. The basis of this rule is that lymphatic spread does not precede invasion across the muscularis mucosae. Concern that surgeons may proceed to radical colorectal surgery upon receiving a report with the diagnosis "carcinoma-in-situ" resulted in preferential use of the terms "high-grade" or "severe dysplasia" for neoplastic lesions lacking evidence of submucosal invasion. Nevertheless, there are instances in which it is difficult to sustain this rule. An example is the finding of intramucosal poorly differentiated or signet-ring cell carcinoma. This is uncommon in the large bowel, but may occasionally be observed in malignant adenomas and with greater frequency in mucosal neoplasia complicating chronic inflammatory bowel disease.

The Western rule for colorectal neoplasia has been a source of inconsistency with respect to the TNM (tumor/node/metastasis) classification. In esophagus, stomach, and small intestine, intramucosal and submucosal carcinoma are T1 lesions [11]. In the colon, intramucosal neoplasia is grouped with Tis lesions. The fact that the TNM system recognizes carcinoma-in-situ under pTis is problematical as many Western pathologists avoid the term. A recent report prepared by the American Joint Committee on Cancer has recommended that colorectal mucosal carcinoma (currently pTis) be stratified as pTie (intraepithelial) and pTim (intramucosal) [12]. This consolidates the official recognition of mucosal colorectal carcinoma in the West, but three problems remain unresolved. These are the diagnostic distinction between high-grade dysplasia and cancer, arbitrary decisions regarding cancer registrations, and the persistence of differing rules for staging neoplasia in different regions of the gastrointestinal tract.

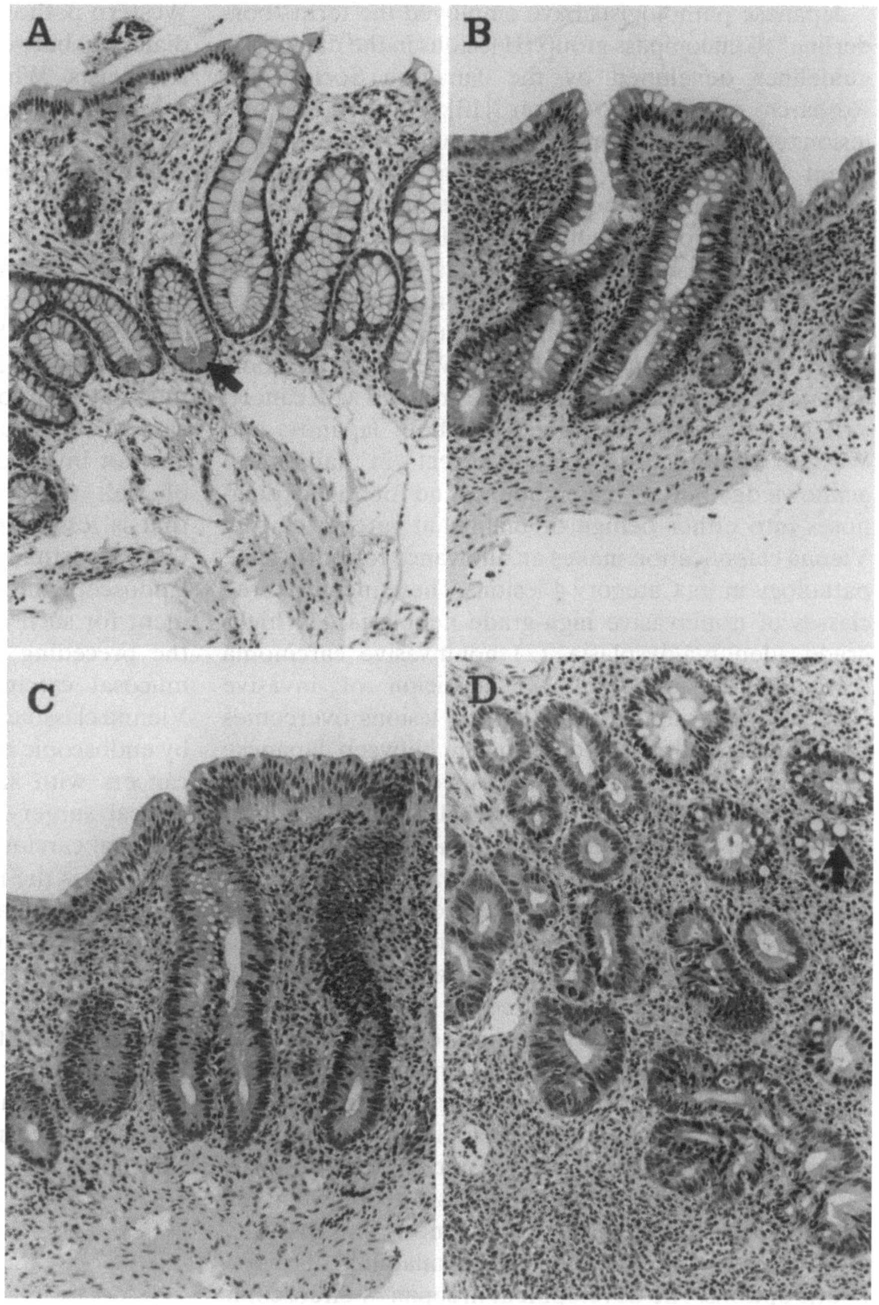

Fig. 1A–D. Illustration of the concept of intraepithelial neoplasia (dysplasia) as distinct from regenerative or reactive change, adenoma, or carcinoma. The material is derived from a colonoscopic series obtained from a subject under surveillance for long-standing ulcerative colitis. **A** Changes of chronic ulcerative colitis with no intraepithelial neoplasia. There is slight crypt irregularity, branching, and Paneth cell metaplasia (*arrow*). **B** Low-grade changes evidenced by nuclear enlargement and palisading, and some loss of goblet cell differentiation. **C** More marked nuclear enlargement and focal loss of nuclear polarity. Pseudostratification of nuclei is conspicuous in the surface epithelium. There is little active inflammation to account for the changes. The changes are borderline between low and high grade. **D** High-grade intraepithelial neoplasia with marked nuclear enlargement, pleomorphism, and loss of polarity. Crypts show irregular branching and budding. Dystrophic or upside-down goblet cells are conspicuous (*arrow*) (Hematoxylin–eosin, ×20)

3. Which Approach is Correct—East or West?

The preceding account demonstrates the reality of a "gray zone" or "borderline" between noncancer and cancer in the gastrointestinal tract. In the West, the concept of borderline lesions is not especially developed in the gastrointestinal tract. An uncertain or indefinite category has been introduced to cover the gray area between reactive change and dysplasia in inflammatory bowel disease, but the term "borderline lesion" is generally understood to span cancer and noncancer. It relates to lesions recognized as neoplastic but of uncertain or limited malignant potential. The Western pathologist dichotomizes gastrointestinal neoplasia into benign or malignant. In the absence of unequivocal invasion, borderline lesions are likely to be classified as benign (dysplasia or adenoma).

Japanese pathologists have employed the term "borderline" to encompass group III lesions in the diagnostic guidelines developed by the Japanese Society for Research on Gastric Cancer [13]. Most borderline lesions equate to adenomas. Gastric adenomas are infrequent lesions in the West. Currently, few Japanese pathologists employ the term "borderline lesion" when reporting gastrointestinal biopsies. Like their Western counterparts, Japanese pathologists split neoplasms into benign (adenoma) versus malignant. Nevertheless, borderline lesions exist and account for the large discrepancy between Japan and the West. In Japan, borderline lesions are more likely to be grouped with cancer.

It may therefore be argued that both Japanese and Western pathologists are incorrect in failing to acknowledge borderline pathology and forcing all diagnoses into either benign or malignant categories. The Vienna classification makes an allowance for borderline pathology in its Category 4 lesions. These include three classes of noninvasive high-grade neoplasia: (1) high-grade adenoma/dysplasia, (2) noninvasive carcinoma (carcinoma-in-situ), and (3) suspicion of invasive cancer. This grouping of borderline lesions overcomes some but not all of the discrepancy between Japanese and Western pathologists with respect to the diagnosis of esophageal, gastric, and colorectal neoplasia.

There are several reasons for attaching a diagnostic label to a tissue sample. The label may influence immediate management, determine prognosis, impact on lifestyle choices by the patient, become a statistic in epidemiological research, or serve as a gold standard in biomedical research. The diagnostic label may need to be modified or qualified according to its intended use. A Japanese diagnosis could be more scientifically correct for the purposes of biomedical research. That is, the label of cancer may be biologically correct. The same diagnostic label could result in unnecessarily radical surgical treatment of a mucosal neoplasm in the West. In fact, the link between diagnosis and management may be influenced by the availability of therapeutic options. The development in Japan of endoscopic mucosal resection has generated a paradoxical situation in which a more aggressive diagnosis (mucosal carcinoma) is followed by conservative surgery when a similar lesion that is diagnosed as high-grade dysplasia in the West may be treated by radical resection.

4. Utility of the Vienna Classification

The Vienna classification was developed to reduce the major diagnostic discrepancy between Japanese and Western pathologists and thereby facilitate meaningful dialogue between pathologists, clinicians, and epidemiologists. While the Vienna classification partially achieves this goal, the five categories do not permit a direct matching with current therapeutic options [14]. Endoscopic mucosal resection is a preferred treatment for small mucosal neoplasms irrespective of the presence or absence of invasion of the lamina propria. The risk of lymph node metastasis for intramucosal carcinoma of esophagus, stomach, and colorectum is 2%–3%, 2%–4%, and 0%, respectively [14]. The risk rises to 37%–52%, 14%–22%, and 3%–18% for submucosal invasion in these respective sites [14]. In the case of intramucosal carcinoma of the esophagus that has not invaded the muscularis mucosae and the case of well to moderately differentiated gastric cancer that is less than 2 cm in diameter and non-ulcerated, there is virtually no risk of lymph node metastasis [14]. Endoscopic mucosal resection is therefore a safe treatment for such early malignant lesions. On the basis of the preceding argument, it is logical to group intramucosal carcinoma with category 4 lesions in the Vienna classification as a category warranting treatment by endoscopic mucosal resection [14]. Most (but not all) cancers with submucosal invasion will require more radical surgery. A second reason for grouping intramucosal carcinoma in the "borderline" Vienna group 4 category is the fact that the histopathological diagnosis of mucosal invasion is highly subjective and prone to interobserver variation. Diagnostic discrepancies would be further reduced if this recommendation were accepted. A third reason would be to eliminate the site differences that currently exist in the TNM system. Specifically, intramucosal esophageal, gastric, and small intestinal carcinoma could then be moved from T1 into Tis, as is the current practice for colorectal intramucosal carcinoma.

5. Limitations of the Vienna Classification

The Vienna classification and its modification discussed above is no more than a method for encoding diagnoses in a way that helps to eliminate differences in reporting practices between Japan and the West. Despite going some way towards achieving this important aim, the Vienna classification does not replace the more traditional forms of diagnosis. While the logic of the approach cannot be denied, a diagnostic group that includes high-grade adenoma, high-grade dysplasia, non-invasive carcinoma, and (in the case of the modified system) intramucosal carcinoma is clearly highly heterogeneous. Apart from providing no distinction between dysplasia (intraepithelial neoplasia) complicating inflammatory bowel disease and adenoma, the Vienna classification does not classify adenomas into tubular, tubulovillous, villous, or serrated. Nor does it recognize subtypes of dysplasia such as intestinalized or nonintestinalized in the case of gastric dysplasia [15]. These points are not faults or deficiences of the Vienna classification but merely reinforce the fact that this classification adds to, rather than substitutes for, existing systems. To meet the deficiencies of the Vienna classification, more detailed and site-specific classifications have been proposed. An example is the Padova classification for gastric dysplasia [16].

Even if intramucosal carcinoma were moved to the group 4 category of the Vienna classification, some discrepancies between East and West would persist. The main explanation for this is the subjectivity of grading adenoma or dysplasia. The level of disagreement is reduced by the use of two grades (low and high) as opposed to three (mild, moderate, and severe), but is not eliminated.

As stated above, grading attempts to define the position of a benign neoplastic process between the extremes of normal (or non-neoplastic alterations) and cancer. However, grading is used in an altogether different way, i.e., to stratify cancers into those with low versus high aggressiveness. For example, an invasive neoplasm showing minimal cytological atypia and architectural complexity with a high degree of cellular differentiation would be classified as a low-grade cancer. The lesion must have existed as a noninvasive neoplasm, yet immediately prior to the onset of invasion it would have been characterized by the same low-grade features as the invasive counterpart. In other words, when the two types of grading are not distinguished, one can have a situation in which a low-grade benign neoplasm can become a cancer without becoming high-grade. This explains why the same lesion can be diagnosed as low-grade adenoma in the West and (non-invasive) carcinoma in Japan.

Examples of cytologically bland colorectal cancers include mucinous, serrated, and DNA microsatellite unstable cancers. These may arise from cytologically bland precursors such as villous and serrated adenomas [17]. Different types of grading system will be required to cope with different pathways of tumorigenesis. Benign neoplasms that are currently diagnosed as low-grade yet carry a high malignant potential may in the future be graded as high-grade on the basis of different (perhaps molecular) features [18].

6. Conclusion

The Vienna classification was developed with the aim of reducing discrepancies between Western and Japanese pathologists reporting on gastrointestinal neoplasia. It should be regarded as supplementary to, rather than replacing, more detailed and site-specific classifications of gastrointestinal neoplasia. The system works by grouping "borderline" lesions into category 4. Despite this, interobserver differences between and within Western and Japanese pathologists continue to be a problem. The persisting problems center on the recognition and diagnosis of intramucosal carcinoma and the distinction between low-grade versus high-grade intraepithelial neoplasia (dysplasia). The first problem can be solved very simply by including intramucosal carcinoma with category 4 lesions. There is no reason for not doing this. The second problem cannot be resolved so easily and requires a greater understanding of the relationships between morphology, molecular biology, and behavior.

References

1. Schlemper RJ, Itabashi M, Kato Y, et al (1997) Differences in diagnostic criteria for gastric carcinoma between Japanese and Western pathologists. Lancet 349: 1725–1729
2. Schlemper RJ, Itabashi M, Kato Y, et al (1998) Differences in the diagnostic criteria used by Japanese and Western pathologists to diagnose colorectal carcinoma. Cancer 82:60–69
3. Schlemper RJ, Dawsey SM, Itabashi M, et al (2000) Differences in diagnostic criteria for esophageal squamous cell carcinoma between Japanese and Western pathologists. Cancer 88:996–1006
4. Lauwers GY, Shimizu M, Correa P, et al (1999) Evaluation of gastric biopsies for neoplasia: differences between Japanese and Western pathologists. Am J Surg Pathol 23:511–518
5. Schlemper RJ, Riddell RH, Kato Y, et al (2000) The Vienna classification of gastrointestinal epithelial neoplasia. Gut 47:251–255
6. Eaden J, Abrams K, McKay H, et al (2001) Inter-observer variation between general and specialist gastrointestinal pathologists when grading dysplasia in ulcerative colitis. J Pathol 194:152–157
7. Rugge M, Farinati F, Baffa R, et al (1994) Gastric epithelial dysplasia in the natural history of gastric cancer: a multicenter prospective follow-up study. Interdisciplinary Group on Gastric Epithelial Dysplasia. Gastroenterology 107:1288–1296
8. Saraga EP, Gardiol D, Costa J (1987) Gastric dysplasia. A histological follow-up study. Am J Surg Pathol 11: 788–796

9. Lansdown M, Quirke P, Dixon MF, et al (1990) High grade dysplasia of the gastric mucosa: a marker for gastric carcinoma. Gut 31:977–983
10. Reid BJ, Weinstein WM, Lewin KJ, et al (1988) Endoscopic biopsy can detect high-grade dysplasia or early adenocarcinoma in Barrett's esophagus without grossly recognizable neoplastic lesions. Gastroenterology 94: 81–90
11. Hamilton SR, Aaltonen LA (2000) World Health Organization classification of tumours. Pathology and genetics. IARC Press, Lyon
12. Compton C, Fenoglio-Preiser CM, Pettigrew N, et al (2000) American Joint Committee on Cancer Prognostic Factors Consensus Conference. Cancer 88:1739–1757
13. Japanese Research Society for Gastric Cancer (1995) Japanese Classification of gastric carcinoma. 1st edn. Kanehara, Tokyo
14. Schlemper RJ, Kato Y, Stolte M (2000) Diagnostic criteria for gastrointestinal carcinomas in Japan and Western countries: proposal for a new classification system of gastrointestinal epithelial neoplasia. J Gastroenterol Hepatol 15:G49–G57
15. Ghandur-Mnaymneh L, Paz J, Roldan E, et al (1988) Dysplasia of nonmetaplastic gastric mucosa. A proposal for its classification and its possible relationship to diffuse-type gastric carcinoma. Am J Surg Pathol 12: 96–114
16. Rugge M, Correa P, Dixon MF, et al (2000) Gastric dysplasia: the Padova International Classification. Am J Surg Pathol 24:167–176
17. Mäkinen MJ, George SMC, Jernvall P, et al (2001) Colorectal carcinoma associated with serrated adenoma—prevalence, histological features, and prognosis. J Pathol 193:286–294
18. Jass JR (2001) Serrated route to colorectal cancer: back street or super highway? J Pathol 193:283–285

III. Early Neoplasia in Barrett's Esophagus

1. Early Neoplasia in Barrett's Esophagus

Manfred Stolte, Michael Vieth, Andrea May, Liebwin Gossner, Irina Dostler, and Christian Ell

1. Introduction

Over the last 10–20 years, the incidence of adenocarcinomas in Barrett's esophagus has increased enormously in many Western countries [1–5]. The increase in these countries is greater than that of all other malignant epithelial tumors, so that the term "new epidemic" has even been applied [6].

The aim of gastroenterologists and pathologists must therefore be to diagnose this neoplasia at as early a stage as possible and thus enable curative endoscopic therapy. A review of the older literature up to the middle of the 1990s leaves the impression that we are far from achieving this objective, since these older publications report mostly advanced Barrett's adenocarcinomas, with the 5-year survival rate varying between 7% and 20% [7].

Over the last 5 years, however, as a result of great advances in diagnostic endoscopy there has been a positive change. Ever more frequently, early-stage neoplasia is being detected endoscopically, diagnosed in biopsy material, and treated via the endoscope [8–11]. Ten years ago, we at the Institute of Pathology of the Bayreuth Hospital diagnosed advanced Barrett's carcinomas almost exclusively. The above-mentioned progress in diagnostic endoscopy has resulted in an increase in the percentage of early neoplasias we have diagnosed over the last 5 years to 50%–60%.

2. How Histology Helps to Improve the Endoscopic Diagnosis of Early Neoplasia in Barrett's Esophagus

Formerly it was believed that "dysplasia" of Barrett's mucosa could be diagnosed only histologically, and therefore quadrant biopsies at intervals of 1–2 cm were recommended [12, 13]. "Dysplasia," however, is defined as unequivocal intraepithelial neoplasia [14]. We therefore earlier postulated that, where something "new" is growing, the surface structure of the mucosa must also be altered, and were of the opinion that, with special endoscopic techniques such as chromoendoscopy and magnification videoendoscopy, such neoplasia could be recognized and submitted to targeted biopsy [15].

With regard to the endoscopic diagnosis of early Barrett's carcinomas, we were initially of the opinion that the macroscopic classification of early gastric carcinoma could also be applied to Barrett's esophagus. Our initial evaluation of the macroscopic types of early Barrett's carcinoma in analogy to early gastric carcinoma in 200 endoscopic mucosectomy specimens, however, then showed that the early carcinomas in Barrett's esophagus often present no uniform macroscopic appearance, but, rather, show a mixed pattern (see Table 1). This is due in particular to the fact that the early carcinoma often does not grow focally, but in a circular fashion over a larger area (see Fig. 1).

On the basis of the macroscopic and histological findings, the following endoscopic presentations can be con-

Table 1. Macroscopic classification of early Barrett's carcinomas in 200 patients, in analogy to the classification of early gastric carcinomas

Barrett's neoplasia	
Type I	11.5%
Type IIa	28.3%
Type IIb	17.7%
Type IIc	3.8%
Type III	1.7%
Mixed type	37.0%

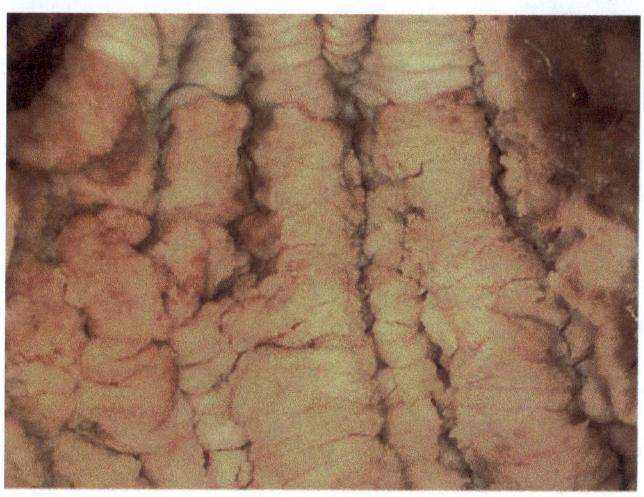

Fig. 1. Operative specimen with a circular growing early mucosal Barrett's adenocarcinoma with irregular surface

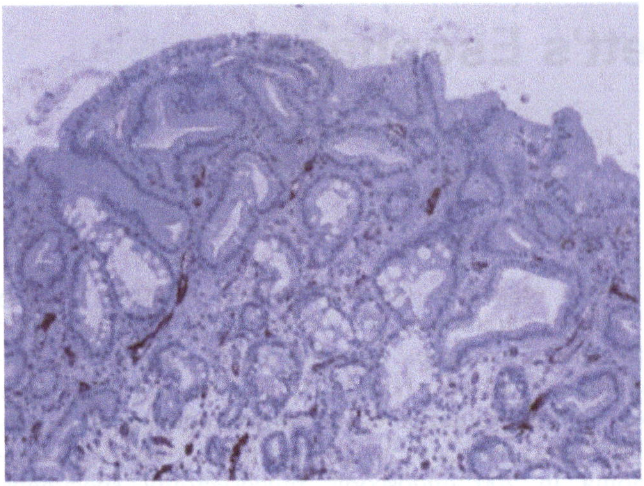

Fig. 2. Normal vascularization of Barrett's mucosa without neoplasia (immunohistochemical marking of the endothelial cells of the capillaries with CD 34 antibody)

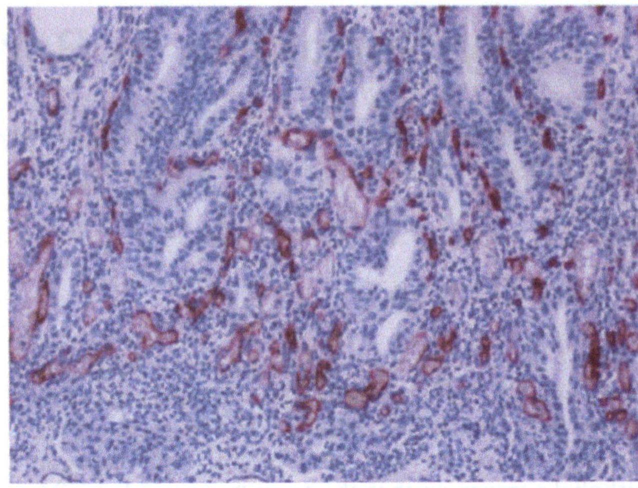

Fig. 3. Increased vascularization of Barrett's mucosa with high-grade intraepithelial neoplasia (immunohistochemistry with CD 34 antibody)

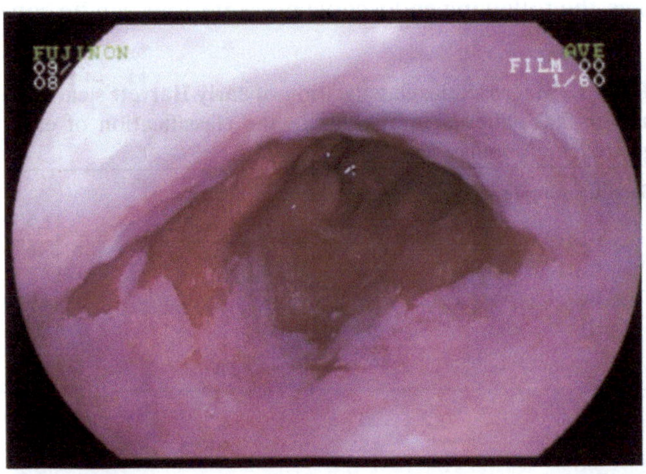

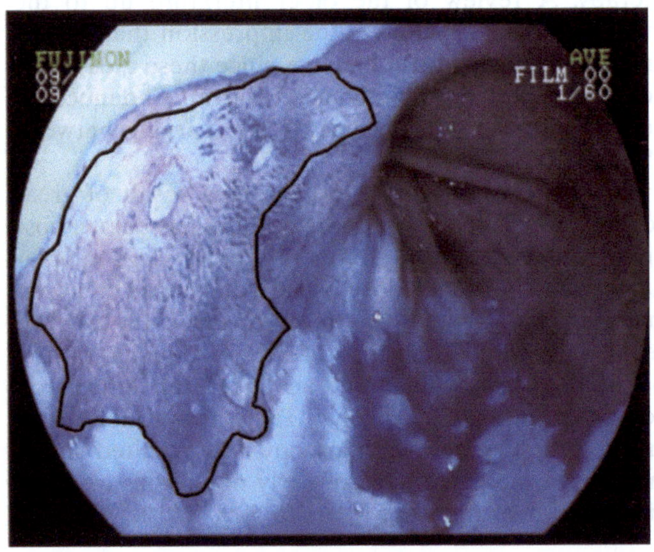

Figs. 4 and 5. Focal adenocarcinoma in a short Barrett's esophagus prior and after methylene blue staining

sidered suspicious for neoplasia and are detectable with the various endoscopic techniques indicated:

1. As a result of the "new growth," the following changes in the surface structure of Barrett's mucosa may occur:
—irregular verrucous or papillary areas, and
—elevations or broad-based polyps.
Such alterations must therefore be detectable with high-resolution video-endoscopy and magnification videoendoscopy.

2. Invasive neoplasia is also characterized by infiltrative and destructive growth. Erosions and ulcers in Barrett's mucosa must be considered as suspicious findings that require targeted biopsy.

3. Neoplasia also leads to the replacement of the goblet cells, which can be visualized with negative methylene blue chromoendoscopy.

4. Neoplasia in Barrett's esophagus induces an increase in angiogenesis (see Figs. 2 and 3), so that during videoendoscopy, a search should also be for foci of increased redness in the salmon-colored Barrett's mucosa.

5. Early carcinomas in Barrett's mucosa reveal considerable disruption of the architecture of the neoplastic tubules (irregular budding and branching). This

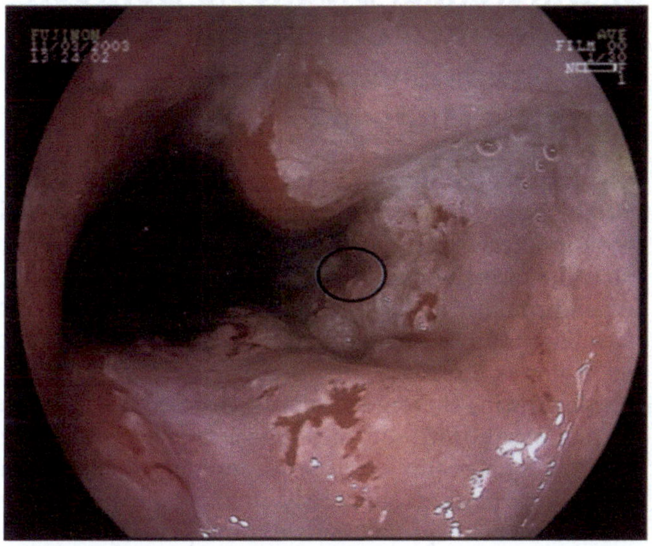

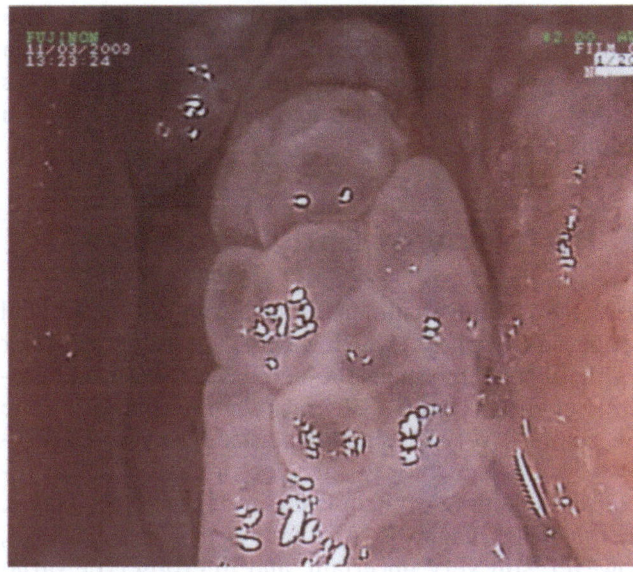

Figs. 6 and 7. High-grade intraepithelial neoplasia in the short Barrett's esophagus: overview and after magnification endoscopy in combination with acetic acid 1.5%

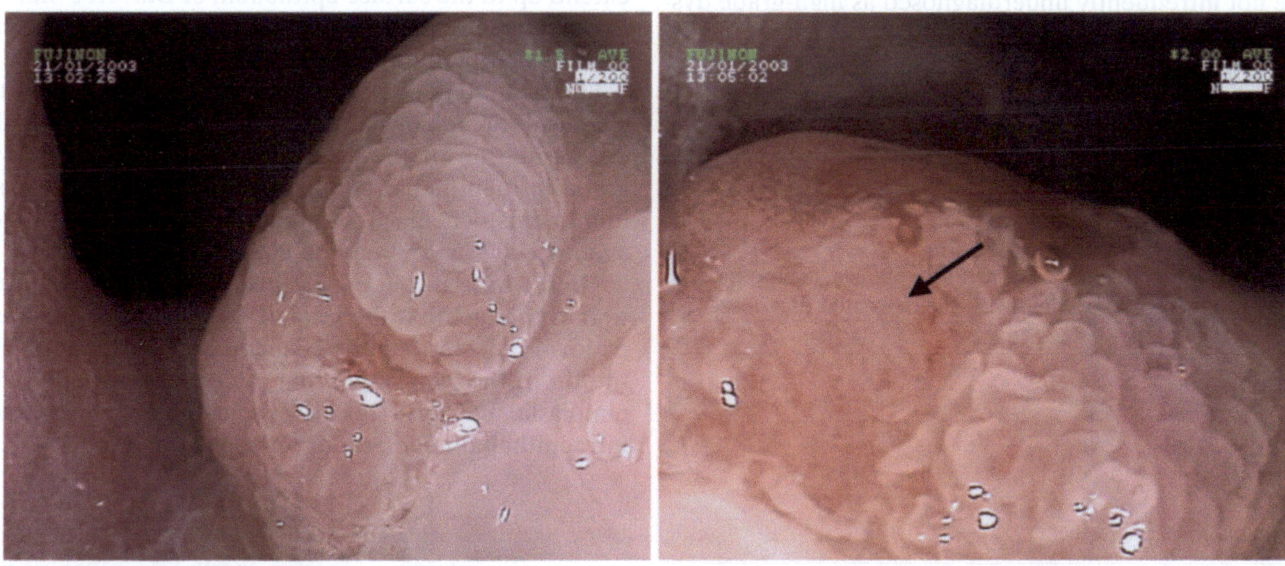

A B

Fig. 8A,B. Early Barrett's adenocarcinoma type IIa after magnification endoscopy with acetic acid 1.5%

histological finding may in future be a "diagnostic search criterion" for new imaging methods such as optical coherence tomography [16, 17] and intravital endoscopic microscopy [18, 19].

6. In addition, early carcinomas are characterized by invasive growth. The best means of detecting this invasive growth and its extent (depth of infiltration) is endosonography carried out with 20 MHz miniprobes [20].

3. Endoscopic Findings in Early Neoplasia in Barrett's Mucosa

According to the above-described morphological patterns discrete changes in color, structure, and mucosal architecture within the Barrett's segment have to be visualized during endoscopy. Small nodules, increased redness, or irregular cobblestone-like pattern are typical for neoplasia in Barrett's. A distorted mucosal pattern or small erosive alterations of the mucosa are also signs for malignant degeneration. High-resolution endoscopy in combination with vital stains such as methylene blue and acetic acid help to delineate such lesions (Figs. 4–8).

4. Histology of Early Neoplasia

Barrett's adenocarcinoma arises from intraepithelial neoplasia (dysplasia) which is classified as low grade or high grade. In this stage, the neoplasia cannot metastasize, but early Barrett's adenocarcinomas limited to the mucosa also very rarely metastasize. The aim of diagnostic endoscopy/biopsy, therefore, must be the histological detection of neoplasia in these early stages. Histological diagnosis of these early neoplasia is, however, still very uncertain, and interobserver variation relatively poor [21–25]. This is also confirmed by the evaluation of our consultational diagnostic work done in 2001 [26]: regenerative changes are frequently overdiagnosed as low-grade dysplasia, and carcinomas are not infrequently underdiagnosed as high-grade dysplasia (see Table 2).

Furthermore, the extremely variable reported prevalence of low-grade dysplasia in numerous publications (see Table 3) indicates that regenerative changes in Barrett's mucosa are obviously overdiagnosed as low-grade dysplasia the world over [27–33].

Table 2. Comparison of Barrett's neoplasia diagnoses submitted for a second opinion with the corrected diagnoses [26]

	Barrett	LGIEN	HGIEN	Ca
LGIEN (n = 89)	75.0%	7.5%	5.0%	12.5%
HGIEN (n = 122)	29.5%	0.8%	13.1%	56.6%
Ca (n = 67)	13.4%	—	—	86.6%

LGIEN, low-grade intraepithelial neoplasia; HGIEN, high-grade intraepithelial neoplasia; Ca, Barrett's adenocarcinoma

Table 3. Differences in the incidence of the diagnosis of a low-grade intraepithelial neoplasia (LGIEN) in published studies

First author [Ref.]	Year	LGIEN
Schnell [27]	2002	67.2%
Sharma [28]	2003	25.0%
Egger [29]	2003	20.2%
O'Connor [30]	1999	17.6%
Fisher [31]	2003	13.5%
Gopal [32]	2003	9.7%
Conio [33]	2003	9.6%
Own material	2003	2.2%

5. Differential Diagnosis Between Regenerative Changes and Low-Grade Dysplasia in Barrett's Mucosa

This differential diagnosis is apparently the most uncertain borderline area in the histological diagnostic workup of Barrett's mucosa. In many cases, back-to-back glands located at the base of Barrett's mucosa with hyperchromatic nuclei and increased mitotic figures are overdiagnosed as low-grade dysplasia (Fig. 9). Back-to-back glands, however, are merely a result of the p-division during the regenerative process [34]. The nuclei in the basal third of the regenerative glands have compact chromatin without prominent nucleoli, the epithelium matures steplessly in the apical direction, and the surface epithelium is normal [35–37].

In low-grade intraepithelial neoplasia (dysplasia) the architecture of Barrett's mucosa with parallel arrangement of glands is largely normal. The neoplastic epithelial cells with basally located, often peg-like nuclei extend up to the surface epithelium of Barrett's mucosa and reveal an abrupt transition to the neighboring Barrett's epithelium (Fig. 10).

Unfortunately, we have no reliable immunohistochemical or molecular-pathological markers for the differentiation of the regenerative changes from low-grade intraepithelial neoplasia. In the individual case, immunohistochemical examinations with an antibody against Ki67 or p53 may be useful [38–40].

On the basis of our experience, we would draw attention to the fact that the reliable biopsy-based diagnosis of low-grade intraepithelial neoplasia may merely be the tip of the iceberg, so that low-grade intraepithelial neoplasia may also be an extension of a high-grade intraepithelial neoplasia or an adenocarcinoma.

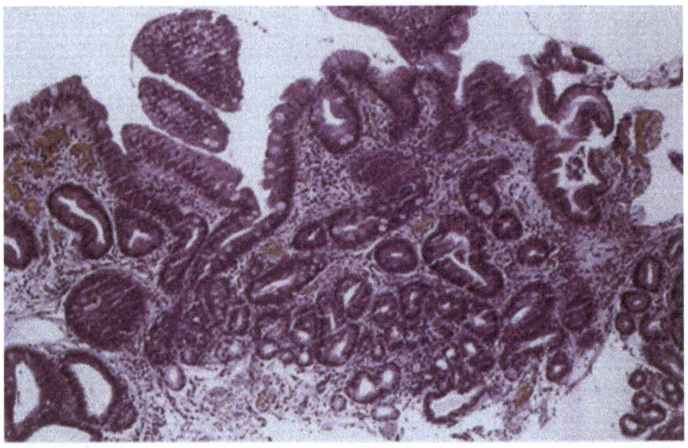

Fig. 9. Regenerative changes in Barrett's mucosa, often overdiagnosed as "low-grade dysplasia"

6. Differential Diagnosis Between Low-Grade and High-Grade Intraepithelial Neoplasia of Barrett's Mucosa

In the case of high-grade intraepithelial neoplasia, too, the normal architecture of Barrett's mucosa is relatively well preserved. As in low-grade intraepithelial neoplasia, the epithelium of Barrett's glands has been replaced by neoplastic epithelium. In comparison with the epithelium of low-grade intraepithelial neoplasia, however, neoplastic epithelium in high-grade dysplasia reveals all the cytological criteria of malignancy. The nuclei show an irregular arrangement (loss of polarity, more marked polymorphism and hyperchromatism with irregularly structured chromatin, with prominent nucleoli and increased pathological mitotic figures [Figs. 11 and 12]).

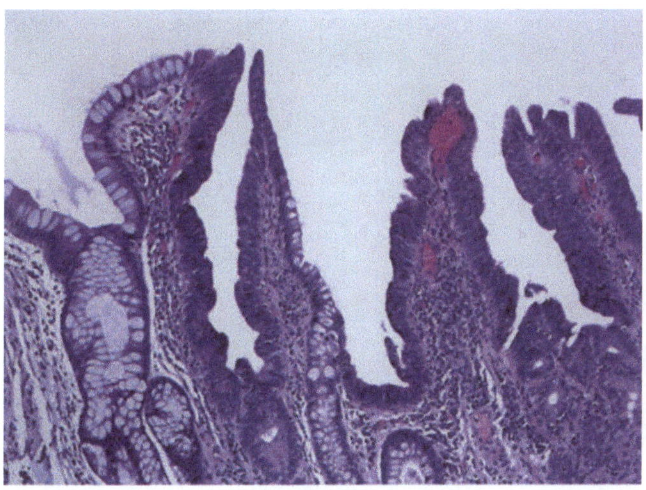

Fig. 10. Low-grade intraepithelial neoplasia ("dysplasia") with extension up to the surface of Barrett's mucosa and abrupt transition to the neighboring epithelium

7. Differential Diagnosis Between High-Grade Intraepithelial Neoplasia and Adenocarcinoma in Barrett's Mucosa

As in the case of high-grade intraepithelial neoplasia, all the above-mentioned cytological criteria of malignancy are also found in well-differentiated Barrett's adenocarcinoma. In addition, invasive growth of the neoplastic tubuli is to be seen. This architectural disruption is interpreted by many American pathologists to be a "partial substrate" of high-grade intraepithelial neoplasia, and not invasive intramucosal carcinoma [41–43]. These pathologists diagnose carcinoma only when there is disruption of the neoplastic glands with single tumor cells within the lamina propria and solid invasive trabecular tumor pegs are found. In our own experience, however, these criteria are to be seen only in moderately or poorly differentiated adenocarcinomas, but not in well-differentiated adenocarcinoma. We are of the opinion that—in analogy to well-differentiated early gastric carcinoma [44–46]—transversally arranged interconnected neoplastic tubuli must be interpreted as invasive growth through the lamina propria. Militating in favor of this interpretation is the fact that these well-differentiated tubular Barrett's adenocarcinomas often fail to show any tumor

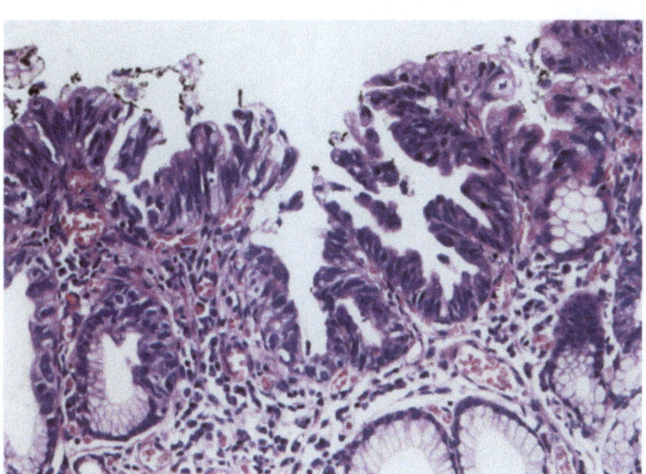

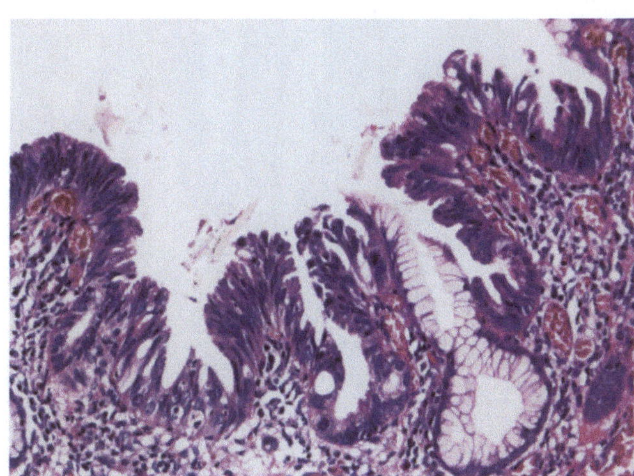

Figs. 11 and 12. High-grade intraepithelial neoplasia of Barrett's mucosa

cell dissociation, even in the invasive front in the newly formed muscularis mucosae, the original lamina propria of the esophageal mucosa, the original muscularis mucosae, and the submucosa, but are here characterized by invasive neoplastic tubuli (Figs. 13 and 14). When confronted by such findings in the endoscopic mucosectomy specimens or surgical specimens, most Western pathologists also diagnose adenocarcinoma—as in the case of well-differentiated tubular adenocarcinoma in the stomach or colorectum. This is also shown by a comparison of the diagnosis of high-grade intraepithelial neoplasia in biopsy material with the definitive diagnosis in the surgical specimen: in 40%–70% of the cases [47, 48], a carcinoma is diagnosed in the surgical specimen, in some cases with evidence of advanced carcinoma [49, 50]. This is not at all surprising, since our experience shows that well-differentiated Barrett's carcinomas often mimic high-grade intraepithelial neoplasia at the surface, while invasive carcinoma is unequivocally diagnosed in the base (Figs. 15 and 16).

For this "borderline area," again, no immunohistochemical or molecular-pathological markers are available for the differential diagnosis between high-grade intraepithelial neoplasia and well-differentiated Barrett's adenocarcinoma. In such a case, the "eye of the pathologist" remains the gold standard [51]. Basically, however, this differential diagnosis is merely "academic," since the consequences to be drawn from a diagnosis of high-grade intraepithelial neoplasia in biopsy material should always be endoscopic treatment.

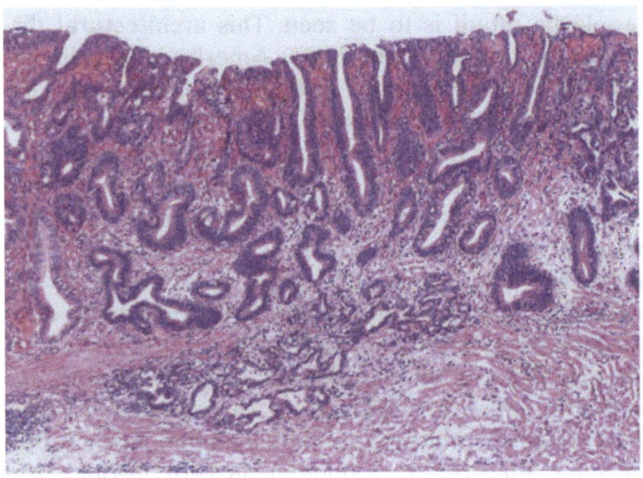

Fig. 13. Barrett's adenocarcinoma with invasion of the muscularis mucosae

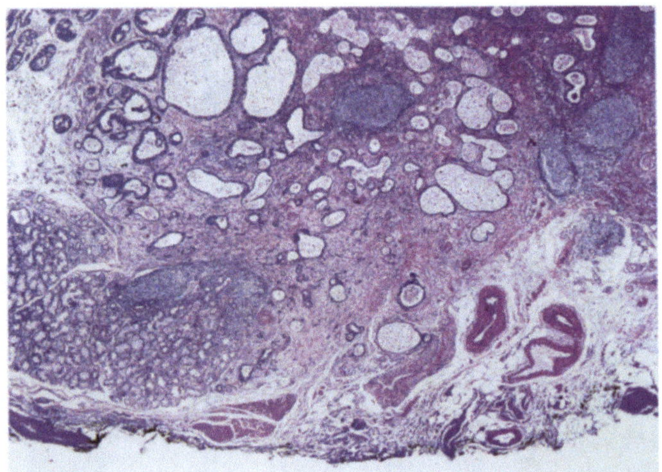

Fig. 14. Barrett's adenocarcinoma with invasion of the superficial submucosal layer

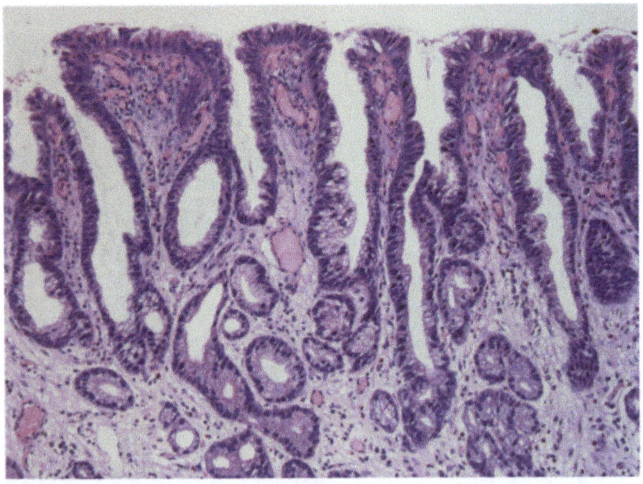

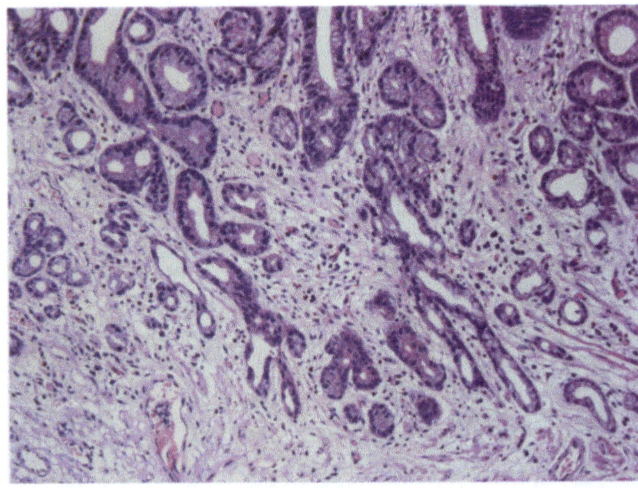

Figs. 15 and 16. Barrett's adenocarcinoma with the appearance of high-grade intraepithelial neoplasia in the upper part of the mucosa

Table 4. Frequency of the histological diagnoses in 1011 endoscopic resection preparations from 399 patients

No neoplasia	2.0%
LGIEN	1.2%
HGIEN	3.2%
pT1-m-Ca	79.7%
pT1-sm1-Ca	6.3%
pT1-sm2-Ca	3.8%
pT1-sm3-Ca	3.8%

n = 399; 1011 endoscopic resections

The fact that the indication for endoscopic resection based on a special gastroenterological diagnostic workup is correct in approximately 90% of the cases is confirmed by our evaluation of endoscopic resection specimens obtained from 399 patients (see Table 4): most neoplasias removed by endoscopic resection were limited to the mucosa, and surgical treatment was necessary in only a few patients in whom the histological workup revealed invasion of the submucosa.

8. Is Endoscopic Resection Adequate Treatment for Early Neoplasia of Barrett's Mucosa?

The justification for the limited endoscopic treatment is provided by six publications on the incidence of regional lymph node metastases in esophagectomy specimens [41, 52–57]. In the case of early carcinomas limited to the mucosa, only two of the seven publications reported finding lymph node metastases, in 2–3% of the cases, while infiltration of the submucosa was associated with an increase in lymph node metastases to between 8% and 56% (see Table 5). In none of these studies was the depth of infiltration in the mucosa and submucosa further differentiated in more detail.

In analogy to the classification of early squamous cell carcinoma [58], we initially differentiate the depth of infiltration of Barrett's adenocarcinomas as follows:

m1 = carcinoma limited to Barrett's mucosa
m2 = carcinoma infiltrating the newly formed muscularis mucosae of Barrett's mucosa
m3 = carcinoma infiltrating the original lamina propria of the esophageal mucosa
m4 = infiltration of the original muscularis mucosae of the esophageal mucosa
sm1 = infiltration of the superficial third of the submucosa
sm2 = infiltration of the middle third of the submucosa
sm3 = infiltration of the deep third of the submucosa

Whether this differentiated classification of the depth of infiltration is of any practical value, e.g., whether m4 carcinomas more frequently metastasize to the lymph nodes than m1 carcinoma, or whether, e.g., in analogy to early gastric carcinoma, sm1 carcinomas relatively rarely metastasize to the lymph nodes, may be answered by the results of our currently ongoing follow-up investigations.

Table 5. Incidence of lymph node metastases (N+) in surgical specimens with Barrett's adenocarcinomas confined to the mucosa (pT1m), and in Barrett's carcinomas infiltrating into the submucosa (pT1sm)

		pT1m		pT1sm	
First author [Ref.]	Year	*n*	N+	*n*	N+
Rice [52]	1997	29	3%	17	8%
Hölscher [53]	1997	10	0%	31	10%
Ruol [54]	1997	4	0%	22	36%
van Sandvick [55]	2000	12	0%	20	30%
Stein [56]	2000	38	0%	56	18%
Dar [41]	2003	20	0%	4	0%
Westerterp [57]	2005	54	2%	66	56%

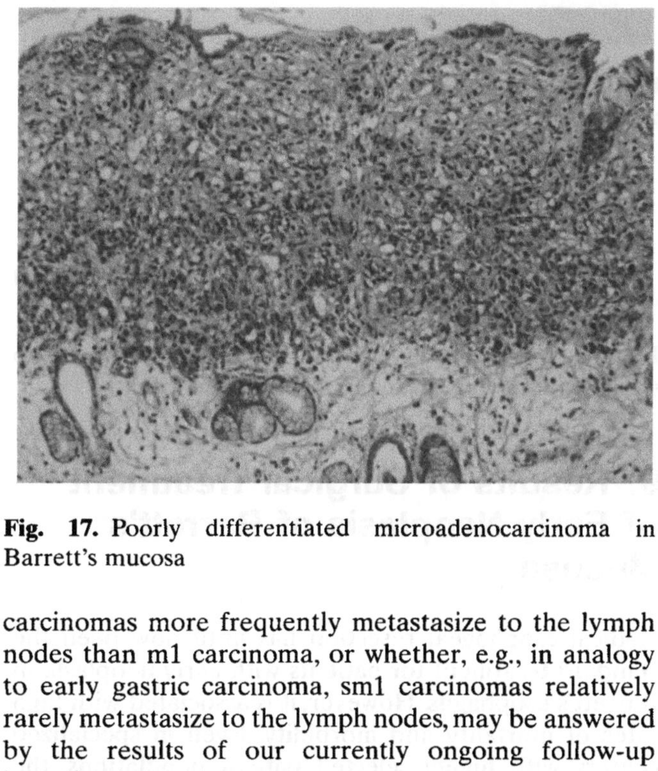

Fig. 17. Poorly differentiated microadenocarcinoma in Barrett's mucosa

As a working hypothesis: in the absence of such data, the risk of metastasis can, for the present, in analogy to early gastric carcinoma, be differentiated as follows:

Low risk
—Depth of infiltration limited to the mucosa (m1 to m4)
—Well to moderately well-differentiated adenocarcinoma (G1, G2)
—No invasion of lymphatic or blood vessels (L0, V0)

High risk
—Depth of infiltration—into the submucosa (sm1 to sm3), or
—Poorly differentiated (Fig. 17) and undifferentiated carcinoma (G3, G4), or

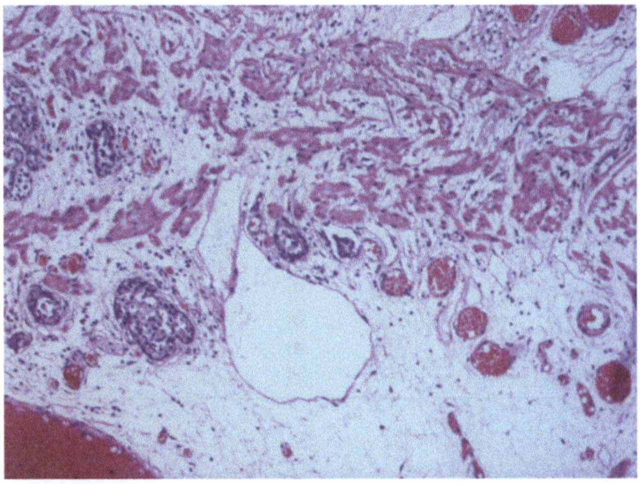

Fig. 18. Barrett's adenocarcinoma with invasion of a lymphatic vessel

—Invasion of lymphatic or blood vessels (L1, V1) (Fig. 18)

Further follow-up investigations will be required to show whether this risk classification is correct.

9. Results of Surgical Treatment of Early Neoplasia of Barrett's Mucosa

Radical esophageal resection has until now been the standard treatment for patients with early neoplasia in Barrett's esophagus. However, it is associated with high rates of mortality and morbidity. Even in specialized centers with highly selected patient populations, the mortality in patients with neoplasias is more than 3%, while morbidity rates of 20%–50% are reported [3, 59]. In patients over the age of 70, the mortality increases to as much as 11% [60]. Another aspect that needs to be taken into account is that patients require at least 9 months postoperatively to achieve a quality of life similar to that which they had before the operation [61]. A further argument in favor of local therapy is the virtually nonexistent risk of lymph node metastases in intraepithelial neoplasias and mucosal early carcinomas [41, 52–57]. It is only when infiltration of the submucosa takes place that lymph node metastases are encountered, in 8%–56% of cases [52–57, 62]. Exact pretreatment staging using chromoendoscopy, miniprobe endosonography, and computed tomography is therefore indispensable [63].

10. Different Endoscopic Resection Techniques

The endoscopic resection (ER) techniques used depend on the anatomical conditions, the macroscopic type of the early carcinoma, and the endoscopist's personal experience. However, ER of intraepithelial neoplasias or early carcinomas in Barrett's esophagus is difficult, as most of the lesions are superficial and lie in an axial hiatal hernia in the area of the esophagogastric junction. In our view, there are two techniques that are particularly appropriate in the esophagus: in protruded lesions, removal after injection under the lesion using the polypectomy technique, with loops adapted to the size of the lesion; in superficial lesions, the "suck-and-cut" technique with a ligation device or cap, which has proven its value.

10.1 Strip Biopsy

In strip biopsy, a diathermy loop is introduced through the working channel of the endoscope and positioned over a protruded lesion, which is fixed by tightening of the loop and slowly detached using an electrical cutting current. This technique can be used in (type I) protruded tumors, but with superficial lesions it is difficult to position the loop, and there may be a risk that the size of the removed specimen will be limited. Nevertheless, this technique has been advocated and has been successfully used in the resection of five superficial early Barrett's carcinomas [64].

Submucosal injection of a solution can lift superficial elevated, flat or shallow depressed lesions (type II) and make it easier to resect them (the "lift-and-cut" technique). In addition to extending the range of target lesions in comparison with simple strip biopsy, this procedure also has other advantages. Injection of a saline–epinephrine solution into the submucosa, for example, lifts the early carcinoma—thereby increasing the distance from the muscularis propria and potentially reducing the risk of perforation. A second advantage of the injection technique may be a reduced risk of hemorrhage, due to the vasoconstriction caused by epinephrine and compression by the injected volume of liquid.

The type of injection solution used has not been standardized. The solution most often used is saline with epinephrine or dextrose in various concentrations. We use 10 ml of a 1:100 000 epinephrine–saline solution. A disadvantage of the epinephrine–saline mixture is its short retention time (3.0 min) in comparison with a 50% dextrose solution (4.7 min) and a 1% rooster-comb hyaluronic acid solution (22.1 min). These data were obtained in an animal-experiment study in the porcine esophagus [65].

10.2 "Suck-and-Cut" Technique

The "suck-and-cut" technique is used in the esophagus more frequently than strip biopsy, due to the anatomical conditions, and our group also uses it almost exclusively. The rationale is that a study by Tanabe et al. [66] demonstrated that endoscopic suck-and-cut mucosectomy in early gastric cancer is more effective than strip biopsy with regard to the largest diameter of the resected specimen, the rate of en bloc resection, and the complication rate.

In the early 1990s, Inoue and Endo developed the cap technique, thereby improving the effectiveness of ER in comparison with simple strip biopsy [67]. In the ER cap technique, a specially developed transparent plastic cap is attached to the end of the endoscope. After injection under the target lesion, the lesion is sucked into the cap and resected with a diathermy loop that has previously been loaded into a specially designed groove on the lower edge of the cap. Since injecting underneath early carcinomas often makes it difficult to distinguish them, prior marking of the lesion, e.g., using electrocautery, is recommended (Fig. 19a–e).

Another resection technique of the "suck and cut" principle is the ligation technique. In this method, the target lesion is sucked into the ligation cylinder, and a polyp is created by releasing a rubber band around it. The polyp is then resected at its base, either above or below the rubber band, using a diathermy loop (Fig. 20a–d). In this technique, the endoscope being used for resection has to be withdrawn again and reintroduced in order to remove the ligation cylinder and introduce the loop. Ligation devices available include, in addition to single-use devices, a reusable ligator [68], with which similar results can be achieved at reduced cost.

A study conducted by our research group compared the two suction mucosectomy techniques—the cap technique and the ligation technique—in the resection of early esophageal neoplasias [69]. In this prospective study, 100 consecutive endoscopic mucosal resections were performed in 70 patients with early esophageal cancer. Fifty resections were carried out with the ligation device without prior injection, and 50 resections using the cap technique with prior submucosal injection with a diluted epinephrine–saline solution. The main criteria were the maximum diameter of the resected specimen, the resection area, and the complication rate. No significant differences were observed between the two groups with regard to the maximum diameter of the resected specimens and the resection area after 24h. There was only a slight advantage for the ligation group in patients who had had prior treatment. One minor bleeding incident occurred in each group, but no severe complications were seen.

In addition to the suck-and-cut and strip biopsy techniques, ER using a double-channel endoscope has also been described [70]. In this method, a grasping forceps is used to pull the target lesion through a diathermy loop that has been introduced through the second working channel. The lesion is then resected with the loop. Due to the large caliber of the endoscope required, double-channel procedures appear to be very difficult, especially at the esophagogastric junction, and may even be almost impossible in the inverted position in short-segment Barrett's neoplasia.

The latest technique is the "en bloc" ER by using "endoknives" as for early gastric cancer. However, for this technique experience in Barrett's esophagus is limited.

11. Endoscopic Resection of Early Neoplasia in Barrett's Esophagus

Our research group has now conducted more than 1500 ERs in the esophagus in a total of more than 650 patients who presented to our institution with early Barrett's carcinoma or high-grade intraepithelial neoplasia (HGIN) between October 1996 and June 2005, and who underwent endoscopic treatment with curative intent. The first major interim report from a prospective series of 64 patients with early Barrett's carcinoma or high-grade intraepithelial neoplasia was published by our group in 2000 [8]. Complete remission was achieved in 82.5% of cases (97% in the low-risk group, 59% in the high-risk group). During a mean follow-up period of 12 months, recurrences or metachronous carcinomas were observed in 14% of the patients, and these again underwent successful endoscopic treatment. The rate of serious and mild complications in this study was 12.5%.

More recent publications by our group have also confirmed the effectiveness of ER in 50 patients with early neoplasias in short-segment Barrett's esophagus [71]. Twenty-eight patients received ER, 13 underwent photodynamic therapy (PDT), and three were treated with argon plasma coagulation (APC). A combination of these therapies was used in six patients. Complete local remission was achieved in 98% of the patients; one patient was switched to surgery after initial ER treatment, as there was submucosal tumor infiltration. In this study, the minor complication rate was again very low, at 6% (bleeding, stenosis), and no major complications were observed.

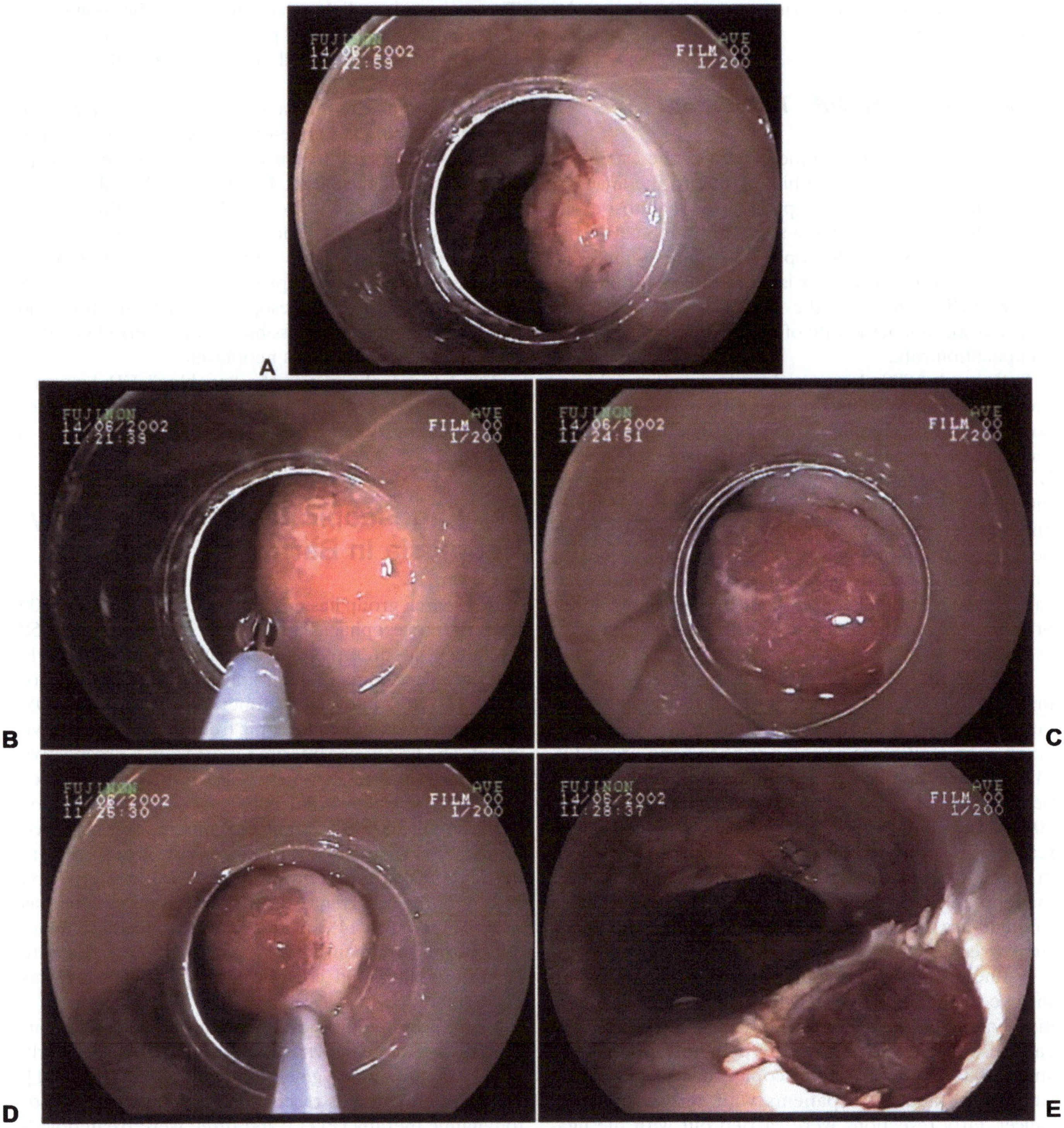

Fig. 19A–E. Endoscopic resection of a type IIa mucosal Barrett's adenocarcinoma using the cap technique

The intermediate results were similarly encouraging (average follow-up period 34 ± 10 months) in 115 patients treated using EMR (*n* = 70), PDT (*n* = 32), and APC (*n* = 3). Multimodal therapy also led to complete local remission in 98% of the patients in this group [9].

Endoscopic resection has also been successfully used by other research groups, although with limited numbers of patients, in the treatment of early malignancies in Barrett's esophagus. In 25 patients with lesions in Barrett's esophagus (13 adenocarcinomas, 4 HGINs), Nijhawan and Wang carried out EMR with diagnostic

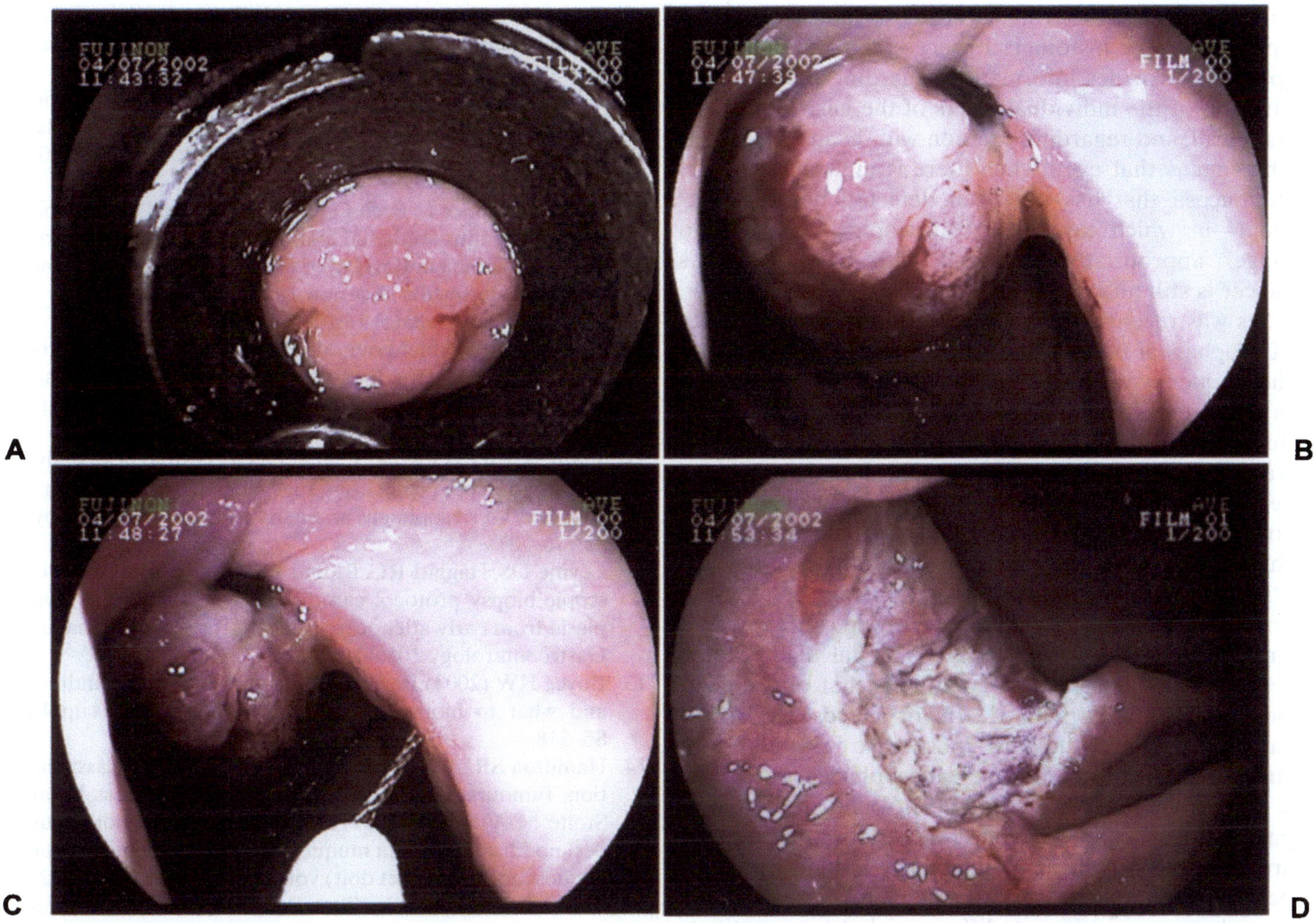

Fig. 20A–D. Endoscopic resection of a type IIa mucosal Barrett's adenocarcinoma with a ligation device

and therapeutic intent [72]. The "lift-and-cut" technique was used in the majority of cases, and the "suck-and-cut" technique with a ligation device was used in only two patients.

In a very heterogeneous group of patients, Waxmann's group carried out 101 ERs in malignant and nonmalignant lesions throughout the entire gastrointestinal tract [73]. The patients also included 12 with lesions in Barrett's esophagus (6 adenocarcinomas, 6 HGINs). The complication rate was 11% and complete remission was achieved in four patients in each group. The literature otherwise only includes a few reports of individual cases. Combination therapy with other local endoscopic procedures appears to be useful and justifiable in individual cases. If evidence of minimal residual carcinoma at the resection margin is found after ER, ablation of the residual tissue using APC or potassium titanyl phosphate (KTP) laser is defensible and useful, in our view. In patients with multifocal intraepithelial high-grade neoplasia, extensive ablation using PDT is indicated as a supplement to ER in individual cases. In 17 inoperable patients with esophageal neoplasia within Barrett's esophagus, Buttar et al. carried out PDT with Photofrin II or hematoporphyrin derivative following ER [74]. After a median follow-up of 13 months, 16 of the 17 patients (94%) were in complete remission. Barrett's epithelium was completely ablated by PDT in only 53% of cases. With the additional PDT, however, stenoses requiring treatment developed in 30% of the patients, and cutaneous phototoxicity in 12%. The conclusion that additional PDT can significantly reduce the rate of recurrence and the rate of metachronous carcinoma cannot be justified on the basis of this study with a limited follow-up period and a small number of patients, without a control group. However, ablation of residual Barrett's mucosa following successful ER treatment does appear to be theoretically useful. On the basis of experience in our own group of patients, this approach appears to reduce the rate of metachronous lesions [75].

In experienced hands, ER is a safe method of resecting dysplastic lesions and early carcinomas of the gastrointestinal tract, and it has distinct advantages in comparison with other local endoscopic treatment procedures (such as thermal destruction and PDT): the opportunity for histological processing of the resected specimen provides information regarding the depth of invasion of the individual layers of the gastrointestinal tract wall, and regarding excision with healthy margins. This means that even when there is infiltration of the submucosa that has not been detected before treatment—in which case local endoscopic therapy is no longer appropriate—a patient with early Barrett's cancer is still able to undergo surgical resection.

As was recently shown, the morbidity and mortality of esophageal resection are significantly dependent on the frequency with which esophagectomy is carried out in each center. When there were more than 20 procedures of this type per year, the surgical mortality was 8%, while in centers conducting less than 10 procedures per year the rate was 21% [76]. In view of the consequent—justified—claim that esophageal resection should only be carried out at high-volume centers, curative endoscopic treatment of early esophageal carcinomas should also only be carried out in centers with a similar frequency to that of the surgical high-volume centers. It is only in these conditions that our conclusion, that patients with HGIN or mucosal Barrett's carcinoma should undergo endoscopic resection with curative intent instead of radical esophageal resection, is defensible. Randomized and controlled studies comparing radical esophagectomy with endoscopic therapy are desirable, but they are difficult to conduct—not least because valid 5-year survival data are now available that show no significant difference between patients who have undergone endoscopic treatment for early Barrett's cancers and the average German population of the same age and sex [77].

References

1. Pera M, Trastek VF, Pairolero PC, et al (1993) Barrett's disease: pathophysiology of metaplasia and adenocarcinoma. Ann Thorac Surg 56:1191–1197
2. Bytzer P, Christensen PB, Damkier P, et al (1999) Adenocarcinoma of the esophagus and Barrett's esophagus: a population-based study. Am J Gastroenterol 94:86–91
3. Conio M, Cameron AJ, Romero Y, et al (2001) Secular trends in the epidemiology and outcome of Barrett's oesophagus in Olmsted County, Minnesota. Gut 48:304–309
4. Powell J, McConkey CC (1990) Increasing incidence of adenocarcinoma of the gastric cardia and adjacent sites. Br J Cancer 62:440–443
5. Vega KJ, Jamal MM (2000) Changing pattern of esophageal cancer incidence in New Mexico. Gastroenterology 95:2352–2356
6. Haggitt RC (1992) Adenocarcinoma in Barrett's esophagus: a new epidemic? Hum Pathol 23:475–476
7. Tytgat GN, Hameeteman W (1992) The neoplastic potential of columnar-lined (Barrett's) esophagus. World J Surg 16:308–312
8. Ell C, May A, Gossner L, Pech O, et al (2000) Endoscopic mucosal resection of early cancer and high-grade dysplasia in Barrett's esophagus. Gastroenterology 118:670–677
9. May A, Gossner L, Pech O, et al (2002) Local endoscopic therapy for intraepithelial high-grade neoplasia and early adenocarcinoma in Barrett's oesophagus: acute-phase and intermediate results of a new treatment approach. Eur J Gastroenterol Hepatol 14:1085–1091
10. Overholt BF, Panjehpour M, Halberg DL (2003) Photodynamic therapy for Barrett's esophagus with dysplasia and/or early stage carcinoma: long-term results. Gastrointest Endosc 58:183–188
11. Vieth M, Ell C, Gossner L, et al (2004) Histological analysis of endoscopic resections specimens from 326 patients with Barrett's esophagus and early neoplasia. Endoscopy; 36:776–781
12. Levine DS, Haggitt RC, Blount PL, et al (1993) An endoscopic biopsy protocol can differentiate high-grade dysplasia from early adenocarcinoma in Barrett's esophagus. Gastroenterology 105:40–50
13. Boyce HW (2003) Barrett esophagus: endoscopic findings and what to biopsy. J Clin Gastroenterol 36(5 suppl): S6–S18
14. Hamilton SR, Aaltonen LA (eds) (2000) WHO classification. Tumours of the digestive system. IARC Press, Lyon
15. Stolte M, Vieth M (2001) Fondement histopathologique des modifications de la muqueuse oesophagienne. Ce que l'endoscopiste peut (et doit) voir. Acta Endosc 31:125–129
16. Pfau PR, Sivak MV Jr, Chak A, et al (2003) Criteria for the diagnosis of dysplasia by endoscopic optical coherence tomography. Gastrointest Endosc 58:196–202
17. Poneros JM, Nishioka NS (2003) Diagnosis of Barrett's esophagus using optical coherence tomography. Gastrointest Endosc Clin North Am 13:309–323
18. Sokolov K, Sung KB, Collier T, et al (2002) Endoscopic microscopy. Dis Markers 18:269–291
19. Inoue H, Igari T, Nishikage T, et al (2000) A novel method of virtual histopathology using laser-scanning confocal microscopy in-vitro with untreated fresh specimens from the gastrointestinal mucosa. Endoscopy 32:439–443
20. Owens MM, Kimmey MB (2003) The role of endoscopic ultrasound in the diagnosis and management of Barrett's esophagus. Gastrointest Endosc Clin North Am 13:325–334
21. Reid BJ, Haggitt RC, Rubin CE, et al (1988) Observer variation in the diagnosis of dysplasia in Barrett's esophagus. Hum Pathol 19:166–178
22. Ormsby AH, Petras RE, Henricks WH, et al (2002) Observer variation in the diagnosis of superficial oesophageal adenocarcinoma. Gut 51:671–676
23. Montgomery E, Bronner MP, Goldblum JR, et al (2001) Reproducibility of the diagnosis of dysplasia in Barrett esophagus: a reaffirmation. Hum Pathol 32:368–378
24. Alikhan M, Rex D, Khan A, et al (1999) Variable pathologic interpretation of columnar lined esophagus by

general pathologists in community practice. Gastrointest Endosc 50:23–26
25. Baak JP, ten Kate FJ, Offerhaus GJ, et al (2002) Routine morphometrical analysis can improve reproducibility of dysplasia grade in Barrett's oesophagus surveillance biopsies. J Clin Pathol 55:910–916
26. Stolte M (2003) Early carcinomas of upper gastrointestinal tract: dignostic problems. Verh Dtsch Ges Path 87:130–136
27. Schnell TG, Sontag SJ, Chejfec G, et al (2001) Long-term nonsurgical management of Barrett's esophagus with high-grade dysplasia. Gastroenterology 120:1607–1619
28. Sharma P, Weston AP, Toalovski M, et al (2003) Magnification chromoendoscopy for the detection of intestinal metaplasia and dysplasia in Barrett's oesophagus. Gut 52:24–27
29. Egger K, Werner M, Meining A, et al (2003) Biopsy surveillance is still necessary in patients with Barrett's oesophagus despite new endoscopic imaging techniques. Gut 52:18–23
30. O'Connor JB, Falk GW, Richter JE (1999) The incidence of adenocarcinoma and dysplasia in Barrett's esophagus: report on the Cleveland Clinic Barrett's Esophagus Registry. Am J Gastroenterol 94:2037–2042
31. Fisher RS, Bromer MQ, Thomas RM, et al (2003) Predictors of recurrent specialized intestinal metaplasia after complete laser ablation. Am J Gastroenterol 98:1945–1951
32. Gopal DV, Liebermann DA, Magaret N, et al (2003) Risk factors for dysplasia in patients with Barrett's esophagus (BE): results from a multicenter consortium. Dig Dis Sci 48:1537–1541
33. Conio M, Blanchi S, Lapertosa G, et al (2003) Long-term endoscopic surveillance of patients with Barrett's esophagus. Incidence of dysplasia and adenocarcinoma: a prospective study. Am J Gastroenterol 98:1931–1939
34. Jankowski JA, Harrison RF, Perry I, et al (2000) Barrett's metaplasia. Lancet 356:2079–2085
35. Faller G, Borchard F, Ell C, et al (2003) Histopathological diagnosis of Barrett's mucosa and associated neoplasias: results of a consensus conference of the Working Group for Gastroenterological Pathology of the German Society for Pathology. Virchows Arch 443:597–601
36. Offerhaus GJ, Correa P, van Eeden S, et al (2003) Report of an Amsterdam working group on Barrett esophagus. Virchows Arch 443:602–608
37. Faller G, Stolte M (2003) Barrett's oesophagus: time for consensus. Virchows Arch 443:595–596
38. Fujii T, Nakagawa S, Hanzawa M, et al (2003) Immunohistological study of cell cycle-related factors, oncogene expression, and cell proliferation in adenocarcinoma developed in Barrett's esophagus. Oncol Rep 10:427–431
39. Kleeff J, Friess H, Liao Q, et al (2002) Immunohistochemical presentation in non-malignant and malignant Barrett's epithelium. Dis Esophag 15:10–15
40. Halm U, Tannapfel A, Breitung B, et al (2000) Apoptosis and cell proliferation in the metaplasia-dysplasia-carcinoma-sequence of Barrett's esophagus. Hepatogastroenterology 47:962–966
41. Dar MS, Goldblum JR, Rice TW, et al (2003) Can extent of high grade dysplasia in Barrett's oesophagus predict the presence of adenocarcinoma at oesophagectomy? Gut 52:486–489
42. Buttar NS, Wang KK, Sebo TJ, et al (2001) Extent of high-grade dysplasia in Barrett's esophagus correlates with risk of adenocarcinoma. Gastroenterology 120:1630–1639
43. Burke AP, Sobin LH, Shekitka KM, et al (1991) Dysplasia of the stomach and Barrett esophagus: a follow-up study. Mod Pathol 4:336–341
44. Takahashi T, Iwama N (1985) Three-dimensional microstructure of gastrointestinal tumors. Gland pattern and its diagnostic significance. Pathol Annu 20:419–440
45. Takahashi T, Iwama N (1984) Atypical glands in gastric adenoma. Three-dimensional architecture compared with carcinomatous and metaplastic glands. Virchows Arch A Pathol Anat Histopathol 403:135–148
46. Borchard F (2000) Forms and nomenclature of gastrointestinal epithelial expansion: what is invasion? Verh Dtsch Ges Path 84;50–61
47. Edwards MJ, Gable DR, Lentsch AB, et al (1996) The rationale for esophagectomy as the optimal therapy for Barrett's esophagus with high-grade dysplasia. Ann Surg 223:585–589
48. Headrick JR, Nichols FC, Miller DL, et al (2002) High-grade esophageal dysplasia: long-term survival and quality of life after esophagectomy. Ann Thorac Surg 73:1697–1702
49. Romagnoli R, Collard JM, Gutschow C, et al (2003) Outcomes of dysplasia arising in Barrett's esophagus: a dynamic view. J Am Coll Surg 197:365–371
50. Collard JM (2002) High grade dysplasia in Barrett's esophagus. The case for esophagectomy. Chest Surg Clin North Am 12:77–92
51. Robert ME (2003) Defining dysplasia in Barrett esophagus. J Clin Gastroenterol 36(suppl 5):S19–S25
52. Rice TW, Blackstone EH, Goldblum JR, et al (2001) Superficial adenocarcinoma of the esophagus. J Thorac Cardiovasc Surg 122:1077–1090
53. Hölscher AH, Bollschweiler E, Schneider PM, et al (1997) Early adenocarcinoma in Barrett's oesophagus. Br J Surg 84:1470–1473
54. Ruol A, Merigliano S, Baldan N, et al (1997) Prevalence, management and outcome of early adenocarcinoma (pT1) of the esophago-gastric junction. Comparison between early cancer in Barrett's esophagus (type I) and early cancer of the cardia (type II). Dis Esophag 10:190–195
55. van Sandick JW, van Lanschot JJ, ten Kate FJ, et al (2000) Pathology of early invasive adenocarcinoma of the esophagus or esophagogastric junction: implications for therapeutic decision making. Cancer 88:2429–2437
56. Stein HJ, Feith M, Mueller J, et al (2000) Limited resection for early adenocarcinoma in Barrett's esophagus. Ann Surg 232:733–742
57. Westerterp M, Koppert LB, Buskens CJ, et al (2005) Outcome of surgical treatment for early adenocarcinoma

of the esophagus or gastro-esophageal junction. Virch Arch 446:497–504
58. Noguchi H, Naomoto Y, Kondo H, et al (2000) Evaluation of endoscopic mucosal resection for superficial esophageal carcinoma. Surg Laparosc Endosc Percutan Tech 10:343–350
59. Heitmiller RF, Redmond M, Hamilton SR (1996) Barrett's esophagus with high-grade dysplasia: an indication for prophylactic esophagectomy. Ann Surg 224:66–71
60. Thomas P, Doddoli C, Neville P, et al (1996) Esophageal cancer resection in the elderly. Eur J Cardiothorac Surg 11:941–946
61. Blazeby JM, Farndorn JR, Donovan J, et al (2000) A prospective longitudinal study examining the quality of life of patients with esophageal carcinoma. Cancer 88: 1781–1787
62. Nigor JJ, Hagen JA, DeMeester TR, et al (1999) Prevalence and location of nodal metastases in distal esophageal adenocarcinom confined to the wall: implications for therapy. J Thorac Cardiovasc Surg 117:16–25
63. May A, Günter E, Roth F, et al (2004) Accuracy of staging in early oesophageal cancer using high resolution endoscopy and high resolution endosonography: a comparative, prospective and blinded trial. Gut 53:634–640
64. Sohendra N, Binmoeller KF, Bohnacker S, et al (1997) Endoscopic snare mucosectomy in the esophagus without any additional equipment: a simple technique for resection of flat early cancer. Endoscopy 29:380–383
65. Conio M, Rajan E, Sorbi D, et al (2002) Comparative performance in the porcine esophagus of different solutions used for submucosal injection. Gastrointest Endosc 56: 513–516
66. Tanabe S, Koizumi W, Kokutou M, et al (1999) Usefulness of endoscopic aspiration mucosectomy as compared with strip biopsy for the treatment of gastric mucosal cancer. Gastrointest Endosc 50(6):819–822
67. Inoue H, Endo M (1993) A new simplified technique of endoscopic esophageal mucosal resection using a cap-fitted panendoscope. Surg Endosc 6:264–265
68. Ell C, May A, Wurster H (1999) The first reusable multiple-band ligator for endoscopic hemostasis of variceal bleeding, nonvariceal bleeding and mucosal resection. Endoscopy 31:738–740
69. May A, Gossner L, Behrens A, et al (2003) A prospective randomized trial of two different suck-and-cut mucosectomy techniques in 100 consecutive resections in patients with early cancer of the esophagus. Gastrointest Endosc 58:167–175
70. Noda M, Kobayashi N, Kanemasa H, et al (2000) Endoscopic mucosal resection using a partial transparent hood for lesions located tangentially to the endoscope. Gastrointest Endosc 51(3):338–343
71. May A, Gossner L, Pech O, et al (2002) Intraepithelial high-grade neoplasia and early adenocarcinoma in short-segment Barrett's esophagus (SSBE): curative treatment using local endoscopic treatment techniques. Endoscopy 34:604–610
72. Nijhawan PK, Wang KK (2000) Endoscopic mucosal resection for lesions with endoscopic features suggestive of malignancy and high-grade dysplasia within Barrett's esophagus. Gastrointest Endosc 52:328–332
73. Ahmad NA, Kochman ML, Long WB, et al (2002) Efficacy, safety, and clinical outcomes of endoscopic mucosal resection: a study of 101 cases. Gastrointest Endosc 55:390–396
74. Buttar NS, Wang KK, Lutzke LS, et al (2001) Combined endoscopic mucosal resection and photodynamic therapy for esophageal neoplasia within Barrett's esophagus. Gastrointest Endosc 54(6):682–688
75. Behrens A, Pech O, May A, et al (2003) Curative endoscopy of early cancer an high-grade neoplasia in Barrett's esophagus: additional endoscopic ablation of Barrett's esophagus can reduce the risk of recurrent carcinomas. Gastroenterology 124:637 (A)
76. Birkmeyer JD, Siewers AE, Finlayson EV, et al (2002) Hospital volume and surgical mortality in the United States. N Engl J Med 346:1128–1137
77. Ell C, May A, Gossner L, et al (2003) Curative endoscopic therapy in early adenocarcinoma of the esophagus. Dtsch Arztebl 100:A1438–A1448

IV. Detection of Early Cancer: Is Endoscopic Ultrasonography Effective?

1. Gastric Cancer

Rikiya Fujita, Hiroshi Takahashi, and Junko Fujisaki

1. Introduction

When early gastric cancer (EGC) was diagnosed for the first time a little more than 40 years ago, abnormal regions were detected by fluoroscopic barium examination and by photographs from a gastrocamera. With regard to the use of endoscopes for diagnosis, the gastrocamera was replaced by the fiberscope in the 1970s. The latter was then replaced with the electronic endoscope in the 1980s. Since the latter half of the 1990s, capsule endoscopes have come into use. In addition to conventional endoscopy, the following endoscopic examinations are now available: chromoscopy, endoscopic ultrasonography (EUS), magnifying endoscopy, and narrow band imaging etc. It is also worth noting that a definite diagnosis of EGC is impossible without biopsy.

The study of EGC was prompted by the fact that the 5-year survival rate of patients with mucosal and submucosal cancers was high. Because mucosal cancer formerly was detected infrequently, "EGC" was defined as mucosal cancer with or without infiltration up to the submucosal layer. A cancer fulfilling the above criterion was defined to be an EGC even though it may have been accompanied by metastases to lymph nodes [JGES (Japan Gastroenterological Endoscopy Society) classification]. This definition was probably derived from the desire to detect as many EGCs as possible. In Japan, the number of EGCs accounts for 60%–80% of the sum of all currently detected cancers. Endoscopic treatment of EGC has also developed from the initial types of treatment, to endoscopic mucosal resection (EMR), and then to endoscopic submucosal dissection (ESD), which now attracts considerable attention in the field of endoscopic surgery. In addition, the laparoscope is used for local resection of cancer in combination with the endoscope. The survival rate of patients with EGC is as high as above 90% after surgical resection. Correct diagnosis of EGC is becoming more and more important not only in Japan but also internationally. There is a trend that early cancers are integrated and classified as superficial carcinomas, since they exist on or in the superficial layer. In "The Paris Endoscopic Classification of Superficial Neoplastic Lesions: Esophagus, Stomach, and Colon" published recently [1], the criteria for the classification of EGC were applied to the classification of early cancers in the esophagus and colon [2]. Cancers in these regions are explained individually as superficial neoplastic lesions (type 0) in the publication.

2. Endoscopic Diagnosis

Lesions can be classified into three fundamental types: protruded type (0-I), superficial type (0-II), and excavated type (0-III). The superficial type is further divided into three subtypes: slightly elevated (0-IIa), flat (0-IIb), and slightly depressed (0-IIc). Some lesions can be divided into classes described by combinations of types and/or subtypes, such as IIa+IIc and IIc+III (see Figs. 1–7).

Because the criteria for the classification described above are subjective, there are surely individual variations in the classification of each lesion among examiners. For instance, type I (protruded type) cannot be definitely differentiated from type IIa (slightly elevated type). To differentiate these two types, it was proposed that the height (2.5 mm) of the closed cups of the biopsy forceps should be used as a standard. Therefore, lesions less elevated than the standard are classified into type IIa and those more protruded than the standard are classified as type I. Even if lesions are considerably protruded, extensive lesions are often classified into type I+IIa rather than into type I when the lesion as a whole is taken into consideration. This may be one reason for individual variations in the classification of lesions. With regard to the classification of EGC, the proportion of patients with type IIc is highest, as shown in Table 1. Patients with type IIc and its combined types account for 75% of all patients suffering from EGC. The proportion of patients with type IIb is increasing slightly, probably because small lesions are detected more easily. In contrast, the proportion of patients with type III (excavated type) has recently decreased.

The following points are used to detect and classify cancerous lesions during endoscopy.

1. Color changes (redness, erosion, discoloration, paleness, milky-colored, etc.) are found in superficial lesions, particularly in depressed lesions (0-IIc). Slightly elevated lesions (0-IIa) can be easily detected by chromoendoscopy. On the other hand, it is difficult to detect flat lesions (0-IIb) based on color changes.
2. Convergence of folds (abnormal folds, enlargement of folds, moth-eaten appearance of folds, thinning of folds, fusion of folds, etc.) are frequently found in excavated lesions (types 0-III, 0-IIc+III) and slightly depressed lesions (type 0-IIc). Because such lesions are often confused with benign ulcer scars, examiners with

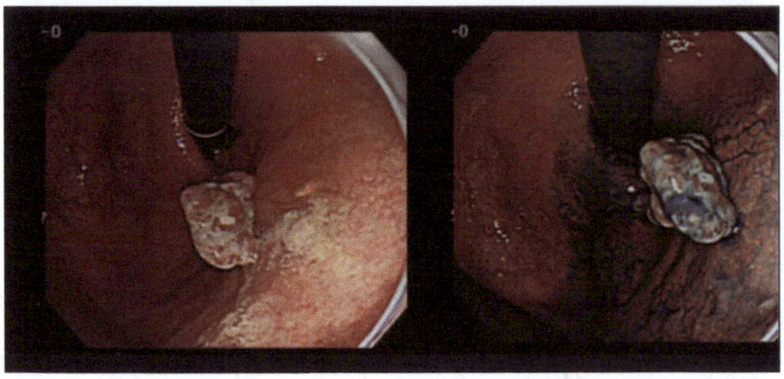

Fig. 1. Early gastric cancer. Well differentiated adenocarcinoma. 0-I protruded lesion

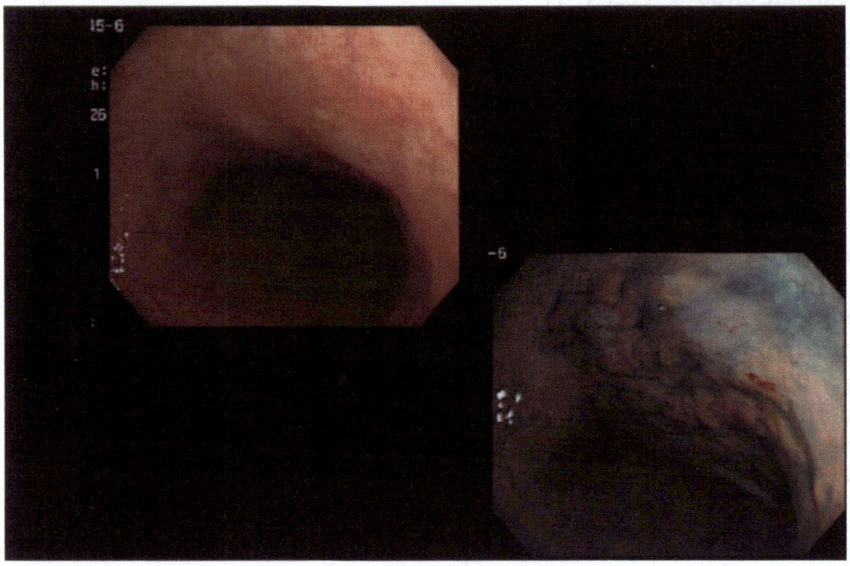

Fig. 2. Early gastric cancer. Well differentiated adenocarcinoma. 0-IIa slightly elevated lesion

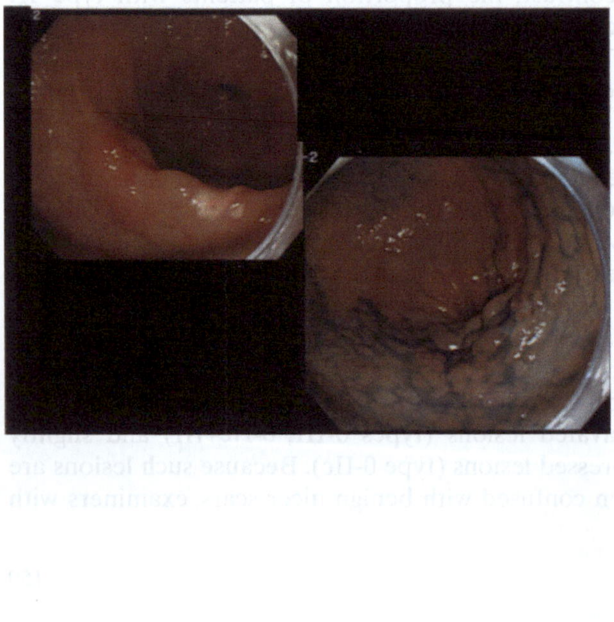

Fig. 3. Early gastric cancer. Well differentiated adenocarcinoma. 0-IIa+IIc slightly elevated and depressed lesion

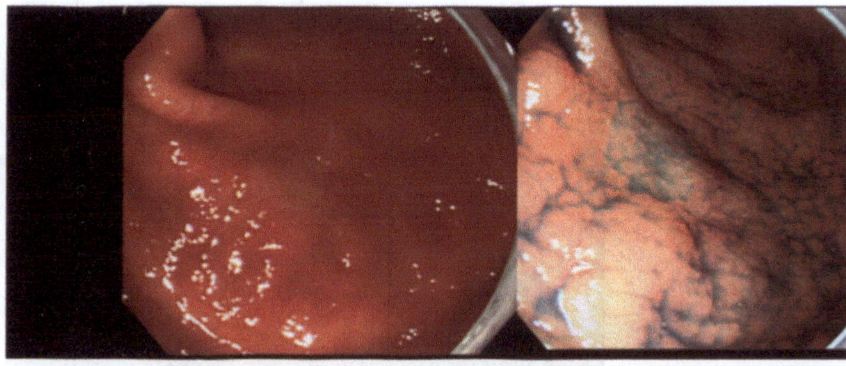

Fig. 4. Early gastric cancer. Poorly differentiated adenocarcinoma. 0-IIb flat lesion

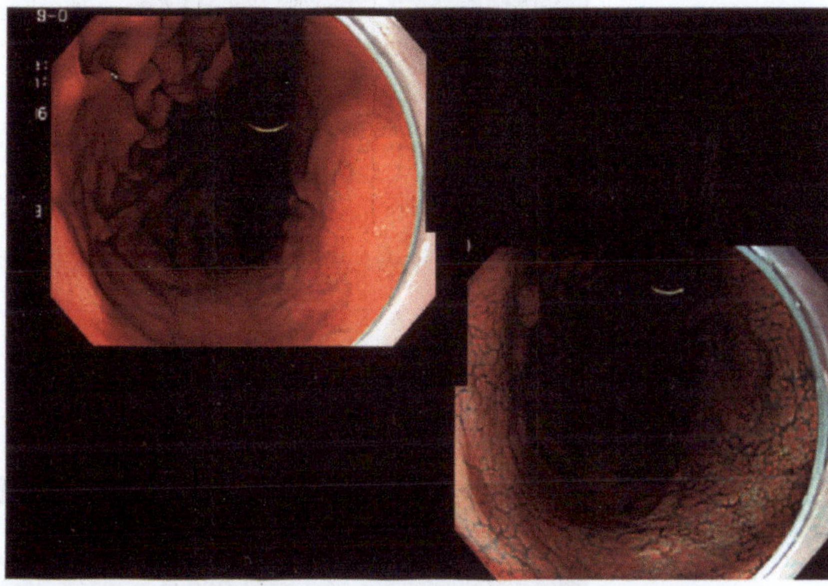

Fig. 5. Early gastric cancer. Poorly differentiated adenocarcinoma. 0-IIc slightly depressed lesion without converging folds

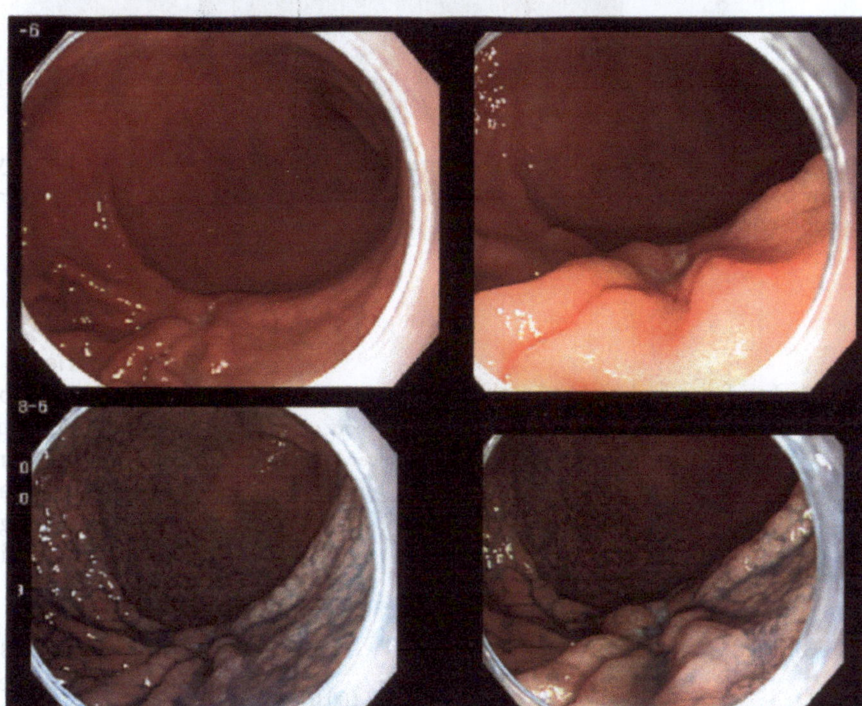

Fig. 6. 0-IIc+III slightly depressed and excavated lesion with converging folds

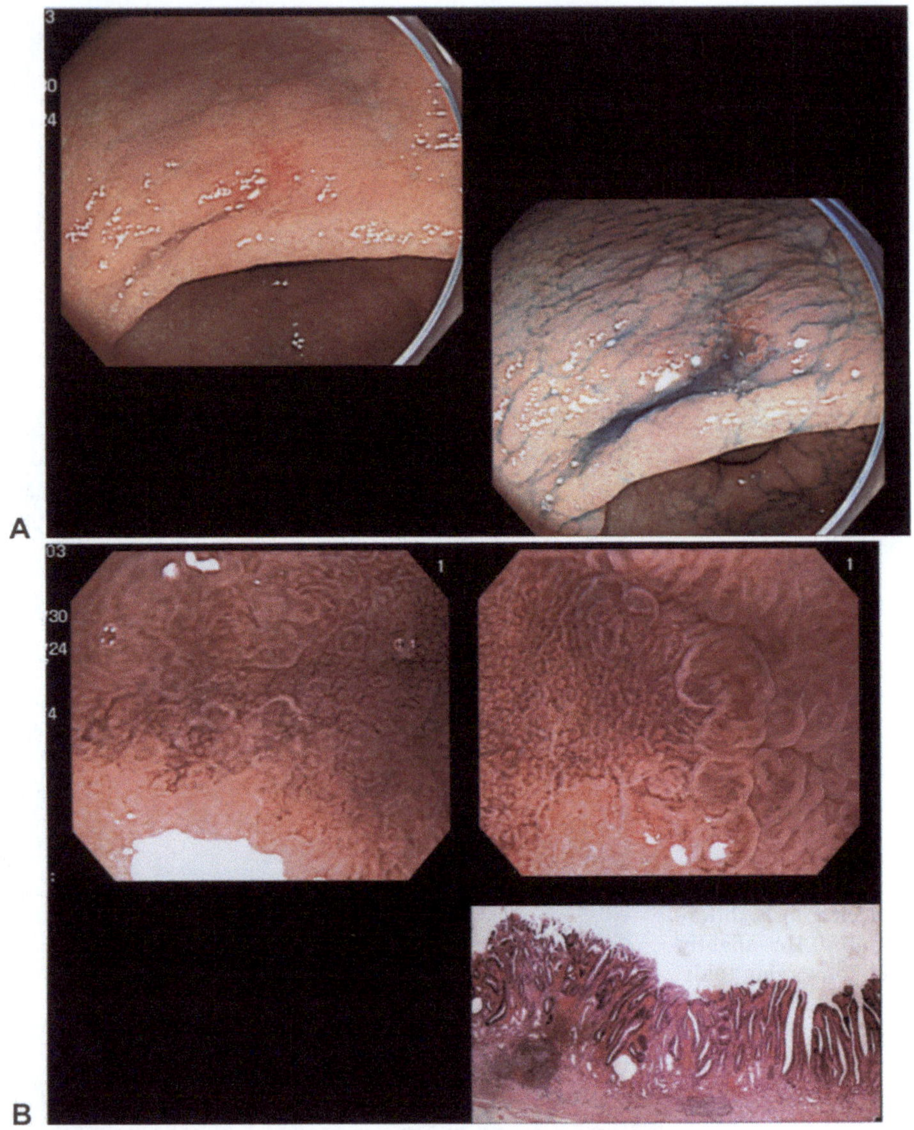

Fig. 7. A Early gastric cancer. Well differentiated adenocarcinoma. 0-IIc slightly depressed lesion with chromoscopy and narrow band imaging (NBI). **B** Endoscopy. Well differentiated adenocarcinoma. 0-IIc slightly depressed lesion with magnifying endoscopy and histopathology

Table 1. Incidence and types of early gastric cancer

Types	1962~71 (Japan survey) N=7,617	1979~2003 (Cancer Institute H) N=4,029
I	14.0%	2.9%
IIa	13.1%	14.1%
IIa+IIc	11.0%	n.d.
IIb	2.6%	8.3%
IIc	55.4%	74.2%
III	4.0%	0.5%
Total	100.0%	100.0%

little experience with EGC fail to detect these lesions. Consequently, biopsies are not performed for these lesions, and cancers easily pass undetected. Chromoscopy performed in combination with conventional endoscopy reveals slight depressions, abnormal changes in folds, and slight elevations more clearly. The rate at which EGC is diagnosed by biopsy ranges from 80% to 90%.

3. Protruded lesions (type 0-I) or slightly elevated lesions (type 0-IIa) can be diagnosed correctly if biopsy of the lesions is made without exception. The rate at which EGC is diagnosed by biopsy is over 95%,

which is higher than the corresponding value for excavated lesions.

4. Minute cancer. Gastric cancers smaller than 5 mm in diameter are called minute cancers. Minute cancers have no characteristic appearance of malignant tumors, such as an irregular margin. Clues to identify lesions of this type are a slightly uneven surface, paleness in color, an irregular pattern, disappearance of superficial blood vessels, and redness. An isolated erosive lesion is a feature of cancer of this type. Minute cancers can be detected and diagnosed with the aid of chromoscopy, magnifying endoscopy or NBI (narrow band imaging) and biopsy.

5. Comparison with histopathology. Well-differentiated and undifferentiated adenocarcinomas have been known to exhibit different endoscopic appearances from each other. Well-differentiated lesions exhibit redness whereas undifferentiated lesions exhibit paleness and discoloration. The former are not sharply demarcated, whereas the latter are well circumscribed. The most serious problem concerning the pathological diagnosis is inconsistency in the diagnostic criteria. Presently, there is international discussion to establish unified criteria. Readers are referred to the corresponding chapters.

3. Chromoscopy

The contrast method using indigo carmine (0.2%–0.5% in concentration) is most frequently applied now. The method is performed as follows. After conventional endoscopic observation, a target point is sprayed with a dye solution through a spraying catheter in such a manner that the solution spreads thinly over a wide region that includes the target point. Simple injection of the solution through the biopsy channel is also possible, but using a spraying catheter is much better. After spraying of the solution, recordings and target biopsy are made as quickly as possible. Although chromoscopy cannot make all invisible sites visible, it is a convenient method to differentiate a target point from the surrounding tissue easily. Particularly, it facilitates to determine a site for biopsy and provides a clear border between pathological and normal sites. The procedure takes only 2–3 min. According to our survey of three institutions, the detection rate of EGC did not increase with the rate at which the contrast method was used in individual institutions.

4. Pitfalls of Biopsy Diagnosis

Detection of cancerous lesions is first required. The rate at which EGCs are diagnosed with biopsy is higher than the rate at which advanced cancers are diagnosed with biopsy. Among EGCs, protruded or slightly elevated cancers are diagnosed at a higher rate than slightly depressed or excavated cancers. If a cancer passes undetected by endoscopy and accordingly biopsy is not performed, the cancer remains unnoticed until the next endoscopic examination. Lesions of type IIb and minute lesions of types IIa and IIc are missed very often.

The level of competence of individual endoscopic examiners also influences the detection rate of EGC. We once compared diagnoses from the endoscopic observation with diagnoses provided by subsequent biopsy in routine examinations in order to assess the differences among examiners in the ability to diagnose EGC. We considered a cancer was missed when the endoscopic diagnosis provided was ulcer scar or erosion and then a cancerous lesion was found on biopsy. On the other hand, we considered that an endoscopic diagnosis was correct when it was a suspected cancer and a cancerous lesion was found on biopsy. As a result of such comparisons, we found that the rate of correct endoscopic diagnosis was distributed between 20% and 100% among individual examiners. The personal variations in the rate of correct diagnosis did not depend markedly on the length of experience. The detection rate among upper gastrointestinal tract endoscopists was higher than the detection rate among other specialists in gastroenterology.

The next problem concerns clinical pathologists. The difference in diagnostic criteria among clinical pathologists in Japan, European countries, and the United States is a concern. Schlemper et al. [3] reported their experience where they requested Japanese, European, and American pathologists to examine and provide a diagnosis for the same histopathological preparations. Diagnoses of the same lesion provided by the pathologists varied widely among cancer and high-grade or low-grade adenoma/dysplasia. As with the revised Vienna classification [4], an effort should be continued hereafter to obtain a consensus about the criteria for biopsy diagnosis. Readers are referred to the corresponding chapters regarding pathological diagnostic standards. The diagnostic standard in Japan is shown below.

Group I: Normal mucosa and benign lesions with no atypia
Group II: Lesions showing atypia but diagnosed as benign (non-neoplastic)
Group III: Borderline lesions between benign (non-neoplastic) and malignant lesions
Group IV: Lesions strongly suspected of carcinoma
Group V: Carcinoma

The Paris classification reported in 2003 [1] was based on the Japanese classification [2].

5. Magnifying Endoscopy

With the aid of magnifying endoscopy, observation of EGC and its differential diagnosis, establishment of a demarcation line for EMR, and examination of cancer recurring after EMR are performed under magnifications of 40–100 power. The rate at which EGC is diagnosed by magnifying endoscopy is not as high as compared with the rate at which early colon cancer is diagnosed under magnified observation. However, it is gradually being accepted that magnifying endoscopy is useful when used in combination with chromoscopy or narrow band imaging. The routine use of magnifying endoscopy does not appear to be necessary. The following types of magnifying endoscope are available now on the market.

Fujinon	EG450ZW5	100 × zoom
Olympus	Q240Z	80 × zoom

6. Narrow Band Imaging

Narrow band imaging (NBI) is a recently developed method. It has attracted considerable attention as a technique that allows the detection of abnormal patterns of superficial capillary vessels. Although this method should be used in combination with a magnifying endoscope, the use of NBI is beginning to be used alone in examination of the esophagus, stomach, and colon. According to our experience, we can differentiate patterns of capillary vessels in the superficial layer of the mucosa. The consistency rate between pathological diagnoses and diagnoses obtained with NBI has been established. NBI is gaining attention as a new method that occupies an important role in optic biopsy.

7. Endoscopic Ultrasonography (EUS)

Nowadays, EUS examination using a miniature probe is performed widely. The 3D (three-dimensional)-EUS recently developed makes it easy to identify the stage of cancer in patients. It should be further determined, however, whether EUS is really indispensable to detect early cancers. Since mucosal cancers treatable with EMR (endoscopic mucosal resection) are equally diagnosed with either EUS or conventional endoscopy, EUS does not seem to be indispensable. The rate at which advanced cancers are diagnosed with EUS is not much different from that at which they are diagnosed with conventional endoscopy. The notion that EUS is truly valuable may not be accepted widely unless EUS makes differential diagnosis among sm1, sm2, and sm3 possible [5] (Table 2).

Table 2. Proportions of correct diagnosis obtained using three-dimensional endoscopic ultrasonography

m cancer	95%	(115/121)
sm cancer	77%	(47/61)
advanced cancer	57%	(12/21)
mp cancer	0%	(0/2)
ss cancer	69%	(9/13)
s cancer	60%	(3/5)
si cancer	0%	(0/1)

References

1. The Paris endoscopic classification of superficial neoplastic lesions: esophagus, stomach, and colon (2003) Gastrointest Endosc 58(Suppl 6):S3–S43
2. Schlemper RJ, Hirata I, Dixon MF (2002) The macroscopic classification of early neoplasia of the digestive tract. Endoscopy 34:163–168
3. Schlemper RJ, Itabashi M, Kato Y, et al (1997) Differences in diagnostic criteria for gastric carcinoma between Japanese and Western pathologists. Lancet 349:1725–1729
4. Dixon MF (2002) Gastrointestinal epithelial neoplasia: Vienna revisited. Gut 51:130–131
5. Ida M, et al (2002) Endosc Digest 14:624–632

2. Colorectal Cancer

Seiji Shimizu and Masahiro Tada

1. How to Detect Early Colorectal Cancer

Early colorectal cancers show diversity in configuration. The Japanese Research Society for Cancer of the Colon and Rectum divides the shapes of early cancers into type I (pedunculated, semipedunculated, and sessile), type II (superficial), and special type. Superficial lesions are subdivided into superficially elevated, flat, and superficially depressed types. This classification is also applied to the description of the shape of adenomas. Of these, the superficially depressed-type lesions are very important because they are often malignant and tend to invade the submucosa despite their small size [1].

Protruding lesions can easily be noticed if endoscopic observation is properly performed. In contrast, superficial ones are easily overlooked if the presence of such lesions is not borne in mind. The first step to detect these lesions is to check trivial mucosal changes. Slight discoloration, hemorrhage, obscured normal vascular pattern, and slight deformation of the colonic wall suggest the presence of such lesions [1]. The next step is dye spraying; by this procedure, the presence of lesions usually becomes apparent.

As with protruding lesions, superficial-type tumors histologically include cancer, adenoma, and hyperplastic polyp. Hyperplastic polyps can be recognized from the endoscopic findings, i.e., small, whitish, round to petal-like, superficial elevations. However, the distinction between adenoma and cancer is difficult to establish by ordinary endoscopic observation even with dye spraying. The introduction of magnifying endoscopy has made it possible to make a diagnosis on the degree of cancer invasion with considerable accuracy [2, 3]. Pretreatment by oral intake of an indigocarmine dye capsule has been reported to be useful for detection of small lesions [4]. Recently, real-time color enhancement of the image of electronic endoscopy has become available (Fig. 1). This may contribute to the detection of superficial-type tumors [5].

2. Significance of Endoscopic Ultrasonography (EUS) in the Management of Early Colorectal Cancers

Since the recognition of the five-layered structure of the intestinal wall by EUS, this modality has been introduced into the diagnosis of colorectal cancers [6, 7]. At first, the usefulness of EUS in local staging was recognized in rectal cancers for determining the surgical procedure. Its application has, however, been focused on early colorectal cancers following the appearance of miniature ultrasonic probes and high-frequency instruments [8, 9].

The development of the endoscopic mucosal resection (EMR) technique has extensively widened the range of endoscopic intervention for early cancers [10, 11]. Mucosal cancers are principally not accompanied by metastasis. However, cancers with submucosal (sm) invasion are known to be accompanied by metastasis in about 10% of cases. Because the curability by EMR depends on the presence of metastasis, its prediction is the critical problem in the management of early cancers. At present, the method to directly detect metastatic lymph nodes has not been established. Accordingly, the possibility of metastasis must be evaluated from the local information.

Based on the fact that the risk of lymph node metastasis increases in proportion to the sm penetration depth, detailed classifications of submucosal invasion depth were devised to discriminate sm cancers with the risk of lymph node metastasis and those without. At first, the thickness of the submucosal layer was simply divided into three layers [11]; but the problem was the difficulty in applying this classification to endoscopically resected materials. Instead, classifications based on the absolute value of sm penetration depth have subsequently been proposed [12]. We have employed the following classification based on the analysis of surgically operated sm cancers: sm1, submucosal invasion within 1000 μm beyond the muscularis mucosae; sm3, invasion close to the muscularis propria; and sm2, invasion between sm1 and sm3. Metastasis is negligible when invasion is sm1. Accordingly, sm1 cancers are considered to be an indication for EMR, while cancers with sm-massive invasion (sm2 and sm3) are principally an indication for surgical resection, although sm2 cancers are technically resectable by EMR.

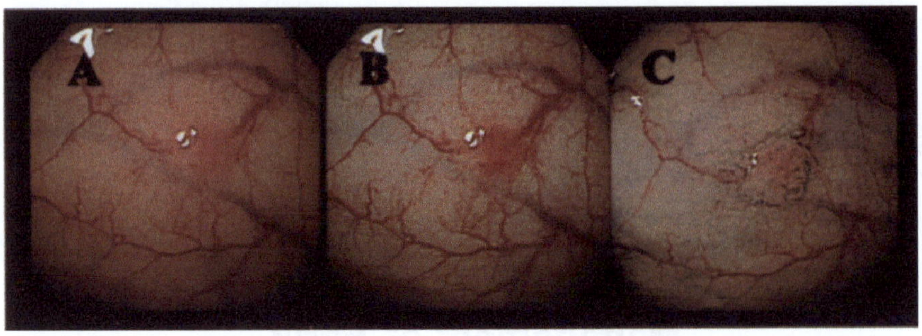

Fig. 1A–C. Color enhancement of electronic colonoscopic image. **A** Original image. **B** Color enhancement image. **C** Ordinary colonoscopic image after dye spraying

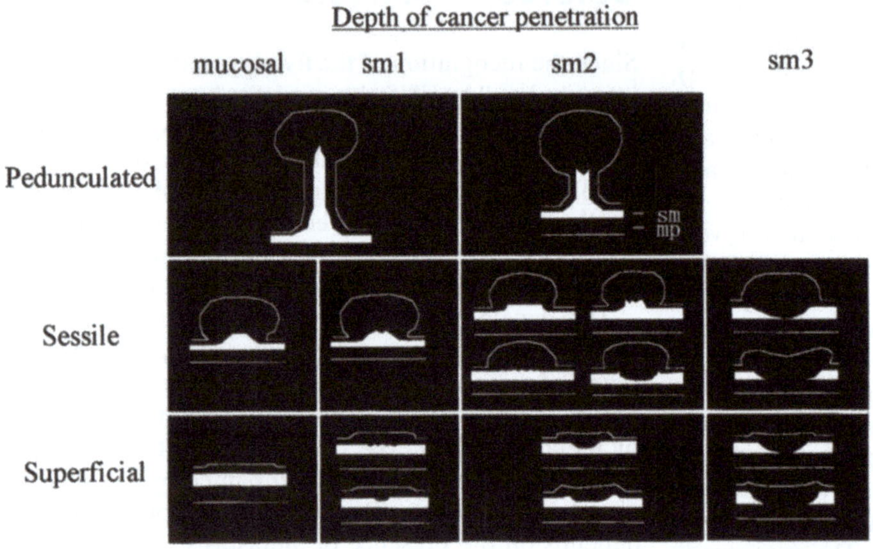

Fig. 2. Schema of endoscopic ultrasonography (EUS) images of early colorectal cancer in regard to the shape and the degree of invasion

The presence of sm-massive invasion can be suspected from ordinary endoscopic findings. They include submucosal tumor-like appearance, deep depression, fold convergence, restricted extensibility of the surrounding wall, and so on. However, the diagnosis is based on indirect information and is difficult if such characteristic findings are lacking.

3. Practical Aspects of Penetration Depth Diagnosis by EUS

By the use of EUS, cross-sectional images similar to histological ones and cancer invasion can be directly visualized. The recognition of the muscularis mucosae is still difficult even with a high-frequency instrument. Accordingly, the extent of sm invasion should be recognized in the context of the various patterns of the submucosal layer in EUS images (Figs. 2 and 3). The distribution of the submucosal layer varies according to the configuration of lesions. In pedunculated ones, the submucosal layer ascends through the stalk to the head portion. In sessile ones, the submucosal layer forms convexly toward the tumor. In superficial ones, the thickness of the submucosa is similar to that around the lesion. When the inner contour of the submucosa can be smoothly traced in EUS images, the lesion can be diagnosed as mucosal. When a defect of 1 mm or less is demonstrated, the penetration depth is diagnosed as sm1. When the continuity of the submucosa is hardly traced but the muscle layer is preserved, the diagnosis of sm3 is made. Intermediate findings suggest sm2 invasion. The diagnosis of penetration depth can be correctly diagnosed only when both the cross-sectional image perpendicular to the lesion and contiguous normal wall are obtained. If such information is not obtained, the examination is considered unsuccessful.

The results of EUS diagnosis of penetration depth in our series of early cancers are shown in Table 1. In determining the indication for EMR, it is necessary to discriminate lesions with invasion of sm1 or less and those with invasion of sm2 or more. The discrimination rate between these two categories is 78.2% with a 7.5 MHz echo-colonoscope and 87.7% with a 20 MHz miniature probe. When the subjects are restricted to the

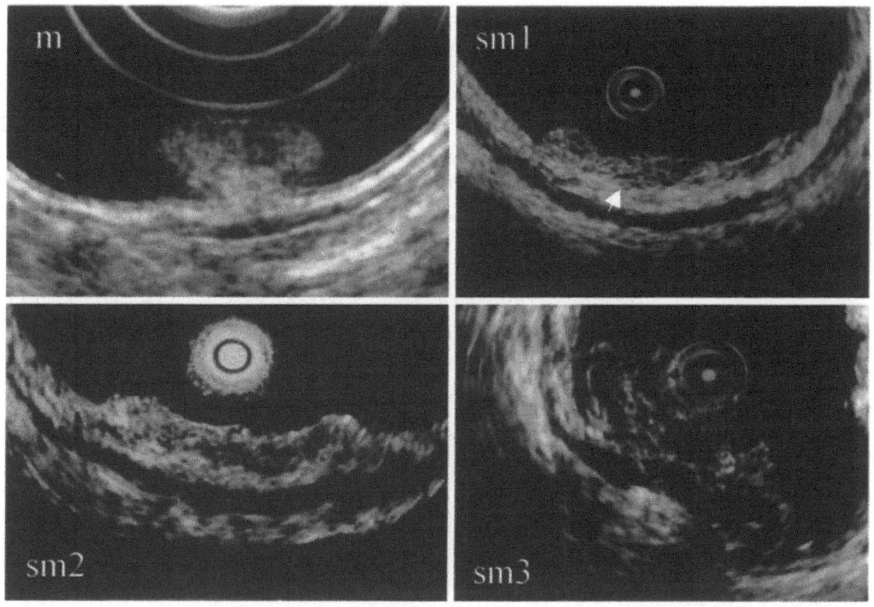

Fig. 3. Actual EUS images of each penetration depth

Table 1. Results of endoscopic ultrasonography (EUS) diagnosis in early colorectal cancers by a 7.5 MHz echo-colonoscope (CF-UM3/20, Olympus) and a 20 MHz miniature probe (UM-3R, Olympus)

Histology	EUS diagnosis						Discrimination between m/sm1 and sm2/sm3	
	m	sm1	sm2	sm3	mp	Failed	In total cases	In successful cases
A. Echo-colonoscope								
m ($n = 65$)	45	2	4	0	1	13	**72.3%**	**90.4%**
sm1 ($n = 10$)	6	2	1	0	0	1	**80.0%**	**88.9%**
sm2 ($n = 27$)	1	0	14	7	1	4	**81.5%**	**95.7%**
sm3 ($n = 22$)	0	0	0	19	1	2	**90.9%**	**100%**
Total ($n = 124$)	52	4	19	26	3	20	**78.2%**	**93.3%**
B. Miniature probe								
m ($n = 60$)	50	1	3	1	0	5	**85.0%**	**90.9%**
sm1 ($n = 10$)	1	5	3	0	0	1	**60.0%**	**66.7%**
sm2 ($n = 20$)	0	0	13	6	0	1	**95.0%**	**100%**
sm3 ($n = 24$)	0	0	0	22	2	0	**100%**	**100%**
Total ($n = 114$)	51	6	19	29	2	7	**87.7%**	**93.5%**

lesions successfully visualized, the rate becomes 93.3% and 93.5%, respectively. This means that both types of instrument have similar diagnostic capability per se, but the rate of successful visualization is superior with a miniature probe. The difference can be explained by the fact that the location of the ultrasound scanner can be more freely selected and that even a minute lesion can be observed endoscopically when using a miniature probe. Consequently, a miniature probe is considered more suitable for evaluating the depth of early cancers except for lesions with considerable thickness. Furthermore, a probe can be inserted through the forceps channel whenever necessary. Similar results have been reported by other investigators. [13] The accuracy rate is higher for superficial-type lesions than for protruded ones (Table 2).

When a discrepancy between the diagnosis by ordinary endoscopy and that by EUS occurs, the more confirmatory of the two modalities should be adopted. When these are properly combined, the diagnostic capability can be improved; the accuracy rate is 93.0% when ordinary endoscopy is combined with a miniature probe, and 88.7% with an echo-colonoscope (Table 3).

Misdiagnoses by EUS derive from various reasons. The factors that influence the diagnosis include the shape, thickness, location of the lesion, presence of vessels, and inflammatory reactions. The taller and thicker a lesion, the more difficult it is to be properly

Table 2. Results of EUS diagnosis with a miniature probe in regard to the shape of early colorectal cancer

Shape of lesion	EUS diagnosis (miniature probe)			Accuracy in successful cases
	Correct	Incorrect	Failed	
Pedunculated ($n = 12$)	10 (83.3%)	0	2 (16.7%)	100%
Semipedunculated ($n = 19$)	16 (84.2%)	1 (5.3%)	2 (10.5%)	94.1%
Sessile ($n = 25$)	20 (80.0%)	3 (12.0%)	2 (8.0%)	87.0%
Superficial ($n = 41$)	38 (92.7%)	3 (7.3%)	0	92.7%
Others ($n = 17$)	16 (94.1%)	0	1 (5.9%)	94.1%
Total ($n = 114$)	100 (87.7%)	7 (6.1%)	12 (10.5%)	93.5%

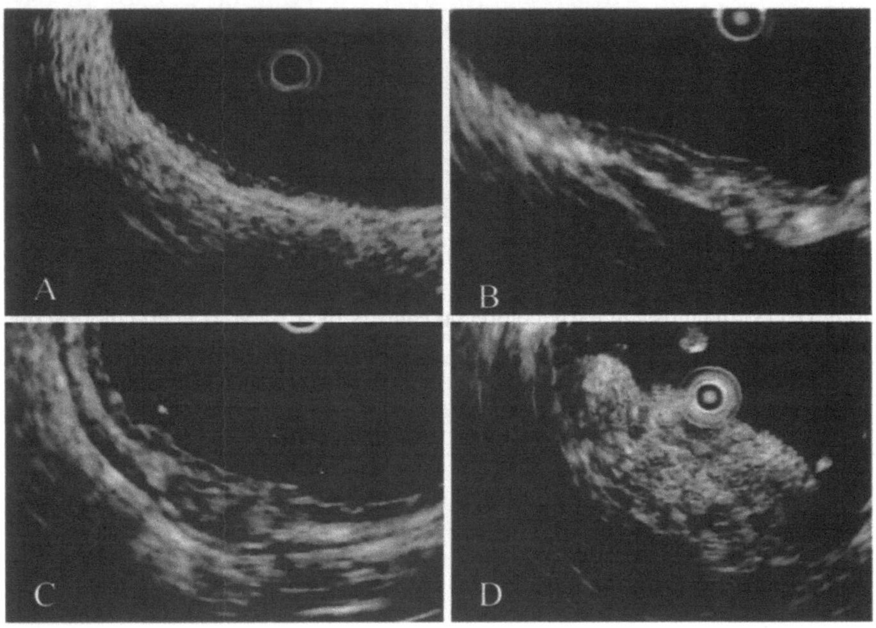

Fig. 4A–D. Correlation between EUS and histology. **A** Lymph follicle. **B** Signet-ring cell carcinoma. **C** Invasion with lymphoid stroma. **D** Mucinous transformation at invasion front

Table 3. Comparison of the diagnostic accuracy between ordinary endoscopy and EUS with a miniature probe

Ordinary colonoscopy	EUS diagnosis (miniature probe)			
	Correct	Incorrect	Failed	Total
Correct	88 (77.2%)	2 (1.8%)	3 (2.6%)	93 (81.6%)
Incorrect	6 (5.3%)	3 (2.6%)	0	9 (7.9%)
Failed	7 (6.1%)	2 (1.8%)	3 (2.6%)	12 (10.5%)
Total	101 (88.6%)	7 (6.1%)	6 (5.3%)	114 (100%)

delineated by EUS. Lesions existing at a flexure or on a fold are also difficult to delineate. The presence of fibrosis and leukocyte aggregation is often the cause of overestimation. In interpreting EUS images, it should be noted that a greater percentage of overstaging than understaging is observed.

Further information derived from EUS concerns the estimation of histology from EUS images (Fig. 4). For example, a small round to oval hypoechoic area often corresponds to a lymph follicle. A larger one may be signet-ring cell carcinoma or invasion with lymphoid stroma; the latter condition is accompanied by a heterogeneous internal structure. Multiple, round, speckled hypoechoic areas may correspond to mucinous transformation. Submucosal fibrosis irrelevant to cancer invasion is visualized as a vague hypoechoic area.

For lesions that can be easily diagnosed as mucosal lesion by ordinary endoscopy, there is no need for EUS. When sm-massive invasion cannot be excluded, EUS should be supplemented. When properly used, EUS is considered a useful tool to evaluate the resectability and curability of early colorectal cancers by EMR.

References

1. Kudo S, Tamura S, Nakajima T, et al (1995) Depressed type of colorectal cancer. Endoscopy 27:54–57
2. Tada M, Kawai K (1986) Research with the endoscope—new techniques using magnification and chromoscopy. Clin Gastroenterol 15:417–437

3. Kudo S, Tamura S, Nakajima T, et al (1996) Diagnosis of colorectal tumorous lesions by magnifying endoscopy. Gastrointest Endosc 44:8–14
4. Mitooka H, Fujimori T, Ohno S, et al (1992) Chromoscopy of the colon using indigocarmine dye with electrolyte lavage solution. Gastrointest Endosc 38:1421–1423
5. Shimizu S (2002) Color enhancement in colonoscopy may be effective for detection of superficial type colorectal tumors. Dig Endosc 14(S1):S62–S64
6. Shimizu S, Tada M, Kawai K (1990) Use of endoscopic ultrasonography for the diagnosis of colorectal tumors. Endoscopy 22:31–34
7. Rosch T, Lorenz R, Classen M (1990) Endoscopic ultrasonography in the evaluation of colon and rectal disease. Gastrointest Endosc 36(suppl 2):S33–S39
8. Shimizu S, Ohtsuka H, Iso A, et al (1989) Preliminary study on the application of a miniature ultrasonic probe for diagnosis of colorectal tumors. J Kyoto Pref Med 98: 1239–1246
9. Martin RW, Silverstein FE, Kimmey MB (1990) Endoscopic ultrasound probes. Gastrointest Endosc 36:40–46
10. Karita M, Tada M, Okita K, et al (1991) Endoscopic therapy for early colon cancer: the strip biopsy resection technique. Gastrointest Endosc 37:128–132
11. Kudo S (1993) Endoscopic mucosal resection of flat and depressed types of early colorectal cancer. Endoscopy 25: 4554–4561
12. Tanaka S, Haruma K, Oh-e H, et al (2000) Conditions of curability after endoscopic resection for colorectal carcinoma with submucosally massive invasion. Oncol Rep 7: 783–788
13. Saito Y, Obara T, Einami K, et al (1996) Efficacy of high-frequency ultrasound probes for the preoperative staging of invasion depth in flat and depressed colorectal tumors. Gastrointest Endosc 44:34–39

3. Esophageal Cancer

Yoko Murata, Masahiko Ohta, Kazuhiko Hayashi, Yoko Hoshino, Yukiko Takayama, Shinichi Nakamura, and Atsushi Mitsunaga

1. How to Detect Early Esophageal Cancer

1.1 What Is Early Esophageal Cancer?

In 2517 cases of superficial esophageal cancer analyzed in Japan, 287 (11.4%) were intraepithelial cancer, 439 (17.4%) were cancer invading the lamina propria or cancer invading the muscularis mucosae, and 1791 (71.2%) were cancer invading the submucosa. Lymph node metastasis comprised 0% for epithelial cancer, 8.7% for cancer invading the lamina propria or the muscularis mucosae, and 36.5% for cancer invading the submucosa [1]. Following these results, in 1999 the definition of early esophageal cancer changed from cancer invading the submucosa to mucosal cancer without lymph node metastasis according to the Japanese Society of Esophageal Disease [2]. Cancer limited to the submucosa was redefined as superficial cancer [2]. This definition appeared practical, because patients with mucosal cancer had a better survival rate, 96.9% for Tis and 91.9% for cancer invading the lamina propria, compared with 66.9% for patients who had cancer invading the submucosa [3]. Therefore, the early stage of esophageal cancer should be defined as cancer limited to the mucosa.

1.2 Classification of the Depth of Cancer Invasion

While the number of mucosal cancers is increasing and resected materials have been analyzed, there are different rates of lymph node metastasis and lymphatic invasion according to the depth of invasion [4]. The rate of lymph node metastasis of cancer limited to the epithelium (m1) is 0%, of cancer invading the lamina propria (m2) 3.3%, of cancer reaching the muscularis mucosae (m3) 12%, of cancer slightly invading the submucosa (sm1) 14%, of cancer invading further than the middle of the submucosa (sm2) 35.8%, and of cancer reaching the proper muscle (sm3) 45.9% [4]. The rates of lymphatic invasion and blood vessel invasion of m1 were 1.0% and 0.3%, of m2 6.5% and 0.4%, of m3 23.1% and 4.3%, of sm1 40.7% and 12.9%, and of sm2,3 52.8%, 67.3% and 22.2%, 32.9%, respectively [4]. Thus, m1 and m2 had a low rate of lymph node metastasis and lymphatic and vessel invasion, so that local treatments such as mucosal resection via endoscopy could be introduced; m3 and sm1 had a low rate of lymph node metastasis but a high rate of lymphatic invasion, so that cases without lymph node swelling could be selected for local treatments, and after lymphatic invasion was recognized in the resected specimen chemotherapy could be performed; while sm2,3 had a high rate of lymph node metastasis so that surgical operation with lymph node dissection could be recommended.

1.3 Symptoms of Early Esophageal Cancer: Detection of Early Esophageal Cancer in Japan

Clinically, in 500 cases of mucosal cancer 56.4% of patients with superficial cancer were asymptomatic, 6.8% of patients had retrosternal pain, and 9% had feelings of stenosis, some involving foreign body sensation, dysphagia, nausea, and so on [3]. Sixty-eight percent of patients had no symptoms or unrelated complaints, and only 37% of cancers were detected based on symptoms [3]. Nabeya reported that 100% of Tis cancers and 44% of mucosal cancers were detected by mass screening or physical checkup [1] and 62% of cancers invading the submucosa were detected based on symptoms. Kodama and Kakegawa also reported that 55% of patients with superficial cancer were asymptomatic [4]. Regarding the detection method, 91% of Tis cancers and 64% of mucosal cancers were detected by endoscopy, but 76% of cancers invading the submucosa were detected by upper gastrointestinal tract X-ray. Koyama reported that m1–m2 cancer that has already been diagnosed by endoscopy can be detected by esophagography in 27% of cases by inexperienced doctors and in 68% of cases by experienced doctors [5]. Most cases of mucosal cancer were asymptomatic and were detected incidentally by endoscopy at the second stage of mass screening or physical checkup. (People are persuaded to have an endoscopic examination when abnormal lesions in the stomach are detected by X-ray examination at the first stage of mass screening.) On the other hand, most cancers invading the submucosa could be detected by X-ray examination.

1.4 Which Active Methods Can Detect Early Esophageal Cancer?

Methods of early esophageal cancer detection in a high-risk group, involving factors such as being more than 55 years of age, of male sex, having a habit of smoking and drinking, having head and neck cancer (esophageal cancer found in 11.8% of patients) [6], achalasia, lye esophagitis, and Barrett's esophagus have been recommended. Endoscopic examination followed by iodine staining has been performed for patients in a high-risk group. Endoscopy followed by iodine staining has a major role in the diagnosis of mucosal cancer. Miyaji et al. reported that esophageal cancer was found in 12.7% of patients with head and neck cancer [7]. Therefore, patients in a high-risk group should undergo endoscopic examination including iodine staining during mass screening.

1.5 Which Endoscopic Findings are Indicative of Early Esophageal Cancer?

First of all, careful examination of the esophagus is necessary when the endoscope is inserted into and withdrawn from the esophagus; the esophageal wall should not be extended too much, while close observation during esophageal movement is also important. Extremely small abnormalities, such as change of color, redness (Fig. 1), abnormal vessels, translucent area, whitish area (Fig. 2), slightly depressed (Fig. 3) and elevated lesions (Fig. 2), granular or rough surface, should be checked and iodine staining performed. For iodine staining, 1.5%–2% iodine solution should be sprayed into the whole esophagus. Esophageal cancer, dysplasia, esophagitis, acanthosis, hyperkeratosis, ulcer, erosion, gastric mucosa, and columnar epithelium lacking glycogen, are not stained by iodine. The size of the unstained

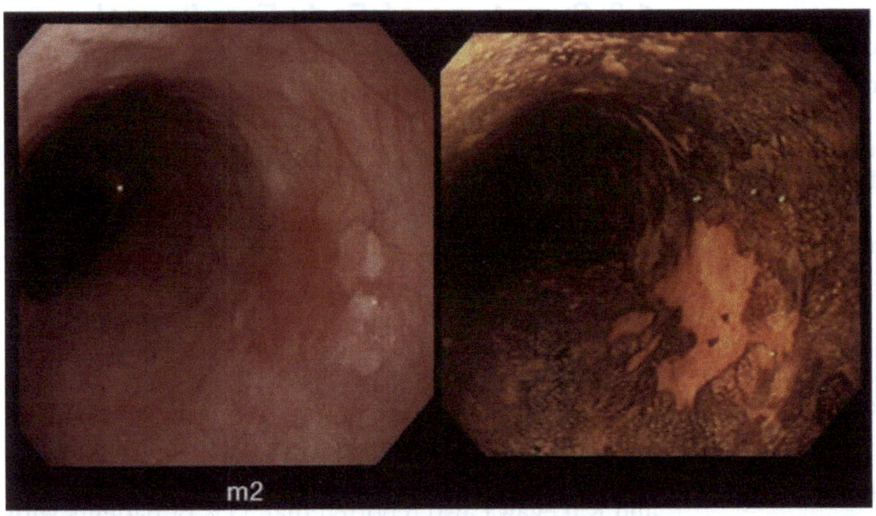

Fig. 1. Type 0–IIc+IIa. A slight depression with redness and slightly whitish elevated lesion is not stained by iodine

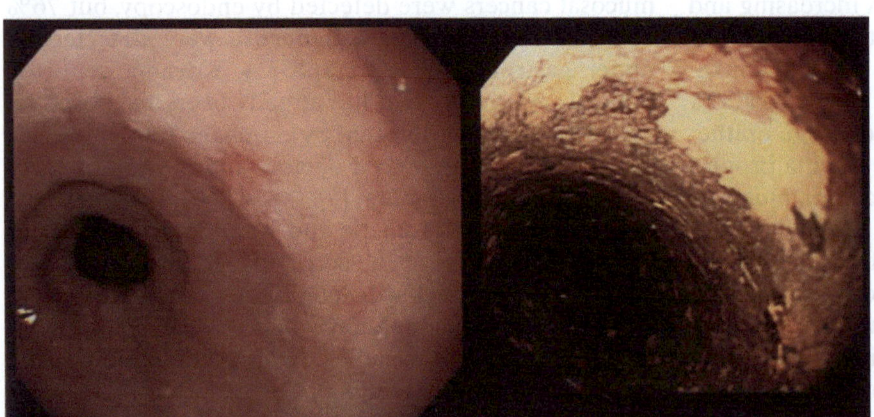

Fig. 2. Type 0–IIa. A slightly elevated and whitish lesion is not stained by iodine

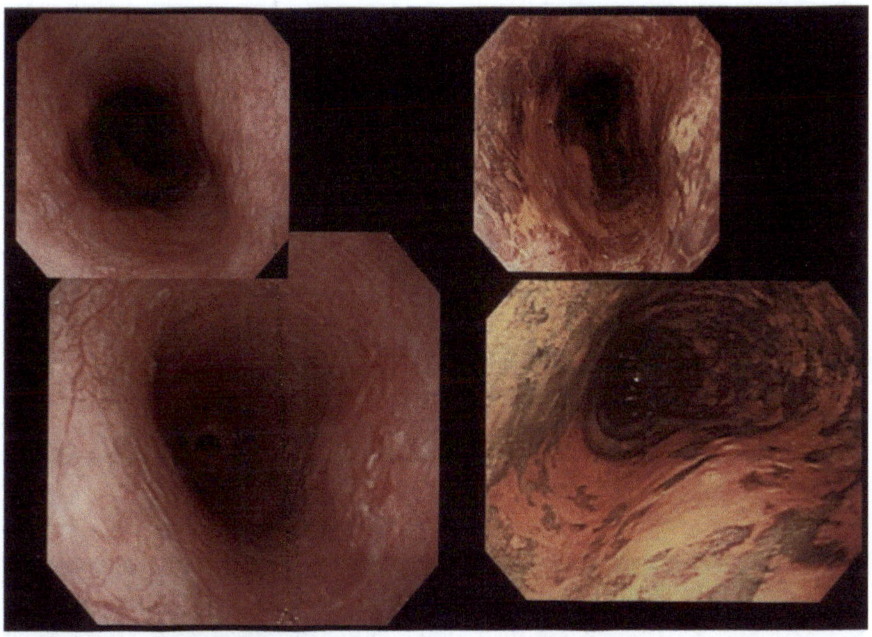

Fig. 3. Type 0–IIc. A slight depression with flat surface is not stained by iodine. There are two lesions in this case

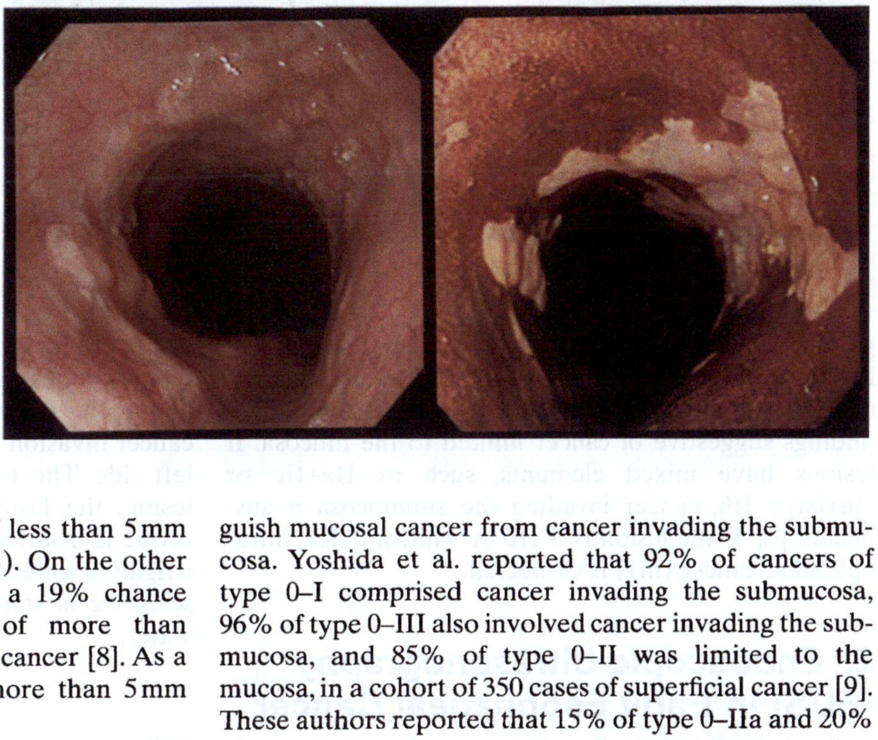

Fig. 4. Type 0–I. A nodular protruding tumor is not stained by iodine

area is important: an unstained area of less than 5 mm has a lower probability of cancer (10%). On the other hand, a 6–10-mm unstained area has a 19% chance of cancer and an unstained area of more than 10 mm has a more than 55% chance of cancer [8]. As a consequence, any unstained area of more than 5 mm should be biopsied.

1.6 Determination of the Depth of Cancer Invasion by Endoscopy

It is helpful to classify the macroscopic type of a lesion, such as protruding type (0–I) (Fig. 4), slightly elevated (0–IIa) (Fig. 2), flat (0–IIb) (Fig. 5), slightly depressed (0–IIc) (Fig. 3), and excavated type (0–III), to distinguish mucosal cancer from cancer invading the submucosa. Yoshida et al. reported that 92% of cancers of type 0–I comprised cancer invading the submucosa, 96% of type 0–III also involved cancer invading the submucosa, and 85% of type 0–II was limited to the mucosa, in a cohort of 350 cases of superficial cancer [9]. These authors reported that 15% of type 0–IIa and 20% of type 0–IIc were cancers invading the submucosa, but all of type 0–IIb were mucosal cancers. Therefore, lesions with protruded or excavated factors relate to cancer invading the submucosa, while superficial lesions associated with color changes tend to be mucosal cancer. Among types 0–IIa and 0–IIc, 15%–20% invade the submucosa. Regarding 0–IIa lesions, diagnostic points indicative of mucosal cancer are a height of the elevated elements of less than 2 mm, a shape that is

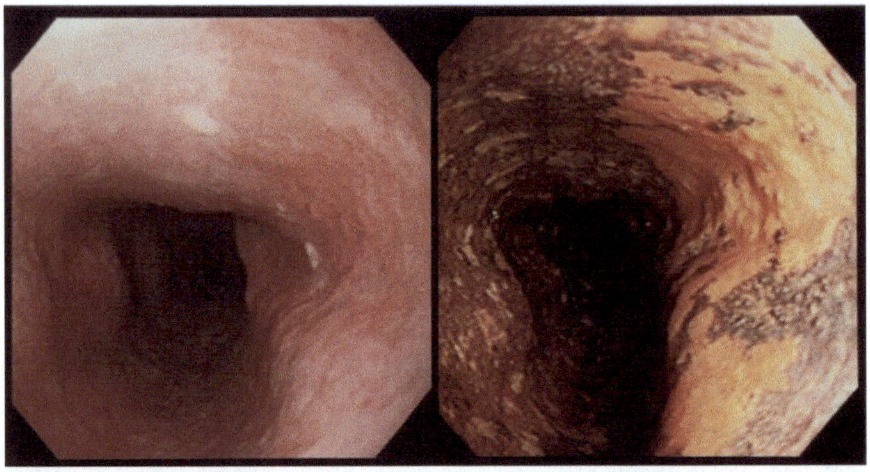

Fig. 5. Type 0–IIb. A slightly red, flat area is not stained by iodine

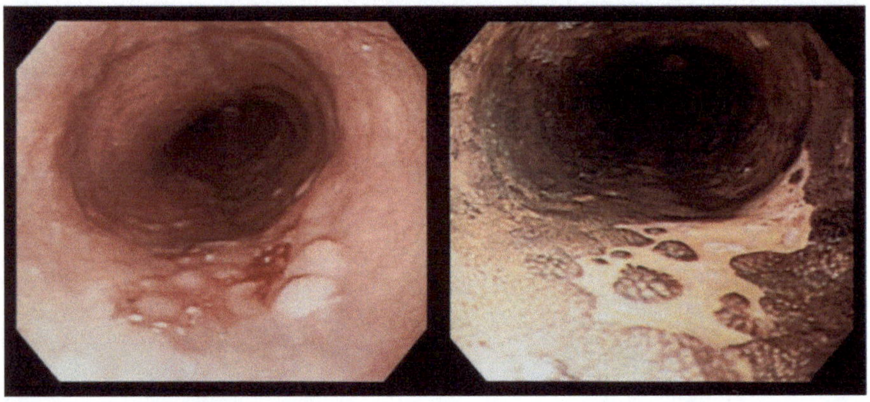

Fig. 6. Type 0–IIc. A slight depression with granular surface is not stained by iodine

granular but not nodular, and a whitish color of the lesion. In 0–IIc lesions, the abscence of a wall and a flat (Fig. 3) or granular (Fig. 6) surface with no nodule are findings suggestive of cancer limited to the mucosa. If lesions have mixed elements, such as IIa+IIc or IIa+large IIb, cancer invading the submucosa is suspected [4]. If the lesion is 0–IIb or whitish 0–IIa, intraepithelial cancer (m1) is suspected.

2. Endoscopic Ultrasonography (EUS) in Early Esophageal Cancer

2.1 What Is the Role of EUS? How to Use EUS

The role of endoscopic ultrasonography (EUS) is not only to determine the depth of cancer invasion but also to detect lymph nodes. Several ultrasonic probes have been developed. Catheter-type probes (30 or 20 MHz, 2.6–2.4 mm in diameter) have been introduced for the diagnosis of superficial esophageal invasion. Conventional probes (7.5 MHz, 12 MHz) are used for detecting lymph nodes in the posterior mediastium and the abdomen. The method of determining the depth of cancer invasion involves the patient lying on his or her left side. The two-channel scope is inserted near the lesion, the lesion is observed, and the catheter-type probe is inserted through the channel while a tube of irrigating water is passed through the other channel. The scanning is started when the lesion is submerged in water.

2.2 Normal Esophageal Wall Structure

The normal esophageal wall is delineated as a structure of nine layers: the 1st and 2nd layer (1, 2/9) comprise the epithelium, and the 3rd (3/9) is the lamina propria. The 4th layer (4/9), the hypoechoic layer, is the muscularis mucosae which is important in distinguishing between cancer involving the lamina propria and cancer invading deeper than the muscularis mucosae. The 5th layer (5/9), the hyperechoic layer, is the submucosa, the

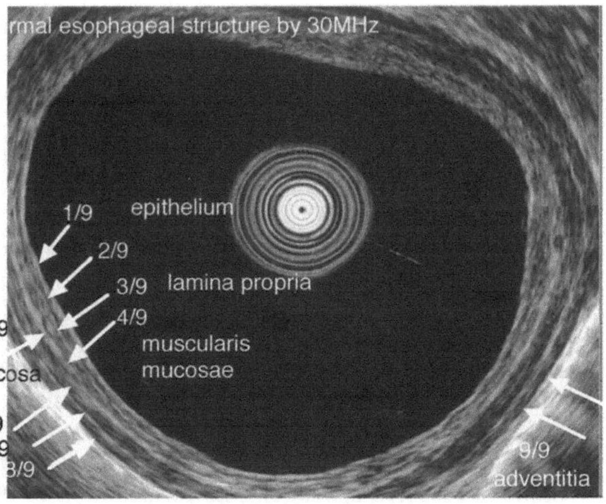

Fig. 7. Normal esophageal wall structure. The 1st and 2nd layers (*1,2/9*) are the epithelium, the 3rd (*3/9*) is the lamina propria, the 4th (*4/9*) is the muscularis mucosae, the 5th (*5/9*) is the submucosa, from the 6th (*6/9*) to the 8th (*8/9*) are the muscularis propria, and the 9th (*9/9*) is the adventitia

6th (6/9) to the 8th (8/9) are the muscularis propria, and the 9th (9/9) is the adventitia (Fig. 7) [10].

2.3 Determination of the Depth of Cancer Invasion: Extent of Accuracy

The depth of cancer invasion can be determined by observing which layers are destroyed or remain normal.

m1: The tumor is limited to the 1st (1/9) and the 2nd (2/9) layers (Fig. 8).
m2: The tumor invades a part of the 3rd layer (3/9); however, the 4th layer (4/9) is preserved under the tumor (Fig. 9).
T1-m3–sm1: The tumor destroys the 4th layer, but the 5th layer (5/9) is preserved under the tumor.
T1-sm2,3: The tumor destroys a part of or whole of the 5th layer, and the 6th layer (6/9) is preserved.

In 113 patients with superficial esophageal cancer, EUS was performed and histological findings were compared with EUS findings. Regarding determination of the depth of cancer invasion, accuracy for m1 was 38%, for m2 95%, for m3 and sm1 62%, and for sm2,3 86%. The overall accuracy was 75%, and the accuracy for determining invasion of less than m2 was 95% (Table 1). Fukuda et al. reported that the accuracy of distinguishing m and sm was 85% [11]. m1 was overestimated as m2 because lymph follicles or lymphocyte infiltration in the lamina propria, which are also observed as hypoechoic areas, made it difficult to diagnose cancer invasion correctly. After the introduction of 30 MHz EUS the muscularis mucosae could be clearly delineated, resulting in an increased accuracy.

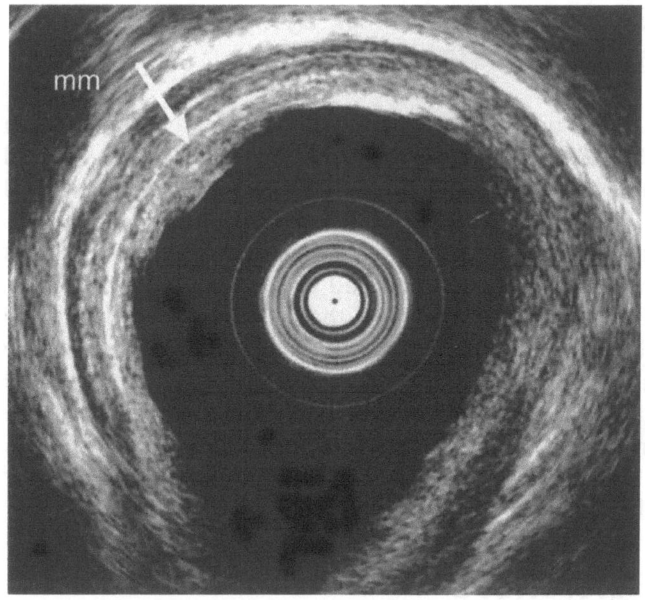

Fig. 8. Cancer limited to the epithelium (m1): *Tis*. The tumor is limited to the 1st (1/9) and the 2nd (2/9) layers (*arrow*)

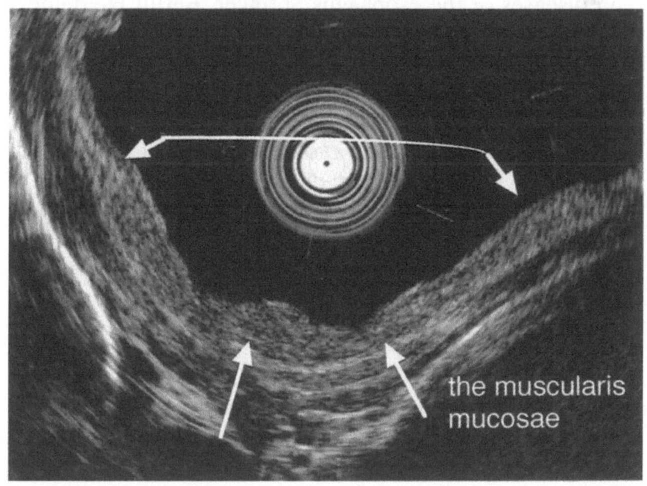

Fig. 9. Cancer invading the lamina propria (m2). The tumor is invading a part of the 3rd layer (3/9); however, the 4th layer (4/9) is preserved under the tumor

Table 1. Relationship between endoscopic ultrasonography (EUS) findings and histologic results in esophageal cancer

EUS findings	Histology			
	Tis	T1lpm	T1mm–sm1	T1sm2,3
Tis	5	1		
T1lpm	8	12		1
T1 mm–sm1		1	8	1
T1sm2,3		3	5	60
T2				8
	5/13	12/17	8/13	60/70
	38%	71%	62%	86%
Overall accuracy				85/113 (75%)
Determination of cancer limited to the lamina propria:				108/113 (95%)

2.4 Determination of Lymph Node Metastasis

Lymph nodes more than 3 mm in diameter located in the posterior mediastium, around the celiac axis, and near the stomach can be delineated by conventional EUS (12 or 7.5 MHz). Endoscopic ultrasonography findings of metastasis were compared with histological results in patients who had undergone a thoracotomy. The sensitivity was 90%, the specificity was 51%, and the overall accuracy was 75%. Since EUS fine-needle aspiration cytology (EUS-FNA) has been performed safely and the accuracy of EUS-FNA for lymph node metastasis has been reported to be around 83%–96% [12], suspected positive lymph nodes in mucosal cancer should be confirmed using EUS-FNA.

References

1. Nabeya K (1993) Early carcinoma of the esophagus. In: Nabeya K, Hanaoka T, Nogami H (eds) Recent advances in diseases of the esophagus Springer, Berlin Heidelbery New York Tokyo, 1993, pp 375–380
2. Japanese Society for Esophageal Diseases (1999) Guide lines for the clinical and pathologic studies on carcinoma of the esophagus. 9th edn. Kanehara, Tokyo
3. Endo M, Yoshino K, Kawano T, et al (1992) Clinical evaluation of mucosal cancer of the esophagus: analysis of 1583 cases of superficial esophageal resected in Japan. In: Nabeya, et al (eds) Diseases of the esophagus. Springer-Verlag, Tokyo, pp 540–545
4. Kodama M, Kakegawa T (1998) Treatment of superficial cancer of esophagus: a summary of responses to questionnaire on superficial cancer of the esophagus in Japan. Surgery 123:432–439
5. Oyama T, Hotta K, Shimaya S, et al (2001) Is esophagography useful for the diagnosis of superficial esophageal cancer? Endosc Dig 13:29–32
6. Makuuchi H, Machimura T, Shimada H, et al (1996) Endoscopic screening for esophageal cancer in 788 patients with head and neck cancers. Tokai Exp Clin Med 21:139–145
7. Miyaji M, Makuuchi H, et al (eds) (1997) Handbook for early esophageal cancer. Chugai Medical, Tokyo, pp 48–47
8. Ide H, Itabashi M (1991) Application of the staining technique in resected specimens: its contribution to the diagnosis of mucosal cancer and slight pathological changes of the mucosa. In: Endo M, Ide H (eds) Endoscopic staining in early diagnosis of esophageal cancer. Japan Scientific Societies Press, Tokyo, pp 47–65
9. Yoshida M, Momma K, Hanashi T, et al (2001) Endoscopic evaluation of depth of cancer invasion in cancer with superficial esophageal cancer. Stomach Intest 36: 295–306
10. Murata Y, Suzuki S, Ohta M, et al (1996) Small ultrasonic probes for determination of the depth of superficial esophageal cancer. Gastrointest Endosc 44:23–28
11. Fukuda M, Hirata K, Natori H (2000) Endoscopic ultrasonography of the esophagus. World J Surg 24: 216–218
12. Barawai M, Gress F (2000) EUS-guided fine-needle aspiration in the mediastinum. Gastrointestinal Endosc 52(Suppl 6):12–17

4. Gastrointestinal Tract Cancer in Europe

Matatoshi Dohmoto

1. Introduction

In this chapter the clinical differences in the diagnosis and endoscopic treatment of gastrointestinal tract carcinoma between Europe and Japan are reviewed.

There is a still little interest in early gastric cancer in Europe today because the frequency is low. Therefore, endoscopic mucosal resection (EMR) and endoscopic submucosal dissection (ESD) methods have not yet become common. So-called EMR methods such as snare EMR, EAM (endoscopic aspiration mucosectomy) and EMR-L (endoscopic mucosal resection using ligation device) as well as associated instruments such as flex [1], hook [2], insulated tip (IT) [3], and triangle-knife [4] are not yet well known.

There is little detection of early cancer in Europe due to the fact that the incidence of gastric cancer is low, and screening examinations for gastric cancer detection are not widespread (Soehendra N, Grund KE, personal communications, 2005). Therefore this field of study is not so active in Europe, and diagnosis of early cancer and endoscopic treatment are not considered paramount.

A suspicious finding on radiological examination necessitates an endoscopic biopsy in any case. X-ray detection of early gastric cancer is not common, however, in consideration of radiation exposure to the X-rays.

On average, 3–9 cases of early gastric cancer per year were diagnosed in five hospitals in Germany and Austria where EMR was performed (Grund KE, Tuebingen; Kaehler GFBA, Mannheim; Hagenmueller F, Hamburg-Altona; Heinermann PM, Salzburg; Soehendra N, Hamburg, personal communications, 2005). The average mortality for gastric cancer (1995–2000) of the 16 developed countries in Europe is very low (12.2 per 100000 population, compared with Japan, 39.8/100000) (Ministry of Health in Japan, Labor and Welfare 2001). This might be the main reason the number of diagnoses and use of endoscopic treatment for early gastric cancer have not increased in Europe.

According to recent research carried out in Japan, most (90%) early cancers are less than 3 cm [5] and the probability of lymph node metastasis of early gastric cancer is 3% for intramucosal carcinoma and 20% for submucous carcinoma [6].

As mentioned elsewhere in this book, the Japanese Gastric Cancer Association proposes indications for en bloc resection by EMR for patients with a low risk of lymph node metastasis as summarized in Table 1. However, there are some of examples of EMR and ESD for early cancers of more than 2 cm [7–9] and for undifferentiated carcinoma [3, 10], which have been reported from Japan. An EMR of an esophageal tumor of 45 mm [11], colorectal tumors larger than 45 mm [12, 13] and a large gastric tumor (130 mm) [14] have also been reported.

2. Diagnosis

A cancer checkup of the digestive tract is rarely paid for by health insurance in Europe. Payment of endoscopic—and X-ray—examinations of a patient without symptoms is difficult. For men older than 50 years in Austria, endoscopic examination is possible once every 5 years (Heinermann PM, personal communication, 2004).

In European hospitals routine chromoscopy, and magnification endoscopy as a routine is still limited [15]. Magnification endoscopy is not yet performed routinely in Japan either.

X-ray examination of the colon and colonoscopy have been done frequently since the advent of the hemo-occult test. Thereby colorectal tumors can be detected at an early stage with consequent reduction in the mortality of colorectal cancer [16–18].

The incidence of colorectal cancer in a control group (856 cases, 11% stage A) was 144 per 100000 population—years in the Nottingham area of the U.K. The median follow-up was 7.8 years. Three hundred and sixty people died from colorectal cancer in the screening group compared with 420 in the control group, i.e., a 15% reduction in cumulative colorectal cancer mortality in the screening group (odds ratio = 0.85 [95% confidence interval 0.74–0.98]) [16] .

There is a higher frequency of colon cancer in Europeans than in Japanese. The Japanese classification of gastric carcinoma is well known as an endoscopic image classification. However, only a few doctors use this classification in their findings. Whether an early cancer or an advanced cancer exists is chiefly diagnosed based on pathology.

Regarding endoscopic diagnosis, a general framework for the endoscopic classification of superficial neoplastic

Table 1. Indications for endoscopic mucosal resection according to the Japanese Gastric Cancer Association guideline [31]

Principals: Tumor with a low risk of lymph node metastasis
Reasonable tumor size and location for one-piece resection

Qualified conditions:
- Differentiated M ca.
- Less than 2 cm in size regardless of macroscopic type
- Without ulcer findings

Expanded indications:
- Differentiated M ca. UL(−), no limit of tumor size
- Differentiated M ca. UL(+) <3 cm
- Differentiated SM1 (<500 µm) ca. <3 cm
- Undifferentiated M ca. UL(−) <2 cm (priority to an operation)

Contraindication:
Operation indication:
Cancers not fulfilling the above conditions after histopathological diagnosis

M ca.: mucosal adenocarcinoma, UL: ulcer or ulcer scar, SM1: superficial submucosal penetration

lesions of the esophagus, stomach, and colon was suggested by the Paris Endoscopic Workshop of 2002 [19].

If specified appearances of superficial neoplastic lesions are used more generally by endoscopists, an improvement in detection rates can be expected.

3. Pathology

Gastrointestinal lesions considered to be high-grade adenoma or dysplasia by Western pathologists using the conventional Western classification are often diagnosed as carcinoma by Japanese pathologists using the Japanese group classification [20]. This may also contribute to the relatively high incidence and good prognosis of gastric carcinoma in Japan when compared with Western countries [21]. To overcome these diagnostic differences, the Padova classification [22], the Vienna classification, and a revision of the Vienna classification have recently been proposed [20]. However, the newly proposed classifications should be used with caution for biopsy specimens, as sampling error may result in an underestimation of the neoplastic grade or depth of invasion [20].

4. EMR Methods

Endoscopic aspiration mucosectomy (EAM), EMRL (endoscopic mucosal resection using ligation device), and the snare method are the mainstream EMR techniques used Europe. Roesch et al. [23] reported endoscopic en bloc resection with IT knives.

Lambert has reported the technique of EMR with an injection into the submucosa to lift the lesion for either cup and aspiration method, or tissue incision with a needle knife [24], but EMR with a hook-knife, flexknife, IT knife, or triangle knife has as yet hardly been reported.

Seewald et al. reported piecemeal EMR by using a simple polypectomy snare without submucosal injection for Barrett's epithelium with early-stage malignant changes. No recurrence, no serious complication, and two strictures were observed [25].

5. Discussion

Preoperative macroscopic endoscopic findings and biopsy diagnosis may lead to suspicion of early cancer. Because early cancer is defined as invasion not reaching the muscularis propria, the final diagnosis is entrusted to pathological examination of the resected lesion [26, 27]. Diagnosis by endoscopic ultrasonography is not considered to be obligatory.

In Europe the average mortality of gastric cancer among the 16 developed European countries is just 12.2 people per 100 000 population (1995–2000), whereas it is more than three times higher (39.8/100 000) in Japan (2001). This is probably the main reason why the number of diagnoses and endoscopic treatments of early gastric cancer have not increased in Europe.

In Europe it is not a common procedure to detect early cancer by a screening examination for gastric and colon cancer, which on the other hand is regularly provided to people more than 40 years old in Japan. However, in Europe circumferential EMR in Barrett's esophagus with high-grade intraepithelial neoplasia has been reported [25, 28, 29] much more often than in Japan where a frequent cancer checkup is available. Furthermore, massive hiatus hernia and Barrett's epithelium are observed daily on endoscopic examination in Europe (author's personal observations).

EMR of early neoplasia in Barrett's esophagus is carried out mainly in Europe. Excision specimens of early neoplasia in Barrett's esophagus were pathologically inspected by Vieth et al. for submucosal invasion, low- or high-grade intraepithelial neoplasia, and infiltration of blood vessels and lymph ducts [28].

More residue and recurrences may occur after piecemeal resection than after en bloc resection [9, 30]. Therefore, the latter is preferred to the former.

In Japan, complete resection is diagnosed from an en bloc resection specimen. Because there is much piecemeal resection in Europe, complete excision is confirmed from the abscission surfaces. On the other hand, a great merit of piecemeal resection is that fewer complications arise than for en bloc excision.

Follow-up of the patient after surgery is not easy in Europe, because for postoperative observation the patient depends mainly on his general practitioner (home doctor). Without doubt the system of health insurance is partially the cause for this situation.

For the choice between endoscopic and surgical therapy, determination of the depth of infiltration by endoscopic ultrasound is essential. In contrast to a surgical operation, endoscopic methods can lower the cost of therapy as well as the rate of morbidity and mortality. However, the endoscopist must consider the possibility of residual disease and recurrence when using EMR and ESD methods for early-stage cancer.

On the whole it does not seem that EMR methods with current instruments can be considered definitive (Soehendra, personal communication, 2004). Regarding complications and suffering of the patient, it will be necessary to review the results of EMR and ESD that involve an especially long time (>1 h) and extensive resection (>5 cm).

References

1. Yahagi N, Fujishiro M, Kakushima N, et al (2002) EMR procedure using an electro surgical snare (thin type). Shokakinaishikyo (Endoscopia Digestiva) 14:187–192
2. Oyama T (2000) Selection of EMR method for esophageal cancer. Shokakinaishikyo (Endoscopia Digestiva) 12:718–719
3. Ono H, Gotoda T, Yamaguchi H, et al (1999) A new method of EMR using an insulation tipped diathermic knife. Shokakinaishikyo (Endoscopia Digestiva) 11: 675–681
4. Sato Y, Inoue H, Furuta T (2003) A New method of EMR using a triangle tip knife. Gastrointest Endosc 45(Suppl 1):531
5. Doi T, Endo H, Hirasaki S, et al (2001) Evaluation from viewpoint of residual and locally recurrent cancer after EMR treatment for early gastric cancer. Rinshohshokakinaika 16:1657–1662
6. Gotoda T, Sasako M, Yanagawa A, et al (2000) Incidence of lymph node metastasis from early gastric cancer—estimation with a large number of cases at two large centers. Gastric Cancer 3:219
7. Inoue H, Sato Y, Kasawa T, et al (2004) Endoscopic mucosa resection using a triangle tip knife. Stomach Intestine 39:53–56
8. Kumai K (2004) Indication of endoscopic submucosal dissection for early gastroenterological cancer: advantages and disadvantages. Endoscopia Digestiva 16:703–708
9. Oyama T, Kikuchi Y, Shimaya S, et al (2002) Endoscopic mucosal resection using a hooking knife. Stomach Intestine 37:1155–1161
10. Fujii K, Ishiguro S, Mano M, et al (2002) Indication for endoscopic mucosal resection (EMR) of undifferentiated type early gastric carcinoma—from a pathological viewpoint. Stomach Intestine 37:1181–1188.
11. Oyama T, Kikuchi Y, Tomori A, et al (2001) Endoscopic mucosa resection using hooking knife for esophageal early cancer. Endoscopia Digestiva 16:1609–1615
12. Uraoka T, Fujii T, Matsuda T, et al (2004) How to perform endoscopic mucosal resection of the large colorectal tumor. Endoscopia Digestiva 16:784–789
13. Jin M, Otaka M, Odashima M, et al (2004) Successful endoscopic en bloc resection of a 50-mm nodule aggregated lesion in the rectum. Endoscopia Digestiva 16: 803–806
14. Oyama T, Kikuchi Y, Hirasawa D, et al (2004) Endoscopic submucosal dissection with the hook knife. Stomach Intestine 39:35–38
15. Lambert R, Rey JF, Sankaranarayanan R (2003) Magnification and chromoscopy with the acetic acid test. Endoscopy 35:437–445
16. Hardcastle JD, Chamberlain JO, Robinson MH, et al (1996) Randomised controlled trial of faecal occult blood screening for colorectal cancer. Lancet 348: 1472–1477
17. Scholefield JH, Moss S, Sufi S, et al (2002) Effect of faecal occult blood screening on mortality from colorectal cancer. Gut 50:840–844
18. Berchi C, Bouvier V, Reaud JM, et al (2004) Cost-effectiveness analysis of two strategies for mass screening for colorectal cancer in France. Health Econ 13: 227–238
19. The Paris endoscopic classification of superficial neoplastic lesions: esophagus, stomach, and colon (2003) Gastrointest Endosc 58(Suppl 6):S3–S43
20. Schlemper RJ, Kato Y, Stolte M (2001) Review of histological classifications of gastrointestinal epithelial neoplasia: differences in diagnosis of early carcinomas between Japanese and Western pathologists. J Gastroenterol 36: 445–456
21. Schlemper RJ, Itabashi M, Kato Y, et al (1997) Differences in diagnostic criteria for gastric carcinoma between Japanese and western pathologists. Lancet 349: 1725–1729
22. Rugge M, Correa P, Dixon MF, et al (2000) Gastric dysplasia: the Padova international classification. Am J Surg Pathol 24:167–176
23. Roesch T, Sarbia M, Schumacher B, et al (2004) Attempted endoscopic en bloc resection of mucosal and submucosal tumors using insulated-tip knives: a pilot series. Endoscopy 36:788–801
24. Lambert R (2003) Treatment of esophagogastric tumor. Endoscopy 35:118–126
25. Seewald S, Akaraviputh T, Seitz U, et al (2003) Circumferential EMR and complete removal of Barrett's epithelium: a new approach to management of Barrett's esophagus containing high-grade intraepithelial neoplasia and intramucosal carcinoma. Gastrointest Endosc 57: 854–859
26. Allgöwer M, Harder M, Hollender LF, et al (1981) Chirurgische gastroenterologie. Springer, Berlin Heidelberg New York, pp 546–547

27. Pichlmayr R, Grotelüschen B (1990) Chirurgische therapie. Springer, Berlin Heidelberg New York, pp 211–213
28. Vieth M, Ell C, Grossner L, et al (2004) Histological analysis of endoscopic resection specimens from 326 patients with Barrett's esophagus and early neoplasia. Endoscopy 36:776–781
29. May A, Gossner L, Pech O, et al (2002) Intraepithelial high-grade neoplasia and early adenocarcinoma in short-segment Barrett's esophagus (SSBE) curative treatment using local endoscopic treatment techniques. Endoscopy 34:604–610
30. Nakamura N, Akamatsu T, Yokoyama T, et al (2002) Treatment for post EMR remnant lesions—limitation of endoscopic retreatment. Stomach Intestine 37: 1195–1200
31. The Japanese Gastric Cancer Association (2004) A guideline of a gastric cancer treatment, Kanehara Shuppan, Tokyo, (2) pp 8–9

5. New Trends in Endoscopic Ultrasonography

Kenjiro Yasuda

1. Introduction

Gastrointestinal carcinoma has been detected and diagnosed by barium meal X-ray study and endoscopic study with or without biopsy study. In particular, early and minute carcinoma can be detected only by endoscopic study. Due to the development and refinement of endoscopy, the diagnosis of early gastrointestinal (GI) carcinoma is now easily accomplished by endoscopic observation and biopsy study. Endoscopic detection of gastrointestinal lesions depends on the recognition of visible mucosal changes. However, the final diagnosis is performed by histopathological study of biopsy materials. Biopsy study is still very important to obtain the correct diagnosis of the lesion as carcinoma, dysplasia, adenoma, and hyperplasia, although it is sometimes possible to diagnose the lesion from the endoscopic investigation of mucosal surface details. In this chapter, endoscopic diagnosis of early carcinoma in the upper GI tract will be described.

2. How to Detect Early GI Carcinoma

Careful observation by endoscopy is important for detecting small lesions. When we focus on small lesions, detecting an abnormal area and performing a biopsy can be effectively carried out. This is easy to say theoretically, but in practice we need to learn the endoscopic observation skills and be familiar with small lesions.

For detection of early carcinoma of the upper GI tract, endoscopists have to learn to recognize early cancer lesions, which are observed with characteristic color changes and an irregular mucosal pattern.

It is useful to employ a dye-spraying method using iodine for esophageal carcinoma and indigocarmine for gastric and colorectal carcinoma. This is a valuable complementary technique but cannot directly detect gastric or colorectal lesions.

Figure 1 shows the early stage of esophageal carcinoma limited to the epithelium with and without iodine spray. The area of the lesion can be clearly detected after dye-spraying. Figure 2 shows a gastric carcinoma limited to the mucosa after spraying with indigocarmine. The shape and irregularity of the lesion are clearly demonstrated.

3. Is Endoscopic Ultrasonography (EUS) Effective?

Endoscopic ultrasonographic diagnosis of early GI tract malignancy is one of the recent clinical topics of importance. We can demonstrate the cross section of the GI wall ultrasonographically by using EUS. Nowadays two types of EUS instruments are available. One is the conventional ultrasound endoscope with a radial scan transducer at the tip of the endoscope, while the other is an ultrasound catheter probe with a small radial scan transducer at the tip, which can be used through the working channel of the endoscope. The gastrointestinal wall can be delineated as five or more layered structures in the water-expanded GI lumen, which correspond well with histological layers. Higher frequency ultrasound scanners such as 20–30 MHz transducers can delineate a more precise picture of the GI wall.

The role of EUS is to evaluate the alteration of the GI wall by carcinoma based on the layered structure of GI wall, but we cannot detect the lesion by EUS except in the rare case of early stage of scirrhous carcinoma. The capability of EUS is to diagnose the depth of carcinoma invasion, which is an important factor in choosing the preferred treatment such as endoscopic resection (ER), laparoscopic surgery, or laparotomy. The diagnostic accuracy of depth of carcinoma invasion is around 80%, when we divide the lesions into mucosal (m) carcinoma, submucosal (sm) carcinoma, carcinoma invading to the muscularis propria (mp), and deeper than the subserosal layer (ss) according to our criteria, which involve three hyperechoic layers of the GI wall.

The accuracy rate of diagnosis of a mucosal lesion, which is a good indication for endoscopic mucosectomy, is 90%. One of the most important diagnostic feats of EUS is to decide the indication for endoscopic treatment at the early stage of GI malignancy. Figure 3 shows EUS pictures of esophageal carcinoma limited to the submucosal layer obtained by an ultrasound probe with a 30 MHz transducer, and Figure 4 shows pictures of a gastric carcinoma limited to the mucosa demonstrated by a 20 MHz ultrasound probe.

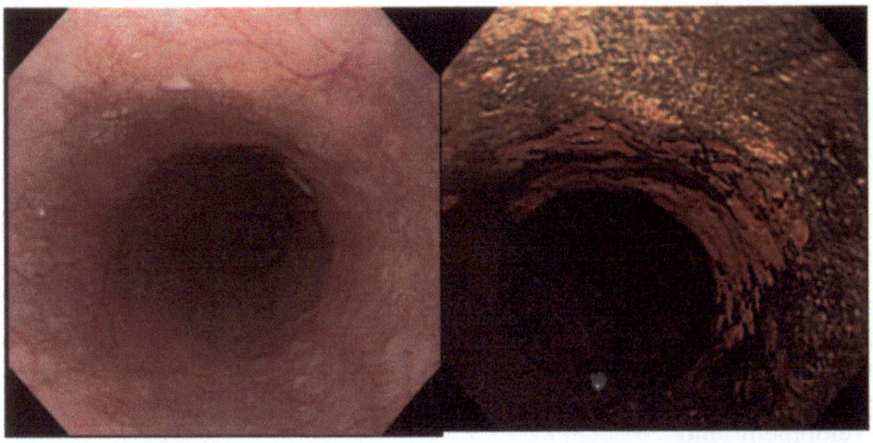

A B

Fig. 1. Esophageal carcinoma limited to the epithelium with (**A**) and without (**B**) iodine spray. The extent of the lesion can be clearly detected after dye spraying (**B**)

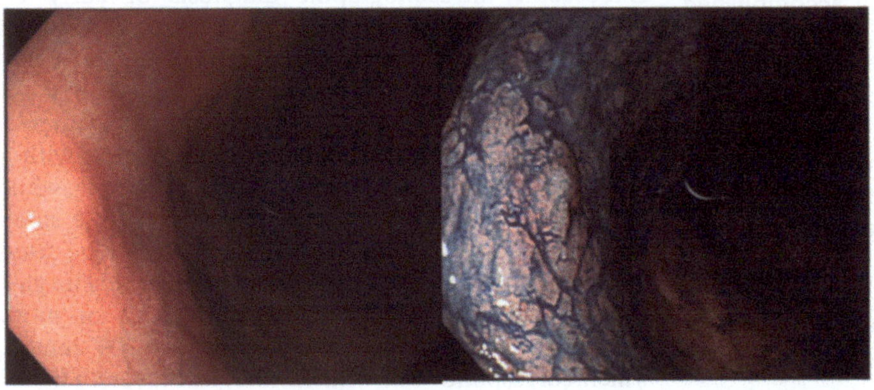

A B

Fig. 2A,B. Gastric carcinoma limited to the mucosa with indigocarmine spraying (**B**). The shape and irregularity of the lesion are clearly demonstrated

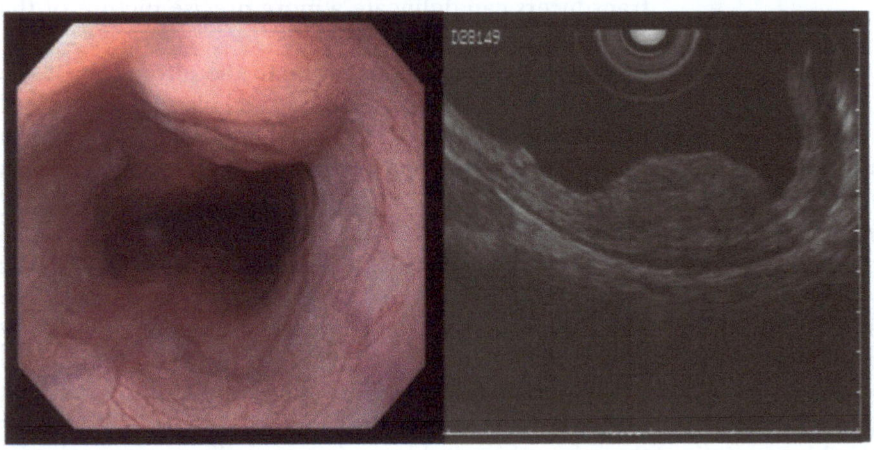

A B

Fig. 3A,B. Endoscopic ultrasonography (EUS) pictures of esophageal carcinoma limited to the submucosal layer obtained by ultrasound probe with a 30 MHz transducer (**B**)

Recently, three-dimensional (3-D) reconstruction of EUS images obtained by a 3-D ultrasound probe has become possible. The significance of 3-D pictures is not only to make the image more easily understood but also to avoid overlooking the lesion. In addition, the therapeutic effect can be evaluated by measuring the mass volume using this method. Figure 5 shows the radial and linear images of gastric carcinoma obtained by 3-D probe and reconstruction of the lesion.

4. Magnifying Endoscopy

Through advances of technology, high-resolution and high-magnification endoscopy with both fiberoptic and video-imaging systems has been developed and improved. There are reports of the diagnostic ability of high-resolution and high-magnification endoscopes. However, it has not been easy to manipulate these endoscopes in ordinary clinical examinations, especially

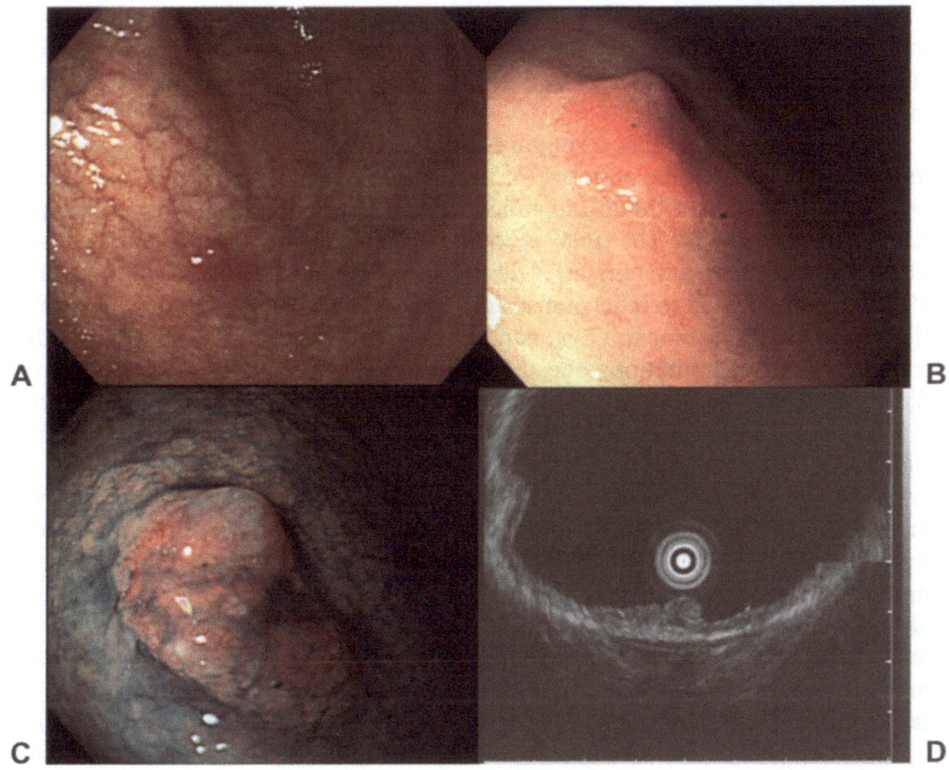

Fig. 4A–D. Early gastric carcinoma type IIa+IIc. **A** Endoscopic finding showing the redness. **B** Close-up view of the lesion. **C** Indigocarmine spraying. **D** Endoscopic ultrasonography pictures of gastric carcinoma limited to the mucosa demonstrated by a 20 MHz ultrasound probe, showing the normal submucosal layer

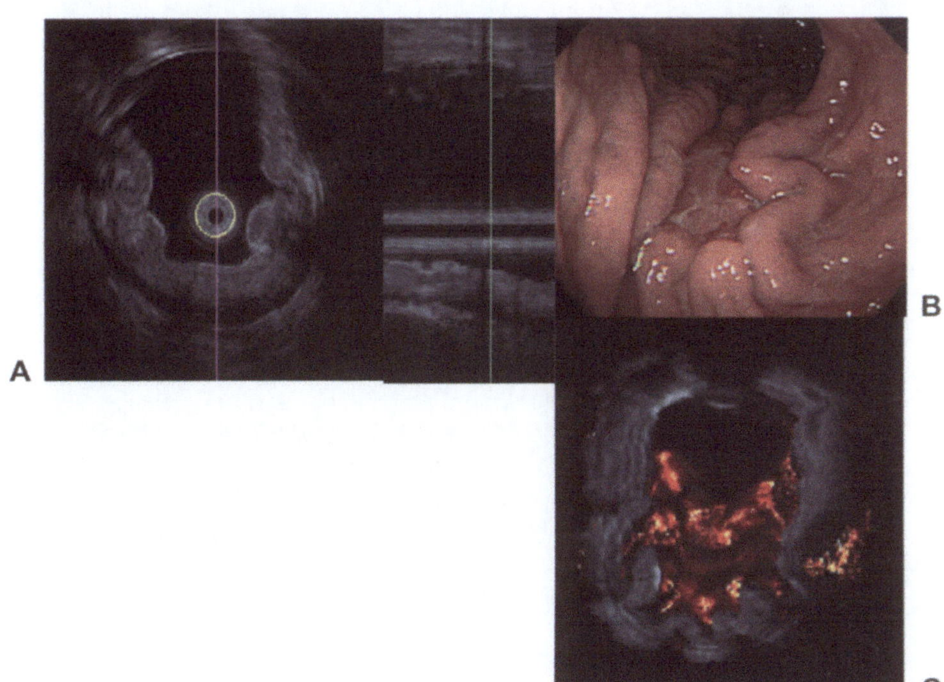

Fig. 5A–C. Three-dimensional (3-D) image of gastric carcinoma demonstrated by ultrasound probe. **A** Radial and linear image (dual planes) obtained by 3-D probe. **B** Endoscopic view. **C** Surface construction of 3-D EUS image

in the upper GI tract, because of the difficulty of focusing due to the movement by respiration and cardiac contractions and the darker imaging view in magnification.

By using new techniques of high-resolution and high-magnification electronic endoscopes, how can we diagnose the GI lesions? High-magnification endoscopes have a long history. The first models, which had a fiberoptic endoscope system, were developed in the late 1960s and attempted to reach a histological diagnosis of the lesions without biopsy. However, handling of endoscopes had some limitations because of the dark visual field and difficulty of focusing.

Progress in the field of electronic endoscopy gives us the hope that high-resolution and high-magnification endoscopes will be developed that are more easily manipulated. The most advanced video endoscope for the upper tract (GF-Q240Z), which can demonstrate magnified images up to 80×, can be used in routine study although the focusing of this model is not so easy at maximum magnification. Nevertheless, this model can provide higher-resolution pictures, easier handling, and satisfactory brightness compared with previous ones.

We can observe the surface mucosal pattern (pit pattern) and capillary structure by using high-magnification endoscopy. Based on the analysis of the mucosal pit pattern obtained by magnification, histological changes of carcinoma, dysplasia, and adenoma can be assessed. However, it is not easy to diagnose the histological changes from the magnified images. In addition, we cannot observe the whole GI wall on the magnified image, even when we have some criteria on magnification image diagnosis. The role of high-magnification endoscopy is thus to magnify the target area when conventional endoscopy has detected some abnormality in ordinary pictures.

Figure 6 shows an example of high-magnification images of an advanced carcinoma in the prepyloric region. Gastric areas can be seen in the normal mucosa; on the other hand, irregular, wider areas and a non-structured surface are observed in the carcinoma (Fig. 6C,D).

Figure 7 shows magnification images of a type IIc, depressed gastric mucosal carcinoma at the greater curvature of the gastric antrum. Magnification images delineate the mucosal lesion with irregularly sized and structured areas.

Figure 8 is a case of type IIa, slightly elevated gastric carcinoma limited to the mucosa at the posterior wall of the gastric body, showing the irregular pit pattern of the mucosal surface.

By gathering many cases and analyzing the images, it should be possible for magnifying endoscopy to help in the assessment of the histological diagnosis.

A B

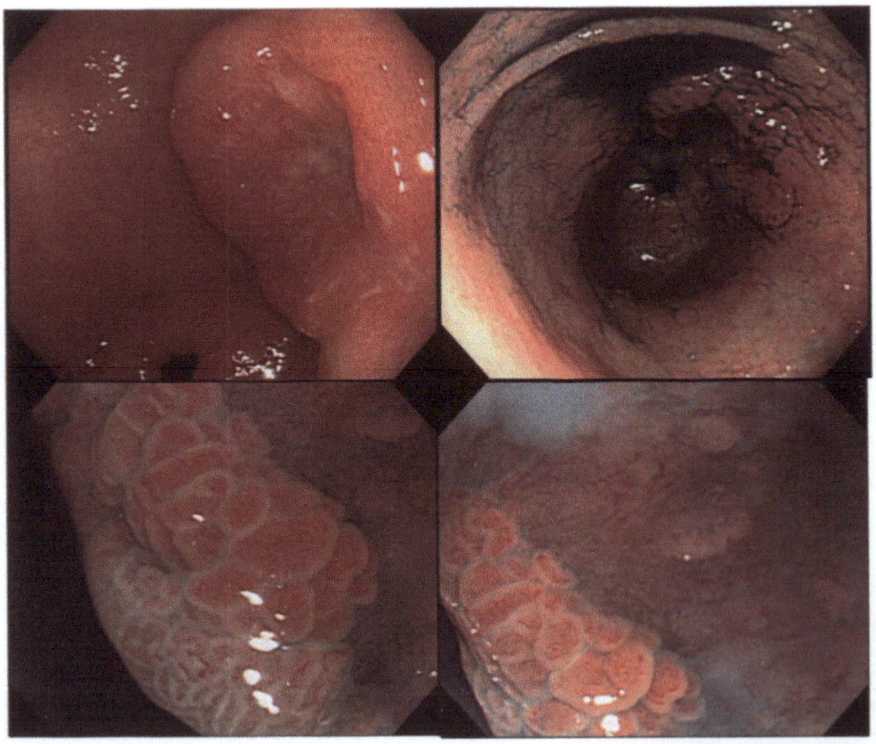

C D

Fig. 6A–D. Advanced gastric carcinoma at the posterior wall of the prepyloric region. **A** Ordinary endoscopic picture of the lesion. **B** Dye-spraying image of the lesion. **C,D** Magnification picture of the border of benign and malignant areas

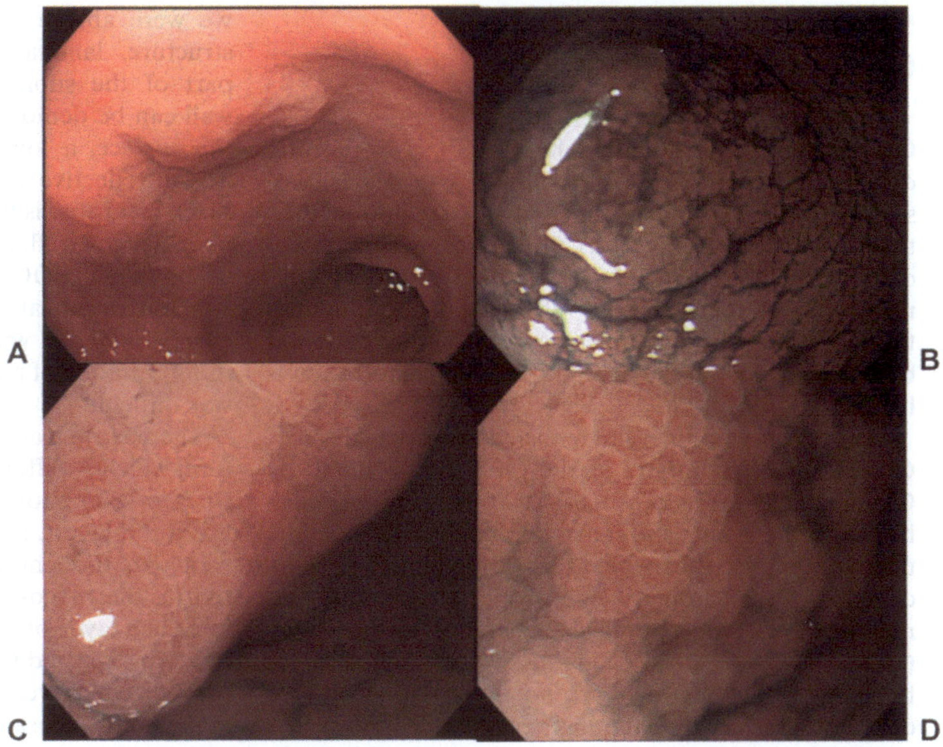

Fig. 7A–D. Gastric mucosal carcinoma (type IIc) in the gastric antrum. **A** Conventional endoscopy picture of the lesion. **B** Close-up view at the site of the cancer showing the irregular areas with dye spraying. **C,D** Magnification images of the malignant depression with dye, showing the irregular mucosal pattern

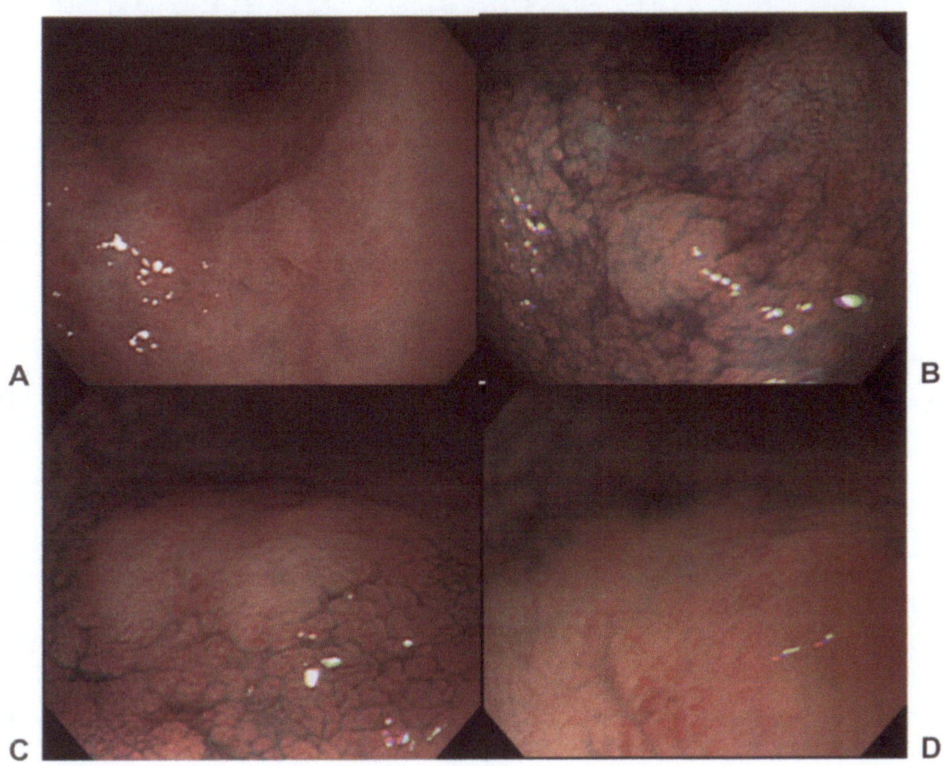

Fig. 8A–D. A case of type IIa, slightly elevated type of gastric carcinoma limited to the mucosa. **A** Ordinary endoscopic view. **B** With dye spraying. **C,D** Magnification images of the lesion showing the irregular pit pattern of the mucosal surface

5. Endoscopic Optical Coherence Tomography

Optical coherence tomography (OCT) is a recently developed technique for demonstrating the cross-sectional images with 10-times higher resolution than that of a 30 MHz ultrasound catheter probe. This system demonstrates the images by using broad-bandwidth illumination and recording the reflection of the illumination. We can observe the microscopic structure of tissues by this method, but the depth of imaging penetration is limited.

We have started to evaluate the clinical application of OCT using a prototype of the OCT probe made by Olympus (Japan) as of August 2000. This probe, which has the same aspect and same view angle of 360° as the ultrasound probe, can be used through the working channel of an ordinary endoscope, so we call this method endoscopic optical coherence tomography (EOCT). For EOCT scanning, water injection or balloon contact methods are not required, as the air does not obstruct the illumination beam.

Examined lesions were demonstrated with high-resolution images, but with poor penetration. The depth of imaging penetration was 1.5–2.0 mm, but we were able to demonstrate the mucosal glandular structure, lamina propria, muscularis mucosae, and part of the submucosa individually. The esophageal wall can be demonstrated as a layered structure. From the surface, a low-reflective homogeneous layer and a high-reflective layer can be seen, behind which is a black layer that is thought to be mucosal muscle and an irregular low-reflective layer of the submucosa. Figure 9 shows an EOCT image of esophageal carcinoma, which demonstrates the thickening of the wall in good correspondence with resected findings. However, the differentiation of normal mucosa and cancerous mucosa was difficult.

The gastric wall is also observed as a layered structure, which is different from that of the esophagus. The surface layer shows the gland structure, behind which are three layers, high-, low-, and high-reflective layers, which are thought to be the lamina propria (high reflectivity), the mucosal muscle (low reflectivity), and the interface layer of the submucosal layer (high reflectivity). We expected OCT to demonstrate the gland structures by which we can differentiate between normal and malignant mucosa. Figure 10 shows the OCT images and mucosectomy specimen of a gastric carcinoma. However, histological diagnosis from OCT images seemed difficult, as we could not analyze the OCT

A

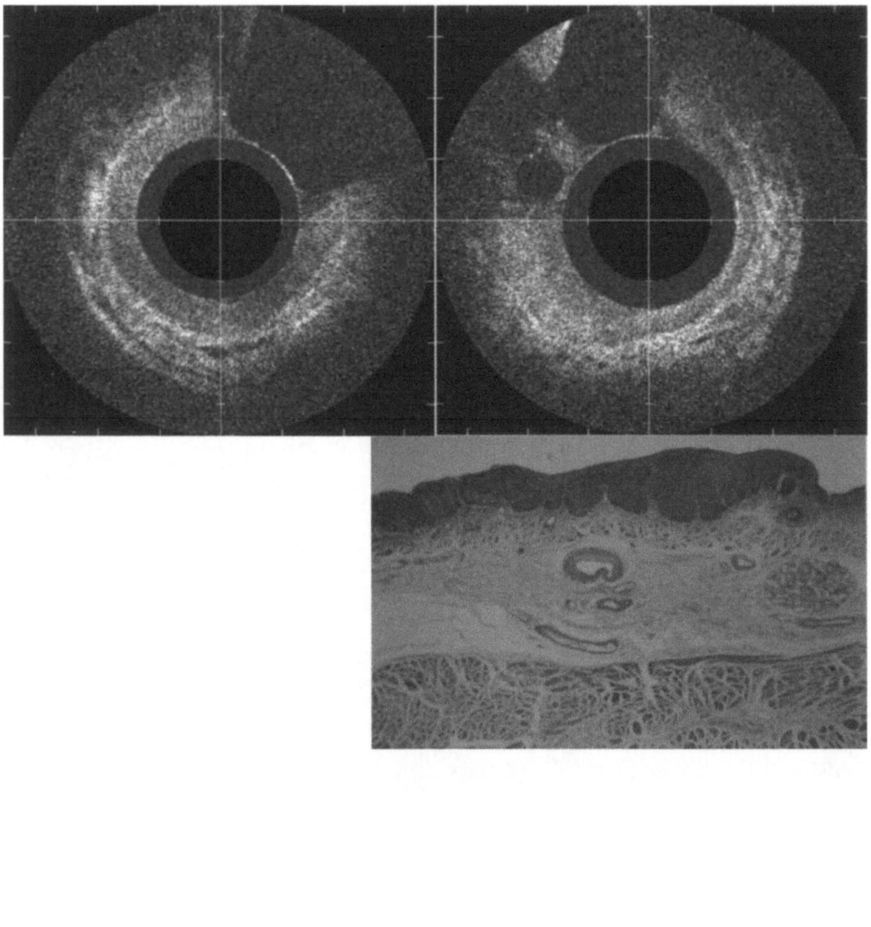

B

C

Fig. 9A–C. Endoscopic optical coherence tomography image of esophageal carcinoma limited to the mucosa. **A** Cross-sectional image of normal esophageal wall. **B** Cross-sectional image of the cancerous region showing the thickening of the wall, in good correspondence with resection findings. **C** Cross-sectional view of resected specimen

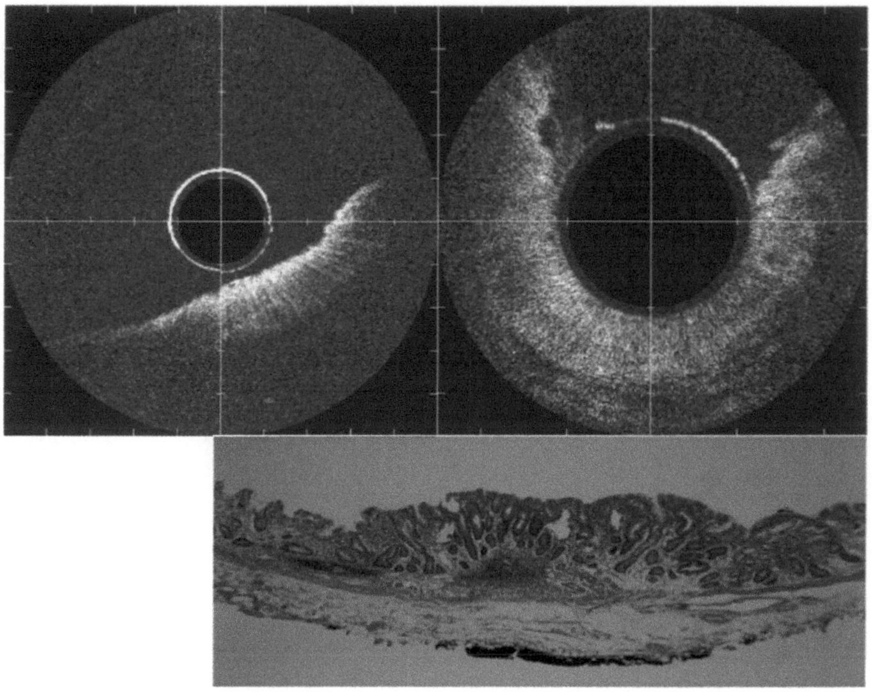

Fig. 10A–C. Endoscopic optical coherence tomography (EOCT) image of gastric carcinoma limited to the mucosa. **A,B** EOCT findings of the gastric mucosal carcinoma showing the gland-like structure. **C** Endoscopic resection specimen showing the well-differentiated adenocarcinoma limited to the mucosa

images of the cancerous region. Further investigation should be performed in this field.

Although the resolution was much higher than that of a 30 MHz ultrasound scanner, penetration of EOCT was too poor to use this method for assessing the depth of tumor invasion. However, by using this particular sophisticated instrument, we can expect to determine the histological nature of tissues in the near future. Endoscopic optical coherence tomography is expected to be a method of optical biopsy study in endoscopic examination in the future.

6. Diagnosis of Early GI Tract Carcinoma in the Future

Presently, the diagnosis of early GI tract carcinoma is performed by endoscopic examination. Universal criteria cannot be established, because the ability to detect and diagnose is dependent on personal capability and experience. Other techniques such as blood tests or gastric juice tests, or gene analysis, might harbor the possibility to detect small GI tract carcinomas, but there are probably some difficulties involved in these diagnostic methods, as we will be unable to know the position of the lesions unless there is direct visualization of the GI lumen.

In the future, use of new EOCT instruments for detecting early and small lesions should become routine. The progress of information technology is so fast and beyond our expectation, so there is hope for detection and differentiation of GI lesions by autodiagnostic endoscopy. We are hopeful that therapeutic procedures for early GI tract carcinoma will be further improved for endoscopists.

References

1. Yasuda K, Nakajima M, Kawai K (1987) Fundamentals of endoscopic laser therapy (ELT) for GI tumors; new aspects with endoscopic ultrasonography (EUS). Endoscopy 19:s2–s6
2. Tio TL, Cohen P, Coene PP, et al (1989) Endosonography and computed tomography of esophageal carcinoma. Gastroenterology 96:1478–1486
3. Yasuda K, Nakajima M, Kawai K (1992) Endoscopic diagnosis and treatment of early gastric cancer using endoscopic ultrasonography (EUS). Gastrointest Endosc Clin North Am 2:495–507
4. Van Dam J (1994) Endosonography of the esophagus. Gastrointest Endosc Clin North Am 4(4):803–826
5. Rosch T (1995) Endosonographic staging of esophageal cancer: a review of literature results. Gastrointest Endosc Clin North Am 5:537–547

6. Kida M, Tanabe M, Watanabe M, et al (1998) Staging of gastric cancer with endoscopic ultrasonography and endoscopic mucosal resection endoscopy. Dig Endosc 30(suppl):A64–A68
7. Yasuda K (2000) Gastrointestinal carcinoma. In: The handbook of endoscopic ultrasonography in digestive tract. Blackwell Science, Japan, pp 54–69
8. Penman ID, Shen EF (2002) EUS in advanced esophageal cancer. Gastrointest Endosc 56:s2–s6
9. Yasuda K (2002) EUS in the detection of early gastric cancer. Gastrointest Endosc 56:s68–s75
10. Yasuda K, Kamaguchi M, Morikawa J, et al (2005) Role of endoscopic ultrasonograhy (EUS) in the diagnosis of early esophageal carcinoma. Gastrointest Endosc Clin North Am 15:93–99

V. Endoscopic Treatment

1. Gastric Cancer

Hiroshi Takahashi

1. Introduction

Endoscopic treatments for early gastric cancers are divided into two groups: mucosal resection methods and coagulation methods (e.g., laser therapies). Mucosal resection methods are usually preferred because through these we can obtain pathological specimens to evaluate. This chapter will present an overview of the current techniques and their future directions.

2. Indication

The indication of endoscopic treatment is limited to gastric cancer without lymph node metastasis. The presence and absence of lymph node metastasis is closely related to the histology, size, and depth of the lesion.

The Japan Gastroenterological Endoscopy Society recommends endoscopic treatment for:

1. Elevated type, differentiated adenocarcinoma of less than 20mm in size, that does not reach deeper than the mucosal layer
2. Depressed type, differentiated adenocarcinoma of less than 10mm in size, that does not reach deeper than the mucosal layer and does not have an ulcer or ulcer scar

3. Choice of Procedure: Endoscopic Mucosal Resection

Endoscopic mucosal resection (EMR) is similar to surgical resection in that we can obtain specimens for pathological examination, while laser therapy and microwave coagulation methods coagulate or vaporize the lesion, leaving no specimens for further examination. Since the latter methods do not allow us to know whether any malignant cells remain, they are not suitable as first choice for curative treatment. The EMR method [1]) is thus preferred, and various techniques have been developed in order to improve the procedure.

3.1 Double-Channel Endoscopy Method

EMR for early gastric cancer can be performed using the method of Tada et al. [2], which requires a double-channel endoscopy that has two forceps channels (Fig. 1). There are two types of endoscopy: front-viewing endoscopy and oblique-viewing endoscopy. Oblique-viewing endoscopy is used for lesions on the posterior wall or in the cardiac region, which are difficult to treat with usual endoscopy. The disadvantage of the double-channel endoscopy method is its uniqueness. This type of endoscopy is rarely available in a usual setting, thus we perform this complex procedure only in highly equipped facilities.

3.2 Single-Channel Endoscopy Method

A more usual endocopic method is cup-fitted panendoscopy that is equipped with a transparent plastic hood at the tip of the endoscope (EMRC) (Fig. 2) [3]. With this method, we are able to use a regular endoscope. After suctioning the lesion into the transparent hood, we cut it off with the snare. The advantages of this method are that we do not need a special endoscope and we can easily reach sites that are less approachable by other EMR methods.

3.3 Endoscopic Submucosal Dissection (ESD)

Current methods such as double-channel endoscopy methods or EMRC have been shown to be effective in treating early gastric cancers, but may not achieve en bloc resection in all cases.

The ESD technique, which makes en bloc resection possible, has been developed in Japan. The actual steps of this procedure are: (a) burn the lesion boundary, marking with the tip of electrocoagulation devices; (b) inject saline or mucinous substances mixed with indigo carmine into the submucosal layer beneath the lesion; (c) precut the rim of the marked lesion; (d) separate the submucosal layer and mucosa with an insulated tip knife (IT knife) [4]) and/or other devices (hook knife, flex knife, snare, etc.); and (e) remove the entire tumor in one piece (en bloc resection). New equipment has been designed to make the ESD technique much safer. An IT

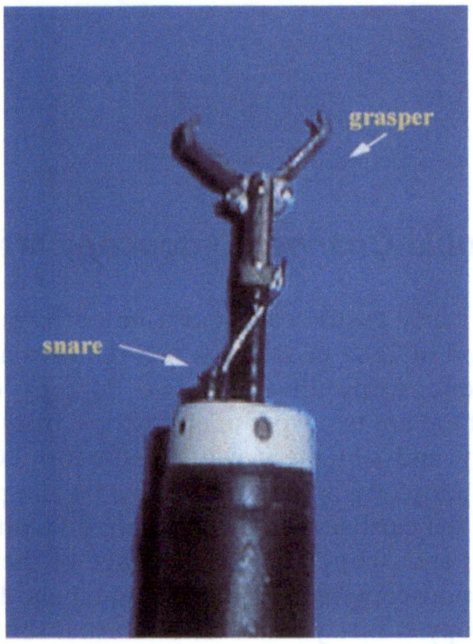

Fig. 1. Endoscopic mucosal resection: double-channel method

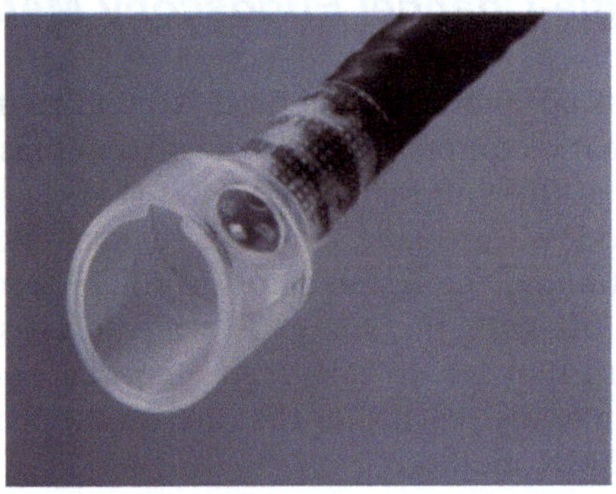

Fig. 2. Endoscopic mucosal resection using cup-fitted panendoscopy: EMRC

knife is a knife that has a ball made of ceramic material at the tip of the high-frequency cutting knife to prevent the knife from penetrating too deeply (Fig. 3).

4. Evaluation of the Procedure

Specimens obtained by EMR should be handled in the following manner. The specimen is spread out, pinned on a flat cork, and fixed in formalin solution. The size of specimen, the size and shape of the tumor, and the margins should be recorded on a schematic diagram. The fixed materials should be sectioned serially at 2-mm intervals parallel to a line that includes the closest resection margin of the specimen (Fig. 4).

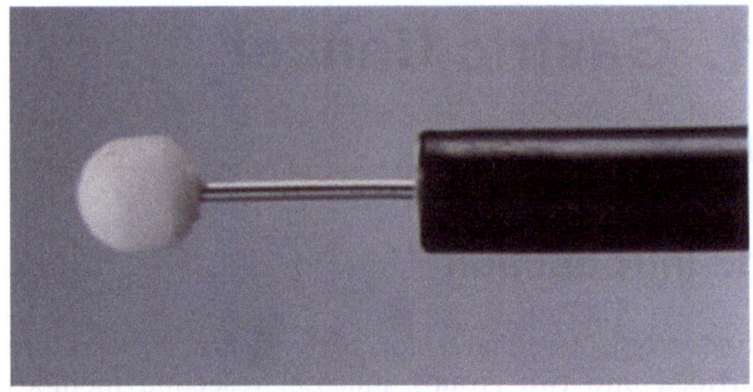

Fig. 3. IT knife (insulation-tipped electrosurgical knife)

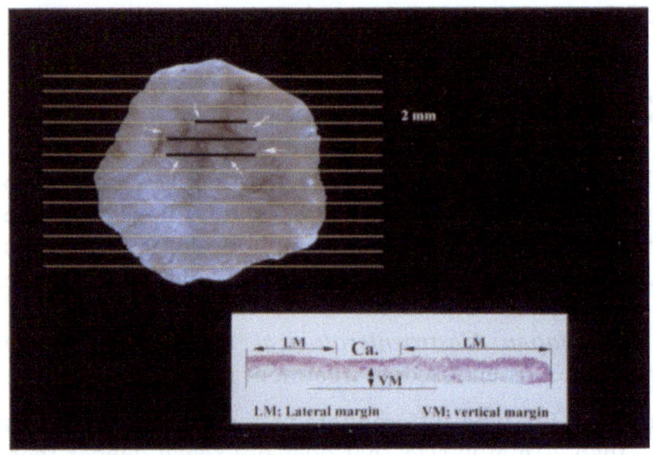

Fig. 4. Histopathological diagnosis

The key point of the evaluation is whether the whole lesion has been resected completely. It is easy to evaluate the en bloc specimen in which the resected specimen has enough distance between the resected margin and the border of the lesion, but the evaluation is rather difficult if we have resected the lesion in separate pieces. The Japanese guidelines for gastric cancer treatments [5] recommend that the results of resections should be evaluated in the following format:

Resection EA:
Depth M (mucosa), histologically pap or tub, no ulcer or ulcer scar in the tumor, vertical margin (VM)(–), no tumor cells within 1 mm of lateral margin (LM), neither lymphatic nor venous invasion

Resection EB:
No margin involvement but not fulfilling criteria for "EA"

Resection EC: VM(+) and / or LM(+)
(LM, lateral margin: VM, vertical margin)

When the lesion is resected in separate pieces, we have usually marked the lesion using a high-frequency knife and/or biopsy scars. However, we are apt to lose track of the site in those cases where a piecemeal resection has been necessary. The use of clips can help us work out the delineation and enables resection of the entire lesion without leaving cancer cells behind [6]. By fixing the colored clips around the lesion before resection, we can deduce the margin of the lesion and whether any residue is left after the procedure. Tani et al. [7] reported that they were able to resect an entire lesion of more than 15 mm in diameter by means of several well-planned partial resections.

5. Results

In a review of 1832 cases of early gastric cancer treated by EMR in 12 facilities [8–11], total removal of cancer was successful in 1353 cases (74%), but in the remaining 479 cases (41%) the tumors could be removed only partially. Of these, 195 patients subsequently underwent surgical resection.

5.1 Partially Resected Cases

The partially resected cases were treated as follows: repeated EMR in 12.7% (61 cases), laser therapy in 12.9% (62 cases), both repeat EMR and laser therapy in 0.8% (4 cases), ethanol injection plus heater probe coagulation in 15.2% (73 cases), and heater probe coagulation in 1.5% (7 cases).

6. Complications

Major complications of EMR are bleeding and perforation. The reported risk of bleeding varies from 1.2% to 11.8% while the risk of perforation is considered to be 0.4%–2.4% [11].

7. Extended Indications for Endoscopic Treatment

Cancers limited to the mucosal layer can be resected by endoscopy, but when we find invasion deeper than the mucosa in the resected specimen, we usually treat them surgically in our facility. However, when the patient's condition does not permit surgery, we can achieve a good outcome by using Nd-YAG laser therapy [12]. Fujisaki et al. [13] reported finding no lymph node metastasis in lesions invading only less than 200 μm into the submucosa. Further research may enable us to better predict the risk of lymph node metastases in various cases, possibly extending the indications for EMR.

8. Problems of Endoscopic Treatment

The most important point we have to be careful about in performing EMR is the possibility of synchronous lesions and metachronous lesions. Synchronous lesions are those that occur in multiple sites at the same time and metachronous lesions are those that occur after a successful resection of the original lesion during the long-term follow-up. Iwanaga et al. [14] reviewed a series of patients who underwent surgical resection and found by thorough pathological examination that 12.8% had synchronous lesions while only 8.6% were recognized before the surgery. In an independent review, Takagi et al. [15] reported that as many as 18.7% of early gastric cancer patients had synchronous lesions. Takekoshi [16] followed up post-EMR cases and reported the frequency of synchronous and/or metachronous lesions as 14.3%, 67% of which were synchronous lesions. In conclusion, even for small cancers that could be successfully removed by EMR, we have to sufficiently explore synchronous lesions and closely follow these up for possible metachronous lesions.

9. Conclusion

Endoscopic mucosal resection has been recognized as a less invasive procedure than surgical resection. We consider that it is important to further evaluate the long-term outcomes.

References

1. Takahashi H, Fujita R, Sugiyama K, et al (1991) Endoscopic therapy of gastric cancer: comparison of endoscopic mucosal coagulation and resection. Dig Endosc 3:215–221
2. Tada M, Shimada M, Yanai H, et al (1984) New technique of biopsy [in Japanese with English abstract]. Stomach Intest 19:1107–1116
3. Takeshita K, Tani M, Inoue H, et al (1997) Endoscopic treatment of early esophageal or gastric cancer. Gut 40:123–127

4. Ono H, Kondo H, Gatoda T, et al (2001) Endoscopic mucosal resection for treatment of early gastric cancer. Gut 48:151–152
5. Japanese Gastric Cancer Association (1998) Japanese classification of gastric carcinoma, 2nd English edition. Kanehara, Tokyo
6. Inatsuchi S, Tanaka M (1994) Clinical evaluation of an improved technique in strip biopsy for gastric lesion [in Japanese with English abstract]. Gastroenterol Endosc 36: 939–948
7. Tani M, Takeshita K, Saeki I, et al (1997) Protection of residue or recurrence following endoscopic mucosal resection for gastric tumorous lesion [in Japanese with English abstract]. Prog Digest Endosc 50:74–78
8. Takekoshi T, Baba Y, Ota H, et al (1994) Endoscopic resection of early gastric carcinoma: result of a retrospective analysis of 308 cases. Endoscopy 26:352–358
9. Tada M, Matsumoto Y, Murakami A, et al (1993) Problems and their solution in curative endoscopic resection of early gastric carcinomas. Endosc Digest 5:1169–1174
10. Takahashi H, Kojima T, Parra A, et al (1997) Clinical evaluation of endoscopic therapy for early gastric cancer. Endoscopy 29:E21
11. Kojima T, Parra-Blanco A, Takahashi H, et al (1998) Outcome of endoscopic mucosal resection for gastric cancer; review of the Japanese literature. Gastrointest Endosc 48:550–555
12. Yasuda K, Miguma Y, Nakajima K, et al (1993) Endoscopic laser treatment for early gastric cancer endoscopy 25:451–454
13. Fujisaki J, Ikegami M, Oota Y, et al (1997) Endoscopic mucosal resection for early gastric cancers: its follow up and management for problematic cases [in Japanese with English abstract]. Prog Digest Endosc 50:70–73.
14. Iwanaga T, Koyama H, Imaoka S, et al (1988) Occurrence of a heterochromous cancer in the remnant stomach following partial gastrectomy in gastric cancer. Gan No Rinsho 34:442–446
15. Takagi K, Ohashi I, Ohta T, et al (1980) Histological transefiguration in gastric cancer [in Japanese with English abstract]. Stomach Intest 15:11–19
16. Takekoshi T (1992) Prognosis of endoscopic resection in early gastric cancer—establishment for radical treatment [in Japanese with English abstract]. Prog Digest Endosc 41:139–143

2. Colorectal Cancer

Masaki Kawahara and Michio Kaminishi

1. Introduction

Recent progress in endoscopic techniques and instruments and interest in the diagnosis of early-stage colorectal cancers has enabled the detection of early colorectal cancers [1]. Early colorectal cancer is defined as "a cancer where the depth of invasion is limited to the mucosal or submucosal layer of the colon and rectum, regardless of the presence of lymph node metastasis" [2]. Although surgical therapy has enabled a high cure rate for early colorectal cancers, increasing evidence suggests that endoscopic treatment can be an effective alternative for localized colorectal cancers without lymph node metastasis or hematogenous spread. As a matter of fact, complete endoscopic resection of mucosal cancer is accepted as a curative procedure because of the absence of a risk of lymph node metastasis. However, the endoscopic resection of submucosal cancers remains controversial, because submucosal cancers have some risk of lymph node or distant metastasis [3]. In cases with metastasis, endoscopic treatment is not curative. Therefore, the indications for the endoscopic resection of early colorectal cancers must be carefully considered.

2. Indications for Endoscopic Treatment

Colorectal cancers may be considered candidates for endoscopic treatment if they can be curatively treated by local resection. These lesions include early colorectal cancers without lymph node metastasis or hematogenous metastasis that are resectable with no possibility of residual tumor on their cut surfaces [4, 5].

Early colorectal cancer can be divided into two categories: mucosal cancer (m-cancer or carcinoma in situ) and submucosally invasive cancer (sm-cancer). In mucosal cancer, all the malignant cells are confined within the epithelial layer and the basement membrane is not involved. Intramucosal cancers do not metastasize, because the lymphatics within the mucosal layer are anatomically sparse. Therefore, endoscopic treatment is generally accepted as adequate. However, sm-cancer has some risk of lymph node metastasis or hematogenous metastasis because of the abundance of lymphatic or venous channels in the submucosal layer.

As for the staging of sm-cancers, the degree of submucosal invasion has been classified into three categories by Kudo and colleagues (Fig. 1): sm1 (invading the superficial one-third of the submucosa), sm2 (invading the middle one-third of the submucosa) [4, 6], and sm3 (invading the deepest one-third of the submucosa). Clinically, sm-cancers have been grouped as sm-slight cancer (sm-s = sm1) and sm-massive cancer (sm-m = sm2 + sm3). Sm-s cancers without venous or lymphatic vessel invasion do not have lymph node metastasis. On the other hand, sm-massive cancers are considered to be associated with a risk for lymph node metastasis. Therefore, the distinction of m- or sm-s cancers from sm-m cancers is clinically important because the decision to perform radical surgery or local excision/endoscopic treatment should be determined on the basis of the risk of lymph node metastasis [4, 6].

3. Recognition of sm-Massive Cancers

As mentioned above, endoscopic treatment for early colorectal cancers is indicated only for mucosal and sm-s cancers, and not for sm-m cancers. Therefore, the recognition of sm-m cancer is important.

3.1 Diagnosis by Conventional Endoscopy

Endoscopically, massive submucosal invasion findings include stiffness, expansiveness, fold convergence, coexisting white spots, ulceration, surface irregularity, and a lack of air-induced deformation. If these findings are detected, the need for curative surgical resection with lymph node dissection should be considered. In addition, morphologically depressed lesions (IIc or IIc+IIa) with a lack of air-induced deformation are usually sm-massive cancers [4, 6].

However, most of these signs are subjective and may be discernible only to specialists. Practically, polyps that are considered to be endoscopically resectable are typical targets of EMR (endoscopic mucosal resection). During endoscopic treatments, sm-massive cancers that cannot be removed endoscopically can usually be dis-

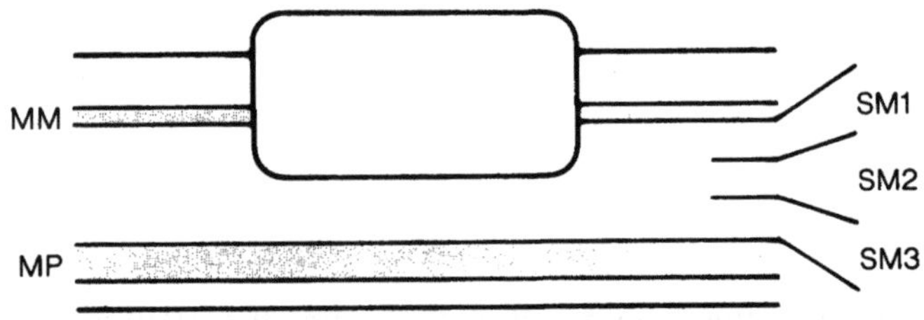

Fig. 1. Classification of the degree of submucosal invasion. Submucosa is divided into three layers equally. *MM*, muscularis mucosae; *MP*, muscularis propria; *SM*, submucosa

Table 1. Classification of the pit pattern of colorectal lesions

Pit pattern	Description	Histology
Type I	Round pits	Normal
Type II	Stellar pits	Hyperplastic
Type III_S	Small tubular pits	Adenoma or noninvasive cancer
Type III_L	Large tubular pits	Adenoma or noninvasive cancer
Type IV	Branched or gyrus-like pits	Adenoma or noninvasive cancer
Type V	Nonstructural pits	Invasive cancer

tinguished. Desmoplastic reactions, which accompany most invasive cancers, fasten the cancer to the underlying submucosal layer, making it difficult to elevate the lesion sufficiently to perform EMR. This phenomenon is widely perceived as the "nonlifting sign" that is visible after the submucosal injection of physiologic saline [7]. Tumors that exhibit a nonlifting sign are thought to be endoscopically unresectable, and surgery is usually indicated.

3.2 Diagnosis by EUS

The evaluation of tumor depth by EUS is accurate and effective when the relationship between the tumor and the colonic wall is clearly interpreted, and m or sm-slight cancer can be distinguished from sm-massive cancer in this manner [8, 9]. In general, the irregular thinning of a layer with a hypoechoic mass is interpreted as the presence of invasion to the corresponding layer, and the disruption of a layer is also interpreted as invasion through the corresponding layer (see Section IV, Chapter 2 by Shimizu for further details).

3.3 Diagnosis by Magnifying Endoscopy

In recent years, magnifying colonoscopes have been used to observe the orifices of colonic crypts (pits) on the tumor surface, and observations of the patterns formed by the pits has improved the accuracy of endoscopic diagnosis of early colorectal neoplasms. Kudo et al. devised a detailed classification based on the mucosal pit pattern [4, 6]. The pit pattern is basically classified into six categories (Table 1). Type V is usually observed in cancerous lesions. As colonic cancer invades the submucosal layer, its surface structure becomes irregular and the regular pit pattern disappears. Type V is subdivided into typeV_I (irregular) and type V_N (nonstructural). The former suggests mucosal or minimally submucosal invasive cancer, while the latter implies deeper invasion (sm2 or sm3). Therefore, lesions with type V_N patterns should be excluded from endoscopic treatment [4, 6].

4. Colonic EMR

Generally speaking, most superficial or sessile lesions of up to 20mm in diameter can be removed by EMR. Larger lesions may best be resected using a piecemeal technique (EPMR: endoscopic piecemeal mucosal resection). The EMR and EPMR techniques are basically the same (Figs. 2, 3).

4.1 Positioning

First of all, EMR must be conducted under a fully controlled colonoscopy. The colonoscope should be held so that the targeting lesion is positioned at the 5 o'clock (lower right) position. Advantageous positioning is best accomplished when the colonoscope shaft is straight, to transmit the torque to the tip.

4.2 Lifting by Injection

Physiologic saline or glycerin (the authors' preference) is injected into the normal submucosal layer on the proximal side of the lesion to lift it above the surrounding mucosa to optimize visuality and faciliate accession. If the lesion is too large to be lifted by a single injection, several injections may be necessary to create an appropriate submucosal bleb, so that the lesion is located on top of the artificial protrusion.

4.3 Snaring and Cutting

Once the lesion is raised high enough, an oval polypectomy snare with spikes is applied over the lesion and the snare is closed firmly until resistance is felt; the lesion should be located in the center of the closed

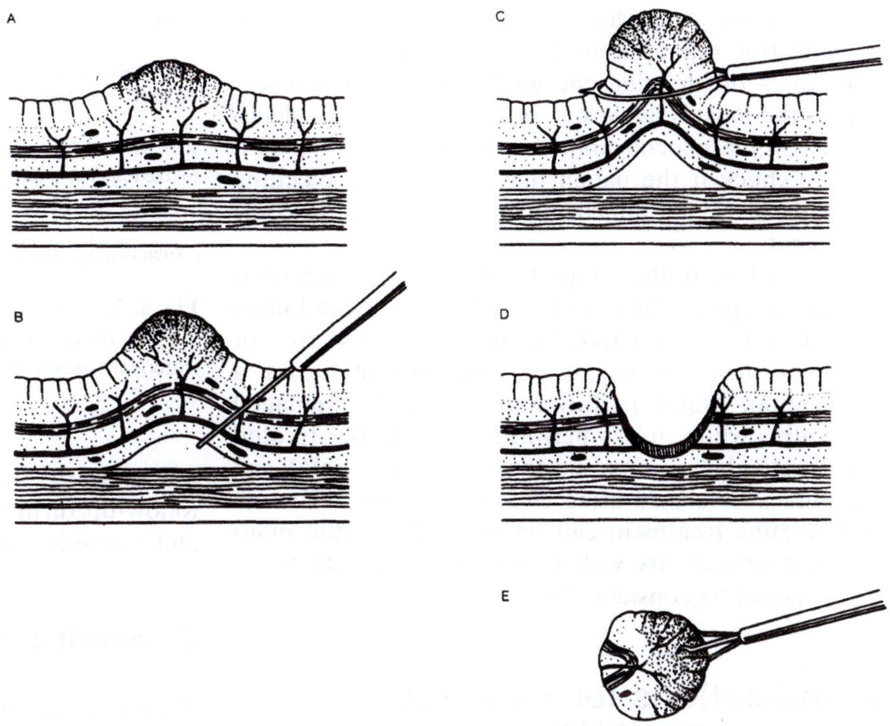

Fig. 2A–E. Technique of endoscopic mucosal resection (EMR). **A** Diagnosis and positioning. **B** Injection into the submucosa. **C** Snaring and cutting. **D** Hemostasis and evaluation of the cut section. **E** Withdrawal of the specimen

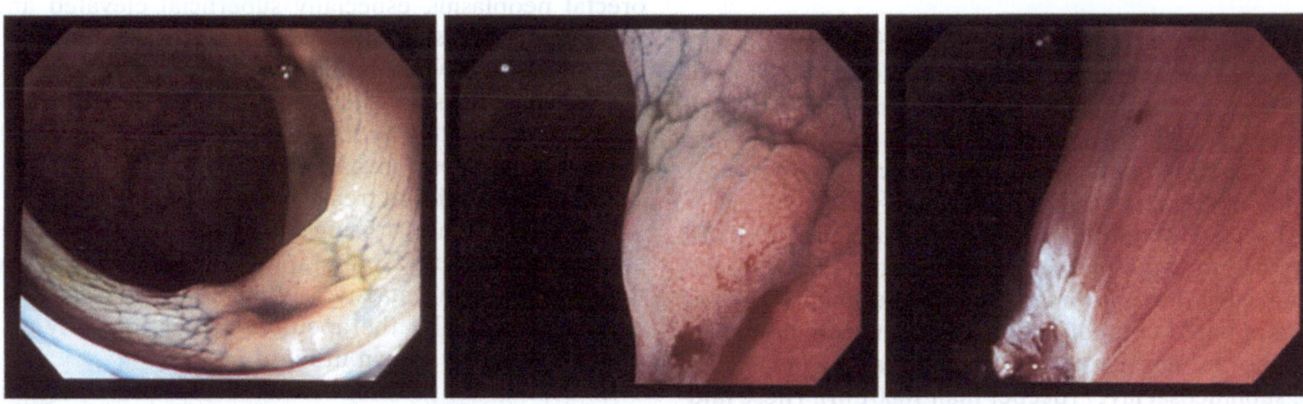

Fig. 3A–C. Endoscopic mucosal resection (EMR) procedure using a magnifying colonoscope. **A** A superficial lesion in the sigmoid colon was detected using chromoendoscopy. **B** The lesion revealed a III_S pit pattern. **C** Resection margins were examined post EMR, which showed a normal pit pattern, indicating complete resection

circle. Applying suction as the snare is closed helps to retain the lesion within the snare. Once the lesion is caught in the snare, the snare is relaxed slightly to prevent involution of the muscular layer. The lesion is then resected using a blend or cutting current.

4.4 Evaluation, Clipping, and Withdrawal

After resection, it is important to confirm whether hemostasis is complete and whether a residual lesion is present at the resection margin. Observation with a magnifying colonoscope is very useful for checking for residual tumors [4, 6, 14]. If the resection is complete and no bleeding is present, the mucosal defect is closed by clipping and the resected specimen is extracted with pentapod-type grasping forceps.

5. Complications

The two main complications of EMR are hemorrhage and perforation. The Japanese Society of Gastroenterological Endoscopy has reviewed the rate of EMR complications. According to their report, the overall complication rate for colonic EMR is 0.14% [15].

In cases of bleeding, the application of endoscopic clips is the most reliable way of stopping arterial bleeding; argon plasma coagulation is also useful. It is necessary to check if the patient has a history of bleeding diathesis or taking anticoagulants prior to endoscopic treatment.

The first sign that a perforation has occurred is abdominal pain. Plain radiographs of the abdomen should be taken to check for the presence of free or retroperitoneal air in patients suspected of having a perforation. Major perforations should be managed surgically, while micro-perforations can be treated conservatively; a minor perforation (small hole) can sometimes be closed using endoscopic clips. Although conservative treatment can be successful in the management of patients with perforations, surgical treatment should be considered in advance.

6. Indications for Additional Surgery after EMR

The incidence of lymph node metastasis in patients with submucosally invasive cancers has been reported to be less than 15%; for cancers with shallow invasion (sm1 carcinomas), the incidence is only 0%–3%. The majority of patients with submucosal cancers do not have lymph node metastasis [3, 16, 17].

The need for additional surgical treatment after EMR may be indicated by the presence of the following histological parameters in the resected specimen: (i) poorly differentiated or undifferentiated adenocarcinoma; (ii) lymphovascular permeation; or (iii) massive invasion of the submucosal layer (deeper than 1000 μm). These findings are considered risk factors for lymph node metastasis by The Japanese Society of Gastroenterological Endoscopy. A radical colectomy with lymph node dissection should be performed in patients with any of these risk factors [18]. Laparoscopic surgery is usually indicated in such cases.

7. Follow-Up after EMR

Patients who have undergone an endoscopic treatment should be followed up with a colonoscopy to evaluate the resected site and check for recurrence. A regular colonoscopic examination is recommended every 6–12 months. In cases with large superficial lesions treated by EPMR, regular follow-ups should be performed earlier and with a shorter interval (such as at 3, 6, 12, and 24

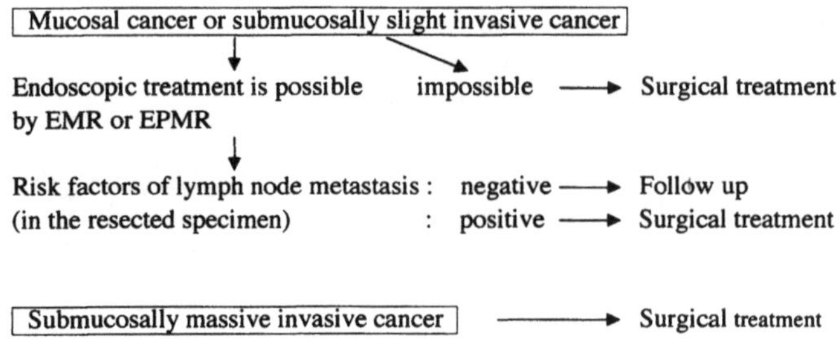

Fig. 4. The strategy for early colorectal cancers. *EMR*, endoscopic mucosal resection; *EPMR*, endoscopic piecemeal mucosal resection

months) [19]. If a residual lesion is detected during follow-up, further endoscopic treatment can be effective and can reduce the recurrence rate.

8. Summary and Future Prospects

Recent advances in endoscopic technology and techniques have enabled endoscopic treatment for early colorectal neoplasms, especially superficial elevated and depressed lesions. Histologically, mucosal cancers or minimally invasive submucosal cancers without lymphovascular invasion and a well-differentiated phenotype can be treated by EMR or EPMR. Cancers with massive submucosal invasion or with adverse histological features should be treated surgically.

Pit pattern analysis using a magnifying colonoscope and endoscopic ultrasonography are useful diagnostic tools for detecting massive submucosally invasive colorectal cancers. The therapeutic strategy for early colorectal cancers is shown in Fig. 4.

In Japan, the cutting EMR technique using an insulation-tipped diathermy knife (IT knife) has become a popular technique for performing gastric resections of early gastric cancers. This technique will also become applicable to colonic EMR in the near future.

References

1. Rembacken B, Fujii T, Kondo H (2001) The recognition and endoscopic treatment of early gastric and colonic cancer. Best Pract Res Clin Gastroenterol 15:317–336
2. Japanese Society for Cancer of Colon and Rectum (1998) General rules for clinical and pathological studies on cancer of the colon, rectum and anus. 6th edn. Kanehara, Tokyo
3. Masaki T, Mori T, Matsuoka H, et al (2001) Colonoscopic treatment. Surg Oncol Clin North Am 10:693–708

4. Kudo S, Tamegai Y, Yamano H, et al (2001) Endoscopic mucosal resection of the colon: the Japanese technique. Gastrointest Endosc Clin North Am 10:519–535
5. Waye JD (2001) Endoscopic mucosal resection of colon polyps. Gastrointest Endosc Clin North Am 10:537–548
6. Kudo S, Kashida H, Tamura T, et al (2000) Colonoscopic diagnosis and management of nonpolypoid early colorectal cancer. World J Surg 24:1081–1090
7. Uno Y, Munakata A (1994) The non-lifting sign of invasive cancer. Gastrointest Endosc 40:485–489
8. Akasu T, Kondo H, Moriya Y, et al (2000) Endorectal ultrasonography and treatment of early stage rectal cancer. World J Surg 24:1061–1068
9. Saito Y, Obara T, Einami K, et al (1996) Efficacy of high-frequency ultrasound probes for preoperative staging of invasion depth in flat and depressed colorectal tumors. Gastrointest Endosc 44:34–39
10. Yoshikawa H, Hidano H, Sakakibara A, et al (1999) Endoscopic resection of laterally spreading tumors of the large intestine using a distal attachment. Endoscopy 31: 426–430
11. Saito Y, Fujii T, Mukai H, et al (2001) Endoscopic treatment for laterally spreading tumors in the colon. Endoscopy 33:682–686
12. Tanaka S, Haruma K, Oka S, et al (2001) Clinicopathological features and endoscopic treatment of superficially spreading colorectal neoplasms larger than 20mm. Gastrointest Endosc 54:62–66
13. Dell'Abate P, Iosca, Galimberti A, et al (2001) Endoscopic treatment of colorectal benign-appearing lesions 3cm or larger: technique and outcome. Dis Colon Rectum 44: 112–118
14. Hurlstone DP, Lobo AJ (2002) Assessing resection margin using high-magnification chromoscopy: a useful tool after colonic endoscopic mucosal resection. Am J Gastroenterol 15:2143–2144
15. Kaneko E, Harada H, Kasugai T, et al (2000) The survey of gastrointestinal endoscopic complications in Japan (1993–1997) (in Japanese). Gastroenterol Endosc 42: 308–313
16. Tung SY, Wu CS (2003) Clinical outcome of endoscopically removed early colorectal cancer. J Gastroenterol Hepatol 18:1175–1179
17. Tung SY, Wu CS, Wu MC (2001) Endoscopic treatment of colorectal polyps and early cancer. Dig Dis Sci 6: 1152–1156
18. Bergmann U, Beger HG (2003) Endoscopic mucosal resection for advanced non-polypoid colorectal adenoma and early stage carcinoma. Surg Endosc 17:475–479
19. Higaki S, Hashimoto S, Harada K, et al (2003) Long-term follow-up of large flat colorectal tumors resected endoscopically. Endoscopy 35:845–849

3. Management of Colorectal Cancer by "Hot Biopsy" and Snare Resection

Yoshihiro Sakai

1. Introduction

Cancer can sometimes be diagnosed on endoscopy, but small carcinomas in adenomas are difficult to detect. When cancer is suspected, resection of the lesion is required either endoscopically or surgically, depending on the estimated depth of invasion in cases of cancer. Endoscopic treatment must be supported by clear-cut evidence that the lesion is superficial and can be completely resected by endoscopic techniques. Endoscopic procedures can be used only when tumor invasion is confined to the mucosa or is estimated to be within 1000 μm from the muscularis mucosae. Magnification and dye techniques are often used to estimate the depth of invasion. Endoscopic ultrasonography (EUS) is also used. With the former technique, lesions invading the submucosa that are exposed and have lost their glandular structure are not indicated for endoscopic therapy. With EUS, lesions in which the third layer is interrupted or the fourth layer is displaced also cannot be treated endoscopically. For convenience, physiological saline solution can be locally injected immediately below the lesion just before endoscopic treatment. The endoscopist then determines whether or not the lesion can be lifted. However, this technique can lead to error because lesions associated with fibrosis resulting from previous biopsy or other causes cannot be lifted. Another potential source of error is that whether or not a lesion can be lifted is often related to the technique and subjective judgment of the endoscopist. Even if the lesion is lifted, sometimes the cancer has invaded deeply in the submucosa close to the proper muscle layer.

2. "Hot Biopsy" for Colorectal Cancer

"Hot biopsy" [1] is used in the management of polyp-like lesions. Part of the lesion is grasped with a hot-biopsy forceps. The lesion is then pulled into the center of the lumen and a high-frequency current, particularly coagulation waves, is applied. In terms of size, lesions indicated for this technique must be able to be grasped by the hot-biopsy forceps and elevated. The shape of the lesion should facilitate concentration of high-frequency current, thereby producing heat. Clinically, pulling the lesion into the center of the lumen causes it to become pendunculated or semi-pendunculated, allowing current to be efficiently applied to the lesion base and the tissue to be retrieved. Even if only small fragments of tissue are collected in the cup of the forceps, the part of the lesion remaining after heat-induced coagulation of the base sloughs off (Fig. 1). Hot biopsy therefore cannot be used to treat sessile lesions or lesions more than 1 cm in diameter. This technique is therefore indicated for small pedunculated lesions less than 5 mm in diameter or small nonpedunculated lesions that have a narrow base.

An advantage of hot biopsy is the ability to repeat treatment within a short period. However, whether the target lesion has been adequately treated cannot be confirmed, leading to an increased risk of recurrence. Lesions containing carcinoma can be evaluated if completely retrieved in the cup of the hot-biopsy forceps. Many lesions cannot fit into the cup of the forceps. In some cases, carcinoma tissue is collected in the cup, whereas in others only the surrounding adenomatous components are collected, increasing the risk of misdiagnosis. In patients with carcinoma, it is an urgent task to estimate the depth of invasion and determine whether the lesion has sloughed off or remains, but histological techniques of verifying the outcome are lacking. If no cancer tissue is retrieved, it is unclear whether the diagnosis of cancer before hot biopsy was incorrect or whether the site grasped by the forceps did not contain cancer tissue. Whether treatment was adequate also cannot be confirmed. Patients treated by hot biopsy must therefore be closely followed up. Distant metastasis is a more important concern than local recurrence. The occurrence of distant metastasis of course precludes radical treatment.

Lesions diagnosed as cancer, including small tumors, should therefore not undergo hot biopsy, even if they are pedunculated or have a constricted base. However, since many small lesions with a fine pedicle or a distinctly constricted base are confined to the mucosa, hot biopsy may be used with caution in selected patients. Because of the risks involved, the use of hot biopsy requires the consent of both the physician and patient.

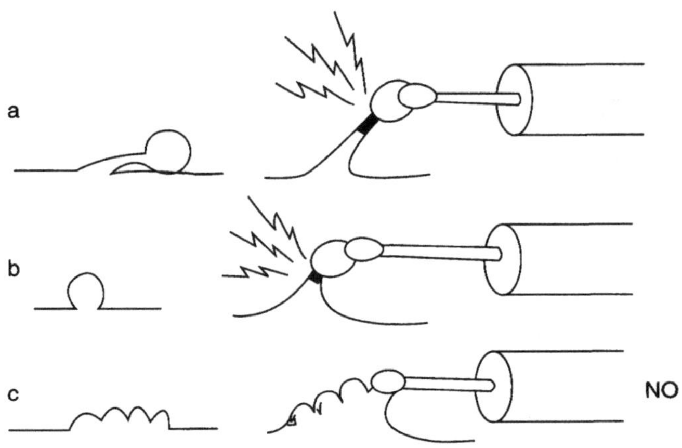

Fig. 1. Indications for hot biopsy technique. Hot biopsy is indicated for **a**, small pedunculated lesions and **b**, small sessile lesions, but not for **c**, large sessile lesions

Table 1. Classification of snare resection

Simple snare resection	
	en bloc
	piecemeal
Combined snare resection[a]	
	en bloc
	piecemeal

[a] including double-snare technique, double-scope technique, preinjection polypectomy or submucosal injection polypectomy, and suction into the hood attached to the scope.

3. Snare Resection for Colorectal Cancer

Snare resection is the procedure of choice for the endoscopic treatment of colorectal lesions diagnosed as cancer. For snare resection high-frequency current is used. The snare is used either alone or with other auxiliary techniques. The former procedure is conventionally referred to as polypectomy, but the term "simple snare resection" is more appropriate because it directly contrasts it with the latter procedure, termed combined snare resection [2] (Table 1). Combined snare resection can be done by two or more basic techniques. A lesion can be lifted with the grasping forceps and encircled with a snare [3] (Fig. 2). Alternatively, two snares can be employed. One snare grasps part of the lesion and the other serves a supplementary role (double-snare technique) [2]. A two-channel scope is required for these procedures. Two separate scopes may also be used. The grasping forceps are inserted via one scope, and the snare is introduced through the other (double-scope technique) [3]. The lesion may also be first grasped with an indwelling snare and ligated. A snare is then placed around the artificially produced constriction. Recently, some investigators have recommended that physiological saline solution is injected into the submucosa immediately below the lesion [4], thereby raising the lesion and facilitating grasping with a snare. This technique is referred to as preinjection polypectomy [5] or subcutaneous injection polypectomy [6]. Recently, this technique became well known as endoscopic mucosal resection (EMR). The original technique was termed endoscopic electroresection [7] and can be traced back to Rosenberg [8].

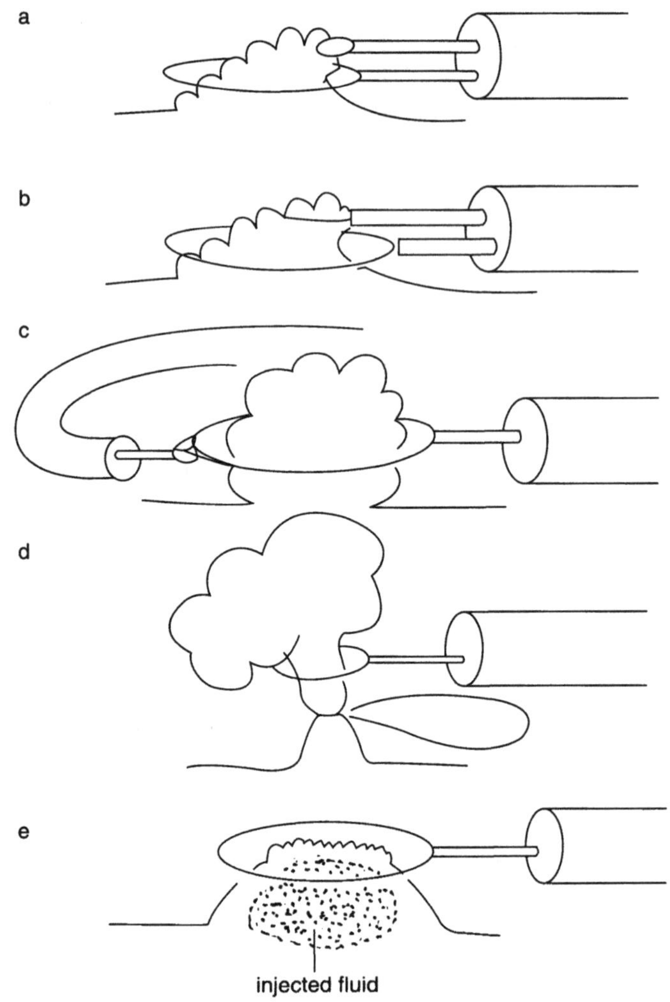

Fig. 2. Various combined snare techniques. **a** Grasping forceps and snare technique. **b** Double-snare technique. **c** Double-scope technique. **d** Detachable snare and snare technique. **e** Preinjection polypectomy (endoscopic mucosal resection, EMR)

Both simple snare resection and combined snare resection can be used to resect lesions en bloc or in a piecemeal fashion. The resection procedure used should be clearly recorded.

In addition to physiological saline solution, epinephrine or dye can be added to the local injection solution.

In general, physiological saline solution is safest and least expensive. A hood can be attached to the scope tip and the lesion encircled with a snare loop. The lesion can then be aspirated into the hood and strangled.

3.1 Simple Snare Resection

Simple snare resection is undertaken with only high-frequency current and a snare. The more familiar term for this procedure is polypectomy. Cancer is frequently present in adenomas measuring more than 1 cm in diameter. Lesions with a relatively fine pedicle have a low risk of submucosal invasion by tumor. Even if such invasion occurs it is usually minimal. This similarly applies to mobile lesions with a distinct constriction. The likelihood of complete resection of cancer is increased by placing the snare at the level of the surrounding mucosa and strangling the lesion. To avoid burns caused by concentration of large amounts of high-frequency current on the muscularis propria, some distance must be physically created between the muscularis propria and the lesion. After strangulation, current should not be immediately applied. First, the lesion should be lifted into the center of the lumen to separate it from the muscularis propria (Fig. 3), or the scope should be pulled distally. Excessive pulling of the scope should be avoided because it can induce peristalsis, or the lesion may be hidden behind the distal semilunar folds. Lesions with a long pedicle that are lifted into the lumen may come in contact with the contralateral mucosa. This causes the high-frequency current to be halved, resulting in low generation of heat at the strangulation site. The time required for resection is prolonged, and the contralateral mucosa adjacent to the lumen may be affected by heat and become purely white. If this occurs, the lesion and snare must be gently moved during the application of current to avoid continued contact with the same site of the contralateral mucosa. Some lesions with a large head cannot be lifted into the center of the lumen. In this case, it is also necessary to slightly change the point of contact with the lesion as described above.

Nonpedunculated hemispheric lesions and sessile lesions are difficult to completely strangle with the snare loop, even when caught by a snare without difficulty. The presence of large amounts of tissue in the loop prolongs the current application time and increases the risk of burning the muscularis propria. Such lesions may also be associated with submucosal invasion. As compared with pedunculated and semipedunculated lesions, determining whether nonpedunculated hemispheric lesions and sessile lesions can be successfully treated endoscopically is more challenging. Endoscopic therapy is not indicated for lesions with a deep central depression and often cannot be used to treat lesions that have narrowing at the border with the surrounding mucosa, large nodules, fold convergence, or surface deformity suggesting mucosal defects. If such findings are unclear, the lesion and surrounding mucosa should be observed at higher magnification or EUS should be performed.

An important goal of endoscopic diagnosis is to determine whether cancer is present. Careful observation of the lesion base can provide vital clues suggesting whether endoscopic therapy is indicated. After resection, all specimens should be retrieved. Evaluation of sections including the resection margin is essential.

To decrease the risk of hemorrhage, coagulation waves are used for the high-frequency current. Nonpedunculated lesions are frequently treated with a blend

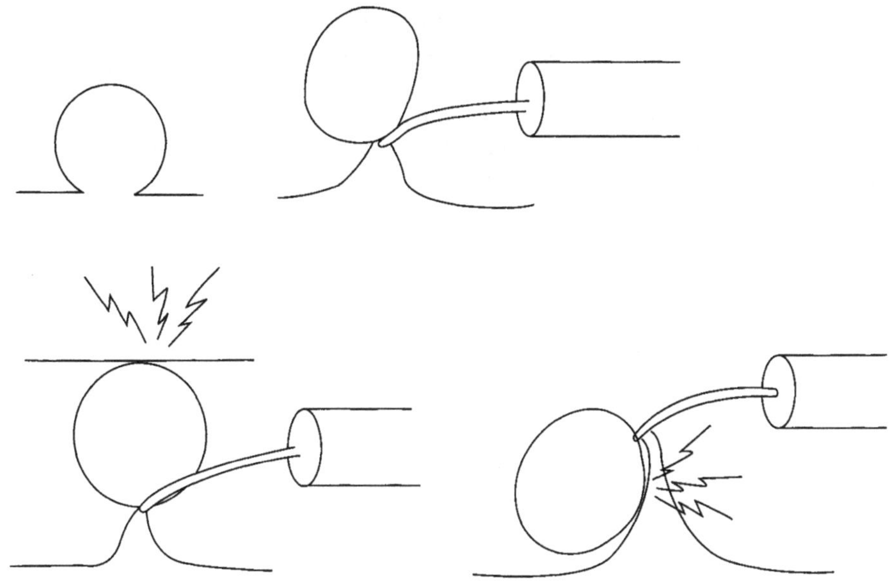

Fig. 3. Simple resection technique and caution during the procedure to avoid excess burn

of coagulation waves and cutting waves. Small amounts of remnant tumor have been shown to slough off due to the burning effect. However, persistence of even small numbers of tumor cells should be avoided.

Additional surgical resection is necessary when the resection margin is tumor positive, the tumor front shows undifferentiated or poorly differentiated carcinoma, or vascular permeation is present [9].

3.2 En Bloc Resection with Local Injection

Local injection ,into the submucosa has three main advantages: (1) the distance between the lesion and muscularis propria can be increased; (2) physiological saline solution acts as insulation; and (3) catching the lesion with a snare becomes easy. Even if insulation is minimal and lesions such as superficial type tumors cannot be ensnared, local injection markedly raises the lesion, facilitating encirclement by the snare loop. Increased distance between the lesion and muscularis propria decreases the concentration of heat on the latter.

In addition to superficial lesions, this technique is also effective for nonpedunculated lesions as described above. It is sometimes used to prevent hemorrhage when resecting large pedunculated lesions.

During local injection, the needle must correctly penetrate to the submucosa. The needle tip should therefore approach the lesion laterally and be inserted with a snap. The recommended angle from the mucosal surface is 30° to 45°. Strong insertion of the needle tip from steeper angles relative to the mucosal surface can result in penetration of the submucosa and muscularis mucosae, as well as penetration of the serosa. Insertion of the needle beyond the intestinal wall results in loss of physiological saline solution, with no change on the mucosal side. When physiological saline solution is injected into the subserosa, a protrusion slowly develops, elevating the lesion. However, the color of the mucosa surrounding the lesion remains unchanged. Correct penetration of the needle into the submucosa and injection of physiological saline causes changes in structure and color tone: a round protrusion develops near the needle tip and a transparent grayish-blue tone appears. By changing the position of the needle during injection, the lesion can be guided to the top of the protrusion. Insertion of the injection needle into the submucosa at the anal side (the side near the scope) of large lesions can cause the lesion to move towards the oral side of the protrusion (Fig. 4). Therefore, the needle should be inserted and physiological saline injected into the submucosa at the oral side of lesions scheduled to be treated by en bloc resection. If the lesion starts to shift to an undesirable site during injection, the needle should be removed and reinserted into an appropriate site.

The snare is used in a conventional manner. It is placed around the lesion, including a small margin of normal mucosa, and the lesion is strangled. The high-frequency current should employ cutting waves for resection of superficial lesions and a combination consisting primarily of cutting waves and including coagulation waves for hemispherical lesions. Strangulation should be stronger than that used with coagulation waves alone, because superficial lesions are supplied by fine blood vessels.

Irrespective of the procedure, bleeding can be effectively managed by clipping. Clips should therefore be available during treatment.

All resected lesions should be retrieved. Superficial lesions should be spread out on cork or rubber plates, pinned in place, and fixed in 10% formalin. Lesions placed directly in formalin curl up, precluding preparation of complete specimens. This can lead to incorrect evaluation of the resection margin or the response to treatment.

3.3 Piecemeal Resection

In principle, lesions should be resected en bloc. To permit non-touch isolation, lesions must not be divided

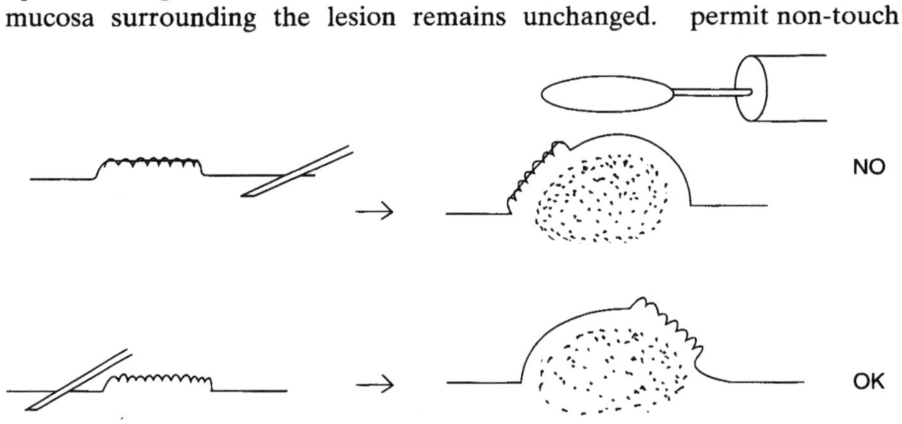

Fig. 4. Suitable site of injection for EMR

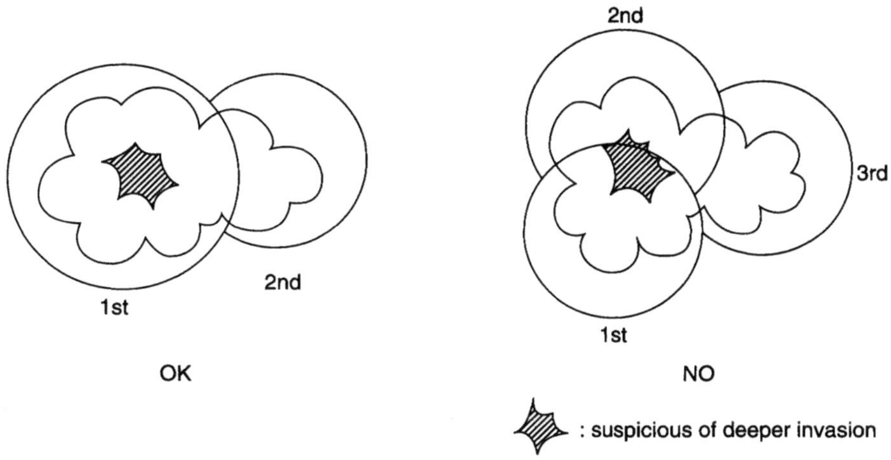

Fig. 5. Planned piecemeal resection and suitable orders

unless absolutely necessary. Tissue retrieved after piecemeal resection performed in a single day usually cannot be treated similarly to specimens obtained by en bloc resection. Piecemeal resection carries an increased risk of error when evaluating tumor spread or properties of the tumor front. During resection of large lesions, the snare may not be able to be removed once the lesion is ensnared, even after the endoscopist realizes that complete en bloc resection is not feasible. These events may necessitate piecemeal resection. Some lesions considered resectable en bloc may be found to be larger than expected after application of current. Undetected parts of lesions can thus lead to remnant tumor. After retrieval, the lesion should be reconstructed as closely as possible. Pieces of the lesion should be pinned in place to maintain their configuration and then fixed in formalin.

Some large lesions undergo piecemeal resection by design. The procedure is similar to that described above. When using a snare, caution is required to avoid division of the lesion along the middle of the tumor (Fig. 5). Large nodules, flat regions differing from the surrounding tumor area, and central depressions are strongly associated with the tumor front. These findings should be included in a single specimen whenever possible.

Piecemeal resection involves the repeated application of high-frequency current to nearly the same site, and large amounts of tissue are present in the snare loop. Resection therefore requires large amounts of heat, even when only cutting current is very strongly concentrated on the target lesion. Consequently, local injection is essential, and the lesion must be drawn into the center of the lumen to adequately separate it from the muscularis propria.

Heat-induced perforation may occur 3–4 days after treatment. Patients must therefore rest after the procedure. Particular caution is required after piecemeal resection.

References

1. Williams CB (1973) Diathermy biopsy, a technique for endoscopic management of small polyps. Endoscopy 5: 215–218
2. Sakai Y (1992) Japanese classification of colorectal carcinoma and tentative classification by Japan Gastrointestinal Endoscopy Society (in Japanese). MB Gastro 9:95–100
3. Takekoshi T, Fujii A, Takagi K, et al (1988) Indication for endoscopic double snare polypectomy of gastric lesions (in Japanese with English abstract). Stomach Intest 23: 387–398
4. Watanabe S, Kishi H, Katagiri K, et al (1990) Endoscopic resection by double colonoscope method for giant colonic polyps (in Japanese with English abstract). Endosc Forum 6:274–278
5. Williams CB (1997) Personal communication
6. Waye JD (2000) Colonoscopic polypectomy. Diagn Ther Endosc 6:111–124
7. Deyhle P, Largiader F, Jenny S, et al (1973) A method for endoscopic electroresection of sessile colonic polyp. Endoscopy 5:38–40
8. Rosenberg N (1955) Submucosal saline wheal as safety factor in fulguration of rectal and sigmoidal polyp. Arch Surg 70:120–122
9. Japanese Society for Cancer of the Colon and Rectum (1997) Japanese classification of colorectal carcinoma. Kanehara, Tokyo

4. Esophageal Cancer: Photodynamic Therapy

René Lambert

1. Early Neoplastic Lesions in the Esophagus

Neoplastic lesions develop in the squamous lining of the esophagus (squamous cell cancer) or in a segment of columnar metaplasia in Barrett's esophagus with a specialized epithelium (intestinal metaplasia). Esophageal adenocarcinoma is increasing in Western countries. At the esophagogastric junction there is often confusion between neoplasia in a short Barrett's esophagus and neoplasia at the cardia.

Precancerous squamous lesions include low-grade dysplasia (LGD) and high-grade dysplasia (HGD). Intraepithelial and intramucosal cancer that have not metastasized to lymph nodes are called early cancer. Submucosal cancer is considered as advanced cancer.

In the columnar metaplastic epithelium, the distinction between LGD and reactive epithelial changes caused by reflux is uncertain [1]. There are conflicting reports on the rate at which LGD progresses to HGD and then to carcinoma. Recent data [2] suggest that the 5-year cumulative incidence of cancer in patients with HGD is low (9%), and the risk of progression to cancer is less in focal than in diffuse HGD [3]. Intramucosal adenocarcinoma corresponds to early cancer.

Japanese authors have described the endoscopic pattern of early squamous cell cancer. In Western countries the detection, definition, and grading of early neoplasia in Barrett's esophagus is still an area of imprecision: neoplastic areas, flat and inconspicuous, easily can go unrecognized. When HGD is detected, foci of early cancer are associated in one third of cases. Chromoscopy with methylene blue helps in the detection of intestinal metaplasia [4], but its contribution to the detection of neoplastic areas (pale color) is debatable. High-rank technology is now being proposed to detect the specialized epithelium or dysplasia in Barrett's esophagus. Magnification, enhanced with acetic acid spraying, has a 100% efficacy in detecting intestinal metaplasia [5]. Based on the fact that the reflectance and fluorescence spectrum are altered in the same way by absorption and scattering in the tissue, a multidisciplinary team has proposed a trimodal spectroscopy [6], which has proved extremely reliable even in the distinction between LGD and HGD when the three methods are combined. Optical coherence tomography, based on the measure of the back-reflection of infrared photons with interferometry, has given a reliable characteristic image of intestinal metaplasia in 121 patients with Barrett's esophagus [7].

2. Principles of Photodynamic Therapy

Photodynamic therapy (PDT) is a tissue-based photochemical reaction in which oxygen is consumed [8, 9]. A photosensitizer absorbs photons with energy matching the level of excitation of the molecule, which passes from a ground state to excited singlet or triplet states (Fig. 1). The singlet state is extremely short-lived and the molecule returns to the ground state after emission of a fluorescent photon. The metastable triplet state (a higher degree of energy) transfers its energy to tissular oxygen forming toxic oxy-products. The reaction is triggered by the monochromatic light from a laser source and the amplitude of the reaction depends on the dosimetry of the photon beam.

The selectivity of the response is influenced by multiple factors: (1) the geometry of irradiation; (2) the concentration of the photosensitizer in the tumor and in the normal tissue—the T/N ratio of concentration is at 2 with hematoporphyrin and may be as high as 6 with new agents; (3) the availability of oxygen, depending on the microcirculation in the tissue.

The energy transfer from the photosensitizer to the tissue target results in cytotoxic oxy-radicals. Most of them are linked to the formation of the hyper-reactive singlet oxygen (issued from the stable triplet oxygen). Cell destruction occurs only for a threshold level of singlet oxygen at 10^9 molecules.

Cell membranes are the principal target of singlet oxygen. The immediate oxidative stress is followed by early apoptosis. The complete destruction of the neoplastic lesion requires a log 6–8 reduction in the number of malignant cells. In theory, this is not achieved with PDT, which achieves a log 2 reduction. The limiting factor in cell killing is the progressive reduction in the availability of oxygen during the reaction. However, other secondary mechanisms kill the spared cells, i.e., ischemia in relation to damaged microvasculature, cyto-

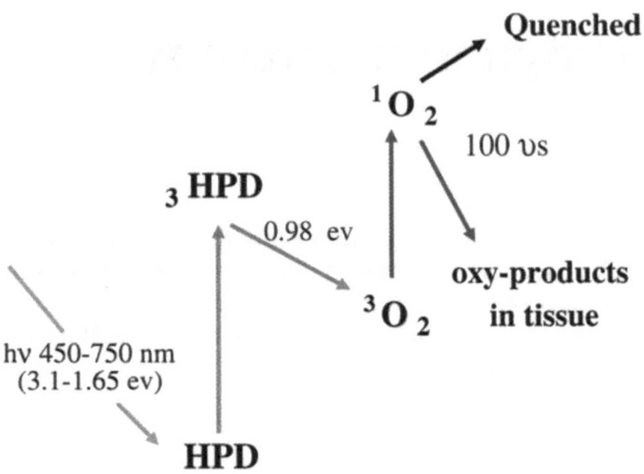

Fig. 1. *Principles of photodynamic therapy (PDT).* The photosensitizer (hematoporphyrin derivative) absorbing the incident photon reaches a transient triplet state and returns then to the ground state. Singlet hyper-reactive oxygen is formed after absorbing energy. The fraction of the metastable singlet oxygen not destroyed by quenching forms toxic oxy products in the tissue. *HPD*, hematoporphyrin derivative

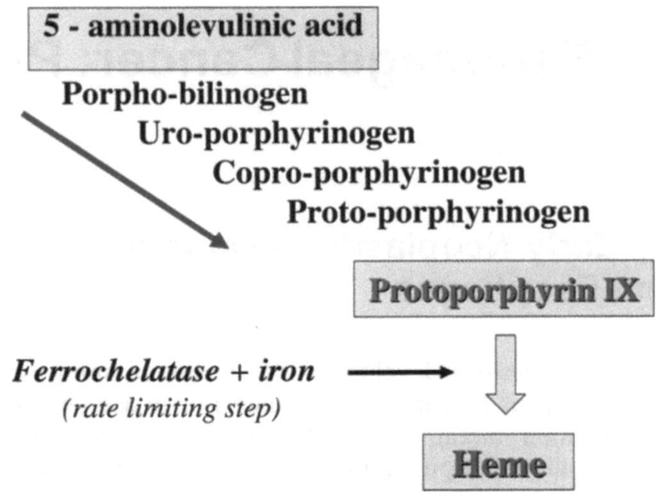

Fig. 2. *Metabolism of 5-aminolevulinic acid* (5-ALA). An exogenous dose of 5-ALA is involved in the metabolic transformation to heme. An accumulation of protoporphyrin IX occurs in the tissue because of the limited output of the final enzymatic step

logical damage by scavenging nitrite oxide, and delayed immune response with tumor antigens presented for recognition to helper T lymphocytes. The antitumor reaction may occur even in areas not reached by the illumination, with unexpectedly good results. Finally, PDT is an endoscopic procedure with tumor destruction and no specimen is available for tumor staging after treatment.

3. Photosensitizers

Photodynamic therapy requires the presence in the tissue target of a photosensitizer agent, a molecule with a resonant macrocyclic ring of alternating single and double bonds (porphyrins or chlorophylls). Exogenous photosensitizers are sprayed directly at the surface of the target, or transferred by the microcirculation, or by intravenous (i.v.) or oral administration. Endogenous photosensitizers are formed locally after administration of a pro-drug.

Most studies have been conducted with porphyrins. The first agent used in clinical studies, HPD or the hematoporphyrin derivative (i.v. dose 2.5–5 mg/kg), is a complex mixture of porphyrins. Photofrin (i.v. dose 1–2 mg/kg, QLT Phototherapeutics, Vancouver, Canada), is a more purified form; the dimeric hematoporphyrin ether (DHE), Photosan-3, is another preparation. All these products are activated by monochromatic red light (630 nm) with a typical dose rate of 100 mW/cm^2.

New synthetic photosensitizers with chemical purity are on trial (lutetium texaphyrin, tin ethyl-etiopurpurin, bacterial chlorophylls, phthalocyanines). m-THPC, or Foscan (i.v. dose 0.15 mg/kg), is a tetra (*m*-hydroyphenyl) chlorin, activated at 514 nm (green light) or 652 nm (red light). The 652 nm wavelength, longer than that used for porphyrins, results in deeper tissue damage (up to 10 mm).

The pro-drug, or endogenous photosensitizer, is 5-aminolevulinic acid (5-ALA). It has been used as a topical agent in dermatology, and more recently in the esophagus (500 mg). The oral route (dose 60 mg/kg) is generally used for digestive tumors. After ingestion the molecule undergoes metabolic transformations up to the heme (Fig. 2). However, the enzyme ferrochelatase, in the presence of iron, is a rate-limiting step. This results in accumulation of the photosensitizer in the tissue target. Protoporphyrin IX is activated by a red light in the range of 630–650 nm, with an optimum at 635 nm.

4. Tissue Target

The efficacy of PDT is influenced by the accessibility of the neoplastic area for illumination with a vector fibroscope. There is no doubt that the depth of penetration of the photons in the digestive wall is a limiting factor. This is why the method is adapted only for the curative treatment of dysplasia and early cancer. There is no sound rationale in using PDT in palliation for debulking advanced cancer.

The concentration of the photosensitizer should be higher in the tumor than in the surrounding normal tissues. The T/N concentration ratio varies with each photosensitizer and is favored if the product is transferred in a lipophilic form. As an example, the tissue concentration of a hexamethyl-5-ALA ester is much higher than that of 5-ALA. The temporal variation in the concentration of the photosensitizer differs in the tumor and in the normal tissue. With hematoporphyrin, the optimal T/N ratio of concentration is at 48–72h; with oral 5-ALA it is at 4–6h.

The T/N concentration ratio varies with the tissular target; selective uptake in the mucosa is an advantage. Photofrin is present in the epithelial cells and also in the lamina propria; the photon beam may reach the submucosa and provoke tissue damage with necrosis, fibrosis, and stricture. Protoporphyrin IX (5-ALA) has an elective affinity for the mucosa; generally it should not be used for lesions over 2mm in thickness.

5. Laser Sources

Initially laser sources from scientific laboratories were used. The dye-laser sources are tunable, within a range of wavelengths depending on the dye used. They are sources pumped either by an Argon gas laser (Spectra-Physics, Mountain View, CA, USA; Coherent, Portland, OR, USA) or by a KTP-Nd:YAG laser that will generate a photon beam at 630nm with enough energy. More recently, material adapted to medical usage has become available. The *Coherent Lambda Plus* laser uses an argon pumped dye-laser and emits up to 2.5W of energy output. The *Lasercope 630* uses a KTP-Nd:YAG to pump the dye-laser, generating up to 7W of energy output. Both are highly expensive. Diode laser sources, now available, represent the future technology; they are not tunable, produce a single wavelength, but are cheap and easily transportable. The *Diomed 630* produces red light at 630nm with an output of 2W and may be plugged in at any source.

6. Operative Procedure

The clinical application of PDT in the esophagus requires light distributors for delivery in the esophagus. The first probes, inserted through the accessory channel of the fibroscope, were flexible glass fibers with a diffuser. Commercially cylindrical diffusers have a diffuser segment at the tip of the fiber and deliver an output of 400mW per cm of diffuser (up to 5cm). Light applicators ensuring a homogeneous and central distribution of light in a dilated esophageal lumen are also proposed; windowed models are adapted to the treatment of sectorial lesions. The devices are available as a bougie (Savary-Gilliard dilator) or as a balloon, and pass through a guide wire [10] (centering Overholt inflatable balloon). Other balloons [11] pass through the accessory channel of the fibroscope.

With Photofrin an i.v. dose of 2mg/kg is slowly injected in a perfusion. The peak concentration is reached in a few hours, but the optimal T/N ratio of concentration is reached at 48–72h and endoscopic exploration with illumination is performed at that time. The delivery of 100–200J/cm^2 with the red photon beam requires 20–30min, according to the size of the lesion. The procedure is conducted under conscious sedation. The endoscopic control at 24h shows inflammation, enanthema, and early necrosis; if the response is not patent a complementary irradiation is still possible. In the next days, inflammation of the esophagus and surrounding mediastinum occurs with increased thickness of the esophageal wall (Fig. 3a,b). The transient necrosis is followed by prompt healing if the neoplastic area is superficial; with lesions reaching the submucosa the necrosis persists longer and a definitive scar occurs (Fig. 4a,b). In some cases a chronic ulcer is observed. From the time of injection of the product, skin sensitization persists for 4–8 weeks so the patient must avoid direct exposure to sunlight. If PDT is integrated in a multimodal protocol, the local tolerance to radiotherapy and to brachytherapy is reduced. With 5-ALA oral, the patient receives 60mg/kg of the product dissolved in orange juice, and endoscopic illumination is performed 3–6h later, just as for Photofrin. The ingestion of the product provokes nausea in most patients for approximately 12h and a transient elevation of aminotransferases for up to 1 week. Endoscopic control at 24h is not helpful (no possible irradiation in complement) and the tissue response is more controlled after 1 week.

The endoscopic evaluation of the initial tumor response takes place at 1 month; the response is classified as complete or incomplete. Some authors attempt to destroy the residual tumor with the Nd:YAG laser or electrocoagulation when the response is incomplete. Alternatively, repeated PDT sessions are performed at 3-month intervals with Photofrin and at 1-month intervals with 5-ALA. Further controls can be repeated at 3 and 6 months, and the follow-up must be prolonged because of a significant rate of recurrence or metachronous lesions after the immediate complete response.

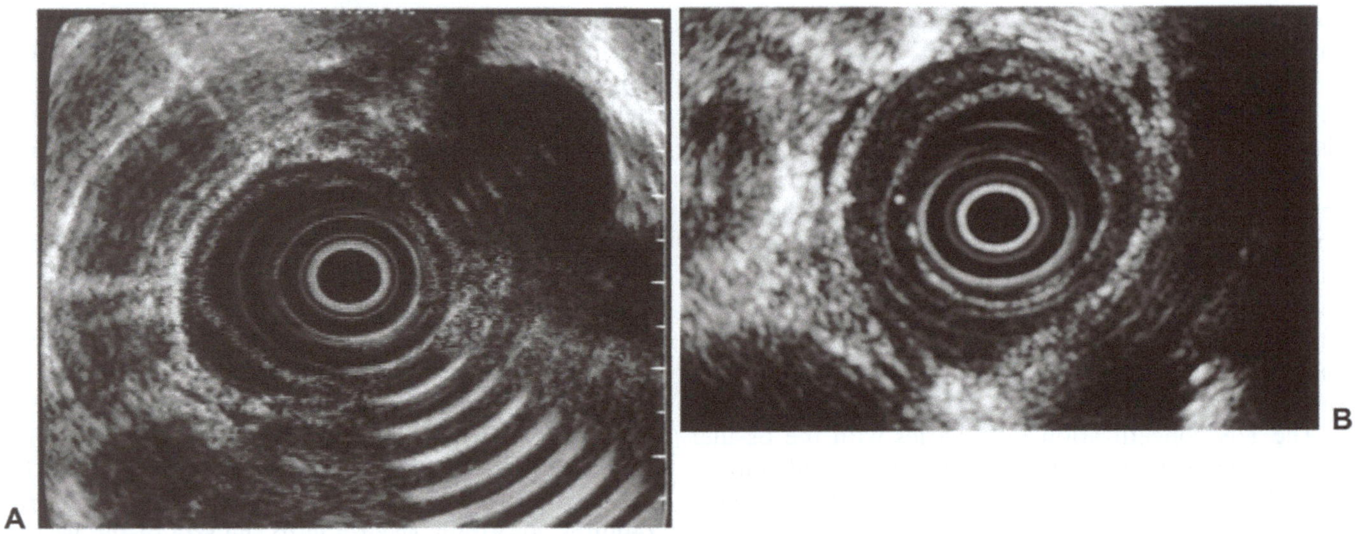

Fig. 3A,B. *Echoendoscopy in PDT.* **A** *Before PDT*: the hypoechoic T1 tumor (*arrow*) is visible opposite the hypoechoic aorta. **B** *After PDT*: diffuse thickening of the esophageal wall; the echoic layers are not delineated

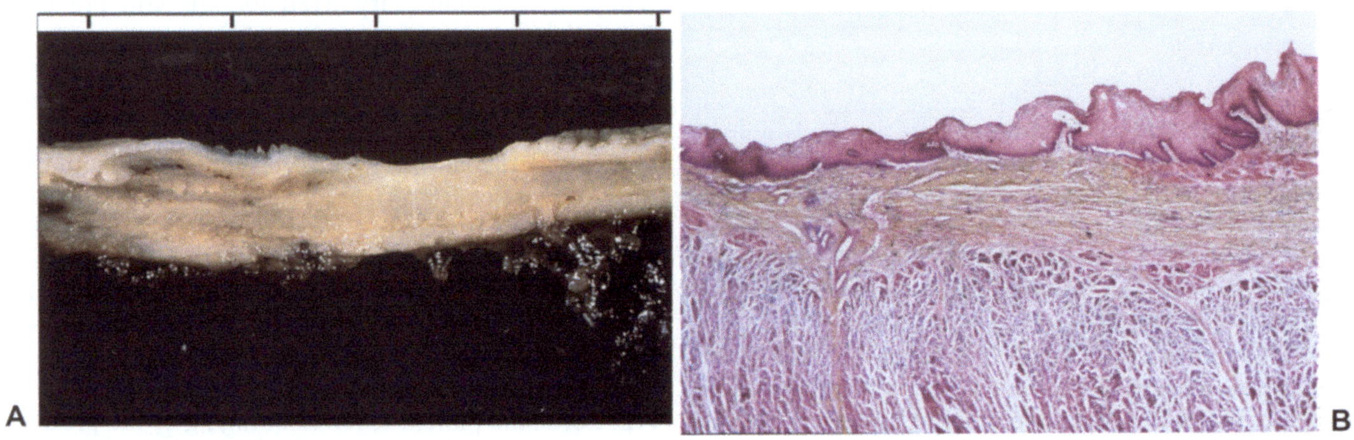

Fig. 4A,B. *Complete response after PDT.* **A** *Semimacroscopic view*: Transverse section of the esophageal wall in a patient submitted to esophagectomy 2 months after destruction by PDT of a T1 squamous cell cancer. The ulcerated area (*arrows*) is healed and covered by a squamous lining. A central scar is visible. **B** *Histology*. The muscularis mucusae (*arrow*) is destroyed under the regenerative squamous epithelium covering the area of treatment

7. Results of Endotherapy with PDT

7.1 In Squamous Cell Cancer

Most results were obtained with hematoporphyrin [12–14]. After the first clinical attempt with the HPD by the group of Dougherty, its application to early esophageal cancer occurred in Japan. Other trials were conducted in Europe (France, Switzerland, Germany). In contrast, in the United States the trials were restricted to palliation of advanced esophageal cancer. Nowadays the focus is only on early cancer. A recent review [12] has accumulated 164 cases of early esophageal cancer. The first series used HPD; then Photofrin and Photosan-3 were used, and more recently Foscan (m-THPC) [12]. Most results are obtained with a variable follow-up (from 1 to 96 months), and evaluation is limited to the initial complete response. The rate of initial complete response in most series is high (70%–90%). The proportion of late recurrences is missing in most series, but is as high as 36% in a series [14] after 12–18 months, justifying a prolonged surveillance protocol. The association of multimodal therapy with radiotherapy or brachytherapy to PDT has shown no substantial benefit. In conclusion, the literature provides substantial evidence that PDT is curative in early esophageal cancer; on the other hand, its position in the treatment of esophageal cancer is still uncertain. Compared with surgical series the number of cases is small, the follow-up is short and irregular, and the absence of post-therapeutic tumor staging in a resected specimen is a major limiting factor.

7.2 In Adenocarcinoma

The trials were conducted in patients with dysplasia or cancer in Barrett's esophagus. Cancer cases were small tumors with a superficial pattern at endoscopy, rather than confirmed early cancer. The first series [15] used HPD or Photofrin. The recent trend is to use 5-ALA for lesions no more than 2mm in thickness, and m-THPC for the other lesions. The results of PDT in Barrett's esophagus, summarized in recent reviews [16, 17], concern the response of nondysplastic areas with metaplasia and the response of neoplastic areas.

The impact on metaplasia has been examined on the basis that after endoscopic destruction, reversal to squamous epithelium occurs during healing in an acid environment, suggesting prevention of the risk of cancer. Results with PDT confirm those obtained with other procedures (contact thermal laser, Argon plasma coagulation). With PDT, metaplasia is eradicated on the surface in about 70% of patients, but there are residual or regrowth columnar glands, covered by the reversed squamous epithelium, with a potential for dysplasia or cancer. Furthermore, there is a toll of endoscopic complications with strictures [15]. In conclusion, the geometry of irradiation during PDT should be limited to the neoplastic area, without treating the surrounding nondysplastic metaplasia.

The results of PDT in HGD have been summarized recently [16, 17]; an initial complete response was observed in 90%–100% of cases. With early cancer the initial complete response has been observed in 60% of cases [16, 18, 19]. The limits of the protocols regarding the length of follow-up, surveillance, and recurrence rate are just as for squamous cell cancer.

8. Complications

Complications [20] include cutaneous photosensitivity with edema, large-scale erythema, blistering, and bullae formation, during up to 8 weeks, with Photofrin; significant toxic dermal side effects occur in 19%. The duration of cutaneous photosensitivity is shorter with m-THPC and even more with 5-ALA (48–72h). Endoscopic complications include frequent and transient side effects (odynophagia and chest pain) and rare severe complications (perforation or bleeding). Pleural effusion, fever, and cardiac arrhythmia have been observed. The major risk is the development of a stricture (15%–58%) during healing.

9. Indications for PDT in Early Esophageal Cancer

The respective indications for surgery or endotherapy in esophageal squamous cell cancer have been analyzed with respect to mucosectomy. The same criteria should apply for PDT; however, the histological control of the resected specimen is absent. This is why echoendoscopy with a high (20 or 30MHz) resolution is recommended before treatment; invasion of the submucosa is a contraindication to the curative option. Extended indications are proposed in patients with a poor performance status. When the lesions fulfill the criteria for curative endotherapy, the alternative is between mucosectomy and PDT.

With squamous cell cancer, the guidelines are clear: a small number of patients with a well-delineated and small mucosal lesion are treated electively by mucosectomy, whereas all other patients should be treated by surgery. Since the extension of the mucosectomy protocol, the elective indications of PDT in patients with a good performance status are scarce. In patients with a poor performance status, extended indications of endoscopic treatment are possible with PDT. This applies to large lesions or multiple foci.

With columnar neoplasia in Barrett's esophagus, the finding of LGD does not justify an early treatment. The first step is a 3-month trial with acid inhibition, followed by repeated biopsies. For HGD, the first attitude is the careful search for an associated area with adenocarcinoma. Echoendoscopy is useful to verify the integrity of the submucosa. The malignant potential of confirmed HGD is debatable, and for most patients surveillance combined with endoscopic treatment is preferred to systematic surgery. The new alternative is therefore between surveillance or surveillance plus endotherapy. The areas with HGD are often flat and poorly delineated; treatment with PDT is easier than with mucosectomy, unless nodular areas are present. The 5-ALA photosensitizer has the advantage of being electively localized in the mucosa, with less risk of damage in the depth of the wall. When early cancer is confirmed mucosectomy is the treatment of choice, but poor risk and extremely aged patients are frequent; in such cases PDT may be proposed. Photofrin or m-THPC are preferred, due to their more aggressive capacity for destruction.

References

1. Spechler SJ (2001) Disputing dysplasia. Gastroenterology 120:1864–1868
2. Schnell TG, Sontag SJ, Chejfec G, et al (2001) Long term non surgical management of Barrett's esophagus with high grade dysplasia. Gastroenterology 120:1607–1619
3. Buttar NS, Wang KK, Sebo TJ, et al (2001) Extent of high grade dysplasia in Barrett's esophagus correlates with risk of adenocarcinoma. Gastroenterology 120:1630–1639
4. Canto MIF, Setrakian S, Willis JE, et al (2001) Methylene blue staining of dysplastic and non dysplastic Barrett's esophagus: an in vivo and ex vivo study. Endoscopy 33: 391–400
5. Guelrud M, Herrera I, Essenfeld H, et al (2001) Enhanced magnification endoscopy: a new technique to identify specialized metaplasia in Barrett's esophagus. Gastrointest Endosc 53:559–565
6. Georgakoudi I, Jacobson BC, Van Dam J (2001) Fluorescence, reflectance and light scattering spectroscopy for evaluating dysplasia in patients with Barrett's esophagus. Gastroenterology 120:1620–1629
7. Poneros JM, Brand S, Bouma BE, et al (2001) Diagnosis of specialized intestinal metaplasia by optical coherence tomography. Gastroenterology 120:7–12
8. Barr H, Dix AJ, Kendall C, et al (2001) Review article: the potential role for photodynamic therapy in the management of upper gastrointestinal disease. Aliment Pharmacol Ther 15:311–321
9. Dougherty TJ, Gomer CJ, Henderson BW, et al (1998) Photodynamic therapy. J Natl Cancer Inst 90:889–905
10. Overholt BF, Panjehpour M, DeNovo RC, et al (1996) Balloon photodynamic therapy of esophageal cancer: effect of increasing balloon size. Lasers Surg Med 18: 248–252
11. Gossner L, May A, Sroka R, et al (1999) A new long range through the scope balloon applicator for photodynamic therapy in the esophagus and cardia. Endoscopy 31: 370–376
12. Radu A, Wagnieres G, van den Bergh H, et al (2000) Photodynamic therapy of early squamous cell cancers of the esophagus. Gastrointest Endosc Clin North Am 10:439–460
13. Çorti L, Skarlatos J, Boso C, et al. (2000). Outcome of patients receiving photodynamic therapy for early esophageal cancer. Int J Radiat Oncol Biol Phys 47: 419–424
14. Sibille A, Lambert R, Souquet JC, et al (1995) Long term survival after photodynamic therapy for esophageal cancer. Gastroenterology 108:337–344
15. Overholt BF, Panjehpour M, Haydeck JM (1999) Photodynamic therapy for Barrett's esophagus. Follow up in 100 patients. Gastrointest Endosc 49:1–7
16. Barr H (2000) Barrett's esophagus. Treatment with 5-aminolevulinic acid photodynamic therapy. Gastrointest Endosc Clin North Am 10:421–437
17. Wang KK (2000) Photodynamic therapy of Barrett's esophagus. Gastrointest Endosc Clin North Am 10: 409–419
18. Gossner L, May A, Sroka R et al (1999) Photodynamic destruction of high grade dysplasia and early carcinoma of the esophagus after the oral administration of 5-aminolevulinic acid. Cancer 8:1921–1928
19. Gossner L, Stolte M, Sroka R, et al (1998) Photodynamic ablation of high grade dysplasia and early cancer in Barrett's esophagus by means of 5-aminolevulinic acid. Gastroenterology 114:448–455
20. Wang KK, Nijhawan PK (2000) Complications of photodynamic therapy in gastrointestinal disease. Gastrointest Endosc Clin North Am 10:487–495

5. Esophageal Cancer: Endoscopic Mucosal Resection

Hiroyasu Makuuchi

1. Early Esophageal Cancer and Endoscopic Mucosal Resection

Endoscopic mucosal resection (EMR) was introduced to the clinical field of treatment for early esophageal cancer in Japan in 1989. This had been developed owing to widespread use of slender panendoscopy and iodine staining throughout Japan [1].

In the United States and European countries, where Barrett's cancer is relatively common, this technique was indicated for such cases.

The surgical treatment for esophageal cancer is extremely invasive regarding operative procedures and impairs postoperative quality of life. So if the cancerous lesion can be resected only by endoscopic treatment and has no lymph node metastasis, this new treatment is recommended as an alternative to invasive surgery. In comparison with other endoscopic maneuvers, EMR allows pathological analysis of the resected specimen; the complete removal of the lesion can be proven by this analysis and, at the same time, the depth of invasion and lymph vessel invasion of cancer can be investigated. In this chapter, the details of EMR are described.

2. Methods of EMR

In general, four different maneuvers of EMR are known to be employed for treatment of early esophageal cancer.

1. Strip biopsy: Under double-channel endoscopy, the lesion is caught by a grasping forceps inserted through one channel, and cut by a snare inserted through the other channel [2].

2. EEMR (endoscopic esophageal mucosal resection)-tube method: Very commonly performed in Japan. After insertion of a silicon-rubber tube into the esophagus, the mucosa containing the lesion is drawn into the tube by endoscopic suction made by an endoscope inserted through the tube, and the lesion is cut by a snare inserted through the side channel of the tube [3]. The complete removal of the lesion and suspected neighboring area is possible by the EEMR-tube 4-step method [4].

3. EMRC (EMR with cap) method: Developed by Inoue et al. [5]. The tip of the endoscope is equipped with a transparent cap and the lesion is cut after drawing the lesion into the cap by suction. This maneuver is widely employed in Europe and the United States.

4. Endoscopic submucosal dissection (ESD) method: Recently developed by Oyama et al. [6]. This enables removal of the lesion containing the mucosa as well as the submucosal layer using a hooked knife, but it requires great skill.

3. EEMR-Tube 4-Step Method [4]

3.1 First Step (Fig. 1)

(a) An endoscope is passed through the EEMR tube (Create Medic, Tokyo, Japan) first, and the endoscope alone is inserted into the esophagus. Iodine staining is carried out to confirm the lesion. An endoscopic puncture needle is inserted through the working channel of the endoscope and the mucosa is punctured approximately 3 mm proximal to the lesion. Saline with indigocarmine is injected into the submucosal layer beneath the lesion to elevate the mucosa containing the lesion entirely.
(b) The EEMR tube is inserted into the esophagus along the endoscope. A slender snare is inserted through the side channel of the EEMR tube and opened above the lesion.
(c) The mucosa containing the lesion is drawn sufficiently into the tube through the open snare by endoscopic suction.
(d) The snare is closed and the EEMR tube is pulled back 3 cm. Then the mucosal lesion is removed entirely by high-frequency current.

3.2 Second Step

The maneuvers mentioned above in the first step are repeated for relatively large residual lesions. Great care should be taken not to draw the area from which the mucosa is already removed into the tube.

3.3 Third Step (Fig. 2)

(a) This third step is suitable for very tiny residual lesions to be removed accurately. The snare is released from the side channel of the EEMR tube and a grasping forceps (alligator jaw forceps) is inserted through the endoscope's working channel.
(b) The forceps is passed through the snare, and the mucosa including the residual lesion is grasped.

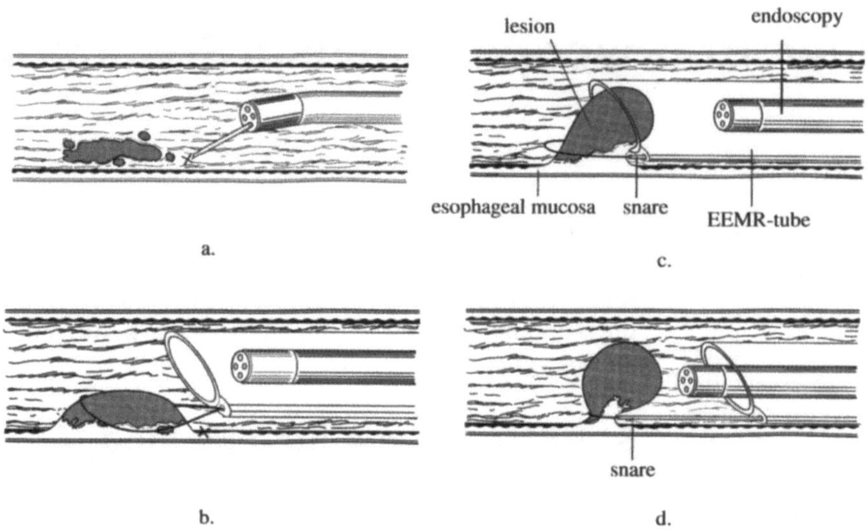

Fig. 1a–d. Endoscopic esophageal mucosal resection (*EEMR*)-tube 4-step method: first step. **a** Saline with indigo-carmine is injected into the submucosal layer beneath the lesion after iodine staining. **b** The EEMR tube is inserted along the endoscopy into the esophagus up to the puncture point. The snare is inserted through the side channel of the tube and opened above the lesion. **c** The mucosa containing the lesion is aspirated into the tube by applying endoscopic suction. **d** The snare is pulled tight and the tube is pulled back. The electric current is passed to resect the mucosa

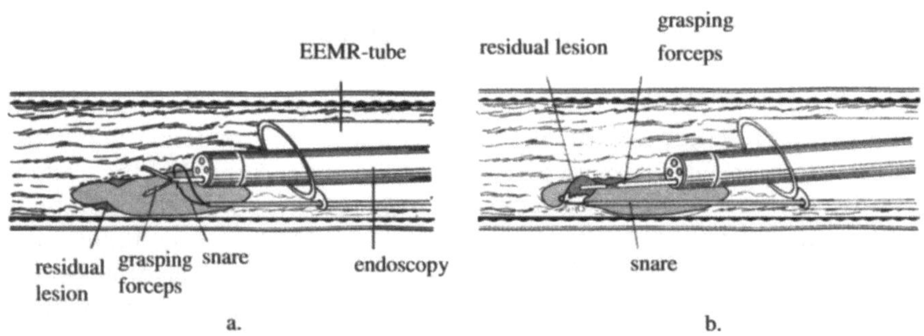

Fig. 2a,b. Endoscopic esophageal mucosal resection (*EEMR*)-tube 4-step method: third step. **a** The snare is inserted through the side channel of the EEMR tube and the grasping forceps is inserted through the working channel of the endoscope. **b** The grasping forceps is passed through the snare and the mucosa with the residual lesion is grasped. The snare is closed and an electric current resects the mucosa

Then the snare is closed and the small area is cut with an electric current.

3.4 Fourth Step

Shreds of mucosa on the boundary of the removal line are treated meticulously with hot biopsy or argon plasma coagulation.

An example of a clinical case is illustrated in Fig. 3.

4. Indications for EMR

The EMR procedure is recommended for early esophageal cancer without lymph node metastasis. This technique is safe without causing major complications and moreover, local recurrence has not been encountered after the procedure if the indication is correct.

4.1 Lesions Without Lymph Node Metastasis

Epithelial cancer, carcinoma in situ (CIS), and mucosal cancer with invasion into the lamina propria (m2) do not have lymph node metastasis. Cancers invading into the muscularis mucosae (m3) and into the upper one third of the submucosal layer (sm1) have lymph node metastasis in nearly 15% of cases. However, when cancer is invading more deeply into the submucosal layer (sm2–sm3), lymph node metastasis is present in more than 40% of cases (Table 1). Therefore, cases of m1–m2 cancer are absolute indications for EMR and m3–sm1 cancers are relative indications.

4.2 The Size of the Lesion

A tumor with a diameter small enough to allow en bloc resection is desirable. If the lesion is smaller than 3 cm

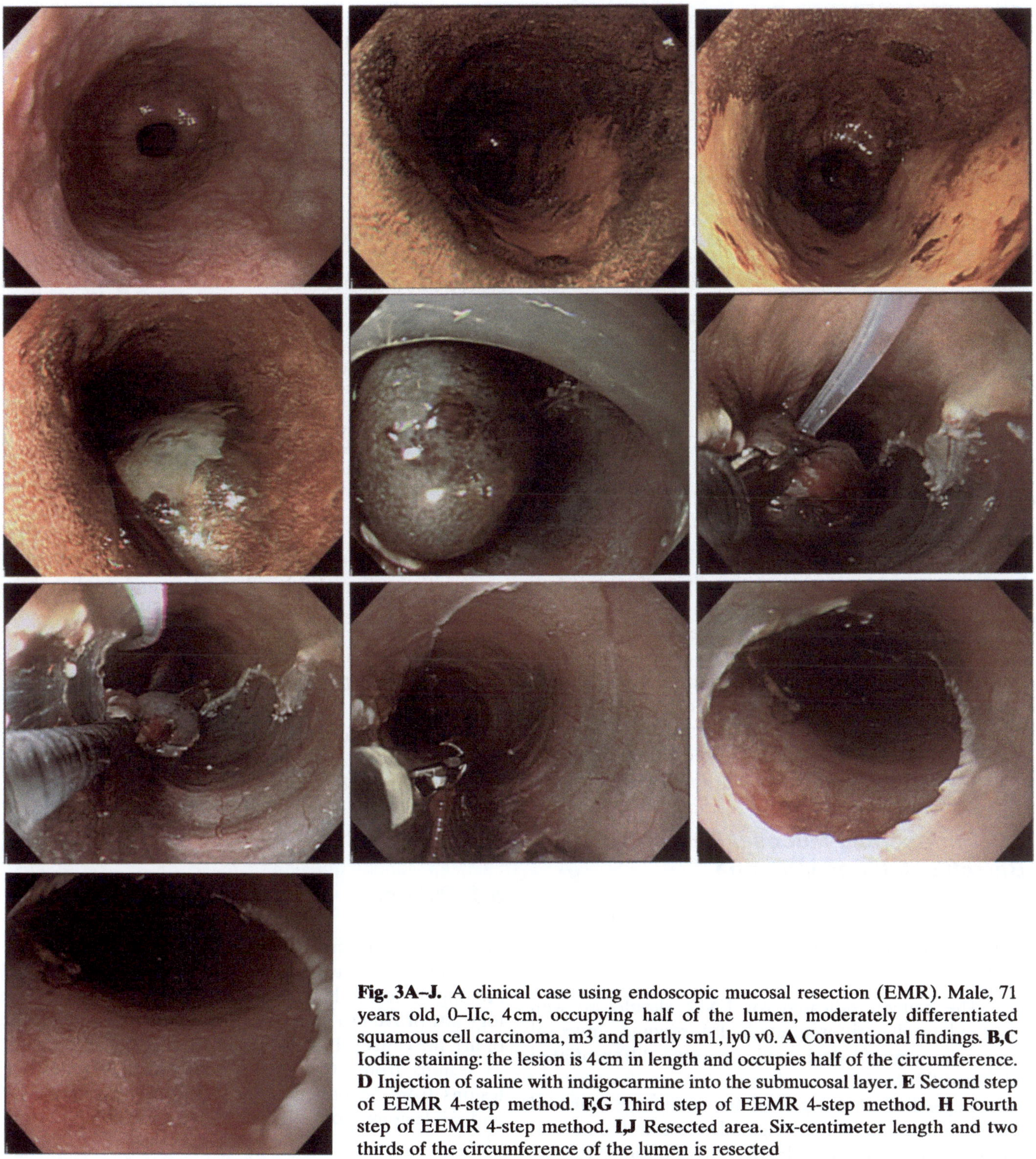

Fig. 3A–J. A clinical case using endoscopic mucosal resection (EMR). Male, 71 years old, 0–IIc, 4 cm, occupying half of the lumen, moderately differentiated squamous cell carcinoma, m3 and partly sm1, ly0 v0. **A** Conventional findings. **B,C** Iodine staining: the lesion is 4 cm in length and occupies half of the circumference. **D** Injection of saline with indigocarmine into the submucosal layer. **E** Second step of EEMR 4-step method. **F,G** Third step of EEMR 4-step method. **H** Fourth step of EEMR 4-step method. **I,J** Resected area. Six-centimeter length and two thirds of the circumference of the lumen is resected

Table 1. Relationship between the depth of invasion of the cancerous lesion and lymph node metastasis and lymph vessel invasion

Depth of invasion	number of cases	lymph vessels invasion	lymph node metastasis
m1	17	0	0
m2	15	0	0
m3	11	6 (54.5%)	1 (9.1%)
sm1	13	8 (61.5%)	2 (15.4%)
sm2	20	16 (80.0%)	8 (40.0%)
sm3	34	28 (82.4%)	15 (44.1%)

Table 2. Relationship between the depth of invasion of Barrett's cancer and lymph node metastasis

Depth of invasion	n(+)	n(−)
Tis (m1)	0	5
T1a (m2, m3)	0	13
T1b (sm)	8	18
T2 (muscularis propria)	5	2
T3 (adventitia)	21	4
Total	34	42

Table 3. Results of endoscopic mucosal resection for esophageal cancer performed in Tokai University from 1989 to 2002

Total cases		551	
Total lesions		790	
Cancer		465 cases	679 lesions
m1, m2		327	480
m3, sm1		118	128
sm2,sm3		20	21
Dysplasia		56 cases	74 lesions
Non-neoplastic tumors		30	37
Operative mortality			0 cases
Postoperative hospital deaths			0
Complications	Perforation		6 cases (0.8%)
	Subcutaneous emphysema		1
	Arterial bleeding		22
	Variceal bleeding		2
	Stricture		10
Follow-up	Local recurrence		17 lesions (2.5%)
	Metachronous multiple cancer		37 cases (8.0%)
	Lymph node metastasis		5 cases
	Distant metastasis (lung, liver)		2 cases

in diameter, en bloc resection is easily performed. Any lesion of a diameter larger than 5 cm has a higher rate of lymph node metastasis. Such a lesion is a relative indication for EMR.

As for the circumferential occupation of the lumen, the lesion should preferably be smaller than two thirds of the lumen of the esophagus. After EMR of a lesion occupying more than two thirds of the lumen there is a tendency for the development of a stenosis.

4.3 Endoscopic Mucosal Resection for Barrett's Adenocarcinoma

Barrett's adenocarcinoma can also be suitable for EMR, but under the following conditions (see Table 2).

1. The cancer indicated for EMR should be well or moderately differentiated. Endoscopic mucosal resection cannot deal with poorly differentiated adenocardinoma.
2. Regarding the depth of invasion, one third of the submucosal layer that originally exists in the normal esophagus is the limit for EMR. This is because tumors invading the submucosal layer more deeply have a tendency for lymph node metastasis.
3. Cancer without lymph vessel invasion is indicated for EMR.

The cancers fulfilling the above points 1–3 are regarded as having no lymph node metastasis.

4. Cancers that are 0-IIa, 0-IIb, or 0-IIc in appearance, with a relatively clear boundary and smaller than 3 cm in diameter, are indicated for EMR.

5. Results of EMR

The outcomes after early esophageal cancer (squamous cell carcinoma) have been reported by several authors. The results described below came chiefly from our institution, which gathered the greatest number of EMR cases with a long follow-up.

5.1 Patients

From 1988 to December 2002, 551 patients underwent EMR in our institution, and 790 lesions were treated. Among these, 679 lesions from 465 patients were pathologically proven to be cancer (480 lesions from 327 cases of m1, m2 cancer; 128 lesions from 118 cases of m3, sm1; 21 lesions from 20 cases of sm2, sm3). Seventy-four lesions from 56 patients were diagnosed as dysplasia and 37 lesions from 30 patients were non-neoplastic (Table 3).

5.2 Complications

5.2.1 Esophageal Perforation

This is the most serious complication after EMR, which must be avoided at any cost but happened in six cases,

0.8% of EMR performances. The causes include (1) adhesion between the mucosa and muscular layer, (2) resnaring a part of the site already removed, (3) resection of a lesion in an esophageal diverticulum, and (4) rough handling of the surgical instruments.

To avoid esophageal perforation, the following steps are recommended.

1. EMR should be discontinued or performed with great care if the lesion fails to be lifted up after injection of saline into the submucosal layer of the lesion.
2. Care must be taken not to apply the snare to exposed muscular layer when the mucosa has already been resected.
3. EMR is contraindicated for lesions in a diverticulum.

The following measures are taken if esophageal perforation occurs, but emergency surgical treatment of perforation is not generally required and conservative care is usually possible. Patients should be observed carefully and the following treatments should be performed: (1) discontinuation of all oral intake, (2) intravenous hyperalimentation, (3) administration of antibiotics, and (4) intermittent aspiration of esophageal lumen through a nasoesophageal tube. Fever resolves within 7 days and the perforation closes in 10–14 days to allow oral intake.

5.2.2 Arterial Hemorrhage

Pulsating or spurting bleeding occurs in about 2.8% of EMR procedures. Bleeding is from a small artery perforating through the muscular layer to the submucosa. Bleeding can be stopped usually by hot-biopsy forceps. A clip is not recommended as it will interfere with the following maneuver.

5.2.3 Esophageal Stricture After EMR

Stenosis can be caused after EMR if mucosa covering more than 75% of the circumference of the esophagus is resected. To prevent severe stenosis in such cases, when stenosis begins to occur prophylactic dilatation is performed with the balloon for endoscopic sclerotherapy attached to the endoscope. If severe stenosis occurs, dilatation is performed with a rigiflex balloon dilator or bougie.

5.2.4 Variceal Bleeding

We performed EMR on five patients with esophageal varices caused by liver cirrhosis after the varix had been eliminated by endoscopic sclerotherapy. In two of these patients, bleeding occurred from the variceal stump during the maneuver. Bleeding was controlled by sclerosant (1% Aethoxysclerol) injection.

5.3 Prognosis

5.3.1 Mortality and Hospital Death

There has been no mortality or hospital death after EMR for esophageal cancer in our institution. To date, no mortality has been reported in Japan.

5.3.2 Local Recurrence

Local recurrence was encountered in 17 lesions (2.5%) after EMR. These lesions were detected by endoscopic follow-up within 1–1.5 years after primary EMR. All these lesions were treated successfully by endoscopic procedures, chiefly EMR, except one patient who required surgical resection.

5.3.3 Metachronous Multiple Cancer

A second primary lesion was detected in another part of the same esophagus in 37 cases (8.0%) more than 2 years after EMR. Multiple cancer is relatively common in esophageal cancer patients. They were all treated by repeated EMR.

5.3.4 Lymph Node Metastasis

Lymph node metastasis after EMR was recognized in five patients after more than 3 years. Three of these were from sm1 and two were from sm2 cancers. Salvage surgical treatment could not be performed except in one case and radiochemotherapy was indicated, although all of them died due to the esophageal cancer.

5.3.5 Distant Metastasis to Lung and Liver

Two patients were found to have distant metastasis after EMR. One patient developed metastasis in the lung and the liver, and the other in the lung. In these cases, primary lung cancer could not be easily ruled out. The primary esophageal cancer of these two patients was m3 cancer.

5.3.6 Five-Year Survival Rate of EMR Cases

The five-year survival rate of cases up to 2001 is 96.1% excluding deaths by other disease or other types of cancer, and 81.7% including all deaths from other causes. For m1 and m2 cancer, the 5-year survival rate is 98.4% excluding other causes of death and 89.5% including all deaths from other causes (Fig. 4).

5.3.7 Results of EMR for m3–sm1 Cancer

We usually perform EMR for m3–sm1 cancer smaller than 4 cm in diameter without a rough mucosal surface. For a lesion of m3–sm1 in its appearance, EMR is first

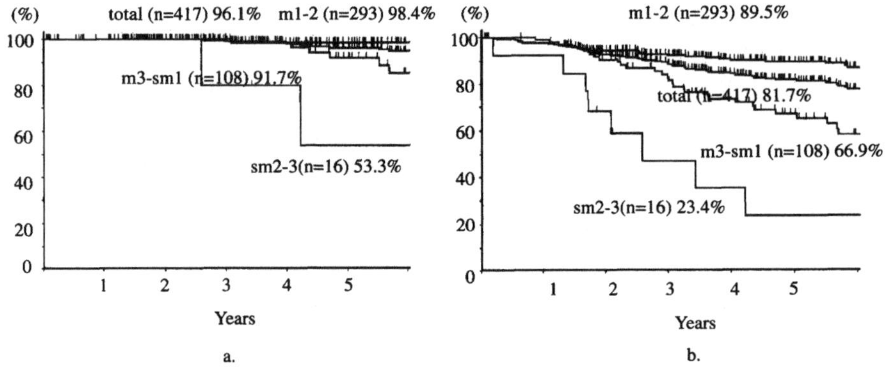

Fig. 4a,b. Five-year survival rate after endoscopic mucosal resection (*EMR*). **a** Excluding other causes of death and death from other cancers. **b** Including other causes of death and death from other cancers

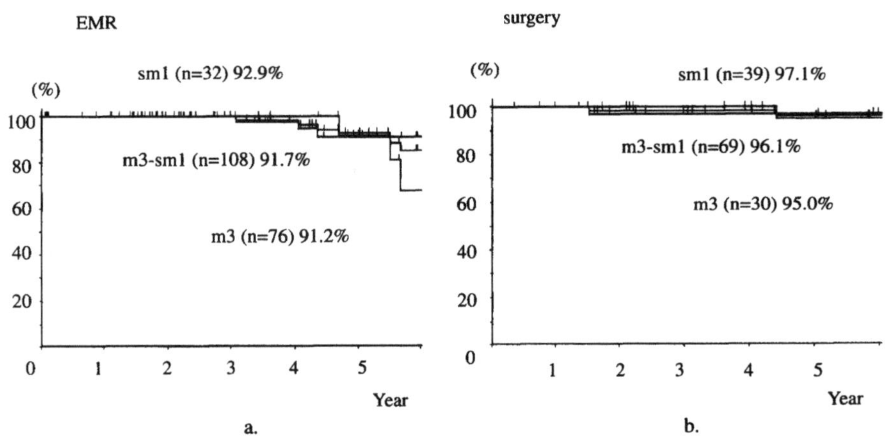

Fig. 5a,b. Five-year survival rate of m3–sm1 cases after endoscopic mucosal resection (*EMR*) or surgical operation excluding other causes of death and death from other cancers. **a** EMR group. **b** Surgical operation group

Table 4. Results of endoscopic mucosal resection for m3–sm1 cases performed in Tokai University from 1991 to 2002

Total cases	113	123 lesions
m3	85	87 lesions
sm1	33	36 lesions
Converted to radical surgery	10	8.5%
Lymph node metastasis	3	2.5%
Distant metastasis (lung, liver)	2	1.8%

performed if possible, and the post-EMR treatment depends on the pathological analysis of the resected lesion. After pathological analysis, the lesions showing lymph vessel invasion (ly(+)), significant infiltration (infγ), or poorly differentiated histological type are further indicated for surgical operation [8].

85 cases (87 lesions) of m3 and 33 cases (36 lesions) of sm1 underwent EMR up to 2002, and 10 patients (8.5%) were further indicated for radical surgery after EMR, judging from the histopathology. Three patients (2.5%) developed lymph node metastasis and two (1.8%) developed distant metastasis (to the lung and the liver) (Table 4).

The 5-year survival rate excluding other causes of death of m3–sm1 patients who underwent EMR up to 2001 is 91.7%. The 5-year survival rate of patients undergoing surgical operation is 96.1%, without significant difference compared with EMR cases (Fig. 5).

6. Endoscopic Mucosal Resection for Barrett's Adenocarcinoma

In Japan, EMR for Barrett's esophageal carcinoma was first performed in 1995 by Zenitani et al. [10], followed by Makuuchi et al. (1997) [8], Oyama et al. (1998) [6], Katayama (1998), and Hoshihara (1999). In the United States and Germany, the number of EMR cases is now greatly increasing [11]. Compared with ablative treatments, EMR is considered to be superior in providing histological confirmation of treatment. High local recurrence rates after EMR for Barrett's cancers have been reported recently, but the accurate diagnosis of the exact area of early cancer and high-grade dysplasia in Barrett's esophagus is extremely difficult even by employment of various chromoendoscopic techniques and magnification chromoendoscopy. Multiple neoplastic lesions seem to remain in Barrett's mucosa even after EMR, which is indicative of its malignant potential. Thirty percent of occurrences of high-grade dysplasia and early adenocarcinoma within 2 years after EMR reported by May et al. [13] can be easily understood.

Argon plasma coagulation and other various laser therapies cannot ablate the lesion as completely as with EMR. The use of EMR for lesions occupying the whole circumference of the lumen causes severe stenosis. Thus, the use of wide EMR combined with mucosal ablation is recommended. Treatment using photodynamic therapy and EMR is controversial in that it is regarded in part only as an experimental therapy indicated only for elderly, poor-risk patients, and is not yet preferred over surgical treatment [14]. However, the argument for EMR as the treatment of choice for Barrett's early cancer and high-grade dysplasia is expected to evolve in a similar way to that extensively discussed in the past, of whether EMR could be an alternative treatment choice for mucosal squamous cell cancer of the esophagus.

Endoscopic mucosal resection has become a treatment choice for early esophageal cancer (mucosal cancer without lymph node metastasis) now, although the endoscopic submucosal dissection method (ESD) has been developed recently. This is a marvelous technique allowing the resection of a comparatively large lesion in one piece, but it demands great skill and requires much time. The EMRC method and the EEMR-tube method do not require any great skill and can be carried out easily. Further development of the ESD method is expected in the near future.

The border of squamous cell carcinoma can be easily identified by iodine staining, but the border of Barrett's cancer is still difficult to be identified, so that further development of chromoendoscopy and diagnosis by magnification chromoendoscopy is also expected in the future.

References

1. Makuuchi H, Machimura T, Sugihara T, et al (1990) Endoscopic diagnosis and treatment of mucosal carcinoma of esophagus (in Japanese with English abstract). Endosc Dig 2:447–452
2. Monma K, Sakaki N, Yoshida M (1990) Endoscopic mucosectomy for precise evaluation and treatment of esophageal intraepithelial cancer (in Japanese with English abstract). Endosc Dig 2:501–506
3. Makuuchi H (1996) Endoscopic mucosal resection for early esophageal cancer: indications and techniques. Dig Endosc 8:175–179
4. Makuuchi H, Yoshida T, Ell C (2004) Four-steps endoscopic esophageal mucosal resection (EEMR) tube method of resection for early esophageal cancer. Endoscopy 36:556–564
5. Inoue H, Endo M, Takeshita K, et al (1992) A new simplified technique of esophageal mucosal resection using a cap-fitted panendoscope (EMRC). Surg Endosc 6:264–265
6. Oyama T, Kikuchi Y, Tomori A, et al (2001) Endoscopic mucosal resection using hooking knife (hooking EMR) for esophageal early cancer (in Japanese with English abstract). Clin Gastroenterol 16:1609–1615
7. Makuuchi H (2001) Endoscopic mucosal resection for mucosal cancer in the esophagus. Gastrointest Endosc Clin North Am 11:445–450
8. Makuuchi H, Shimada H, Chino O, et al (1998) Possibility of endoscopic mucosal resection in patients with m3 and sm1. Stomach Intest 33:993–1002
9. Makuuchi H, Shimada H, Chino O, et al (2002) Long term prognosis of m3, sm1 cancer of the esophagus—comparison between EMR and radical surgery cases. Stomach Intest 37:53–63
10. Zenitani A, Ishioka T, Masamune K, et al (1995) A case of superficial cancer developed in Barrett's esophagus. Stomach Intest 30:1445–1450
11. Ell C, May A, Gossner L, et al (2000) Endoscopic mucosal resection of early cancer and high-grade dysplasia in Barrett's esophagus. Gastroenterology 118:670–677
12. Pech O, May A, Gossner L, et al (2003) Long-term results of local endoscopic therapy for intraepithelial high-grade neoplasia and early adenocarcinoma in Barrett's esophagus. Gastrointest Endosc 57: AB100
13. May A, Gossner L, Pech O, et al (2002) Local endoscopic therapy for intraepithelial high-grade neoplasia and early adenocarcinoma in Barrett's oesophagus: acute-phase and intermediate results of a new treatment approach. Eur J Gastroenterol Hepatol 14:1085–1091
14. Roul A, Zaninotto G, Costantini M, et al (2004) Barrett's esophagus; management of high-grade dysplasia and cancer. J Surg Res 117:45–51

VI. Natural Course of Early Cancer

1. Gastric Cancer

Junji Yoshino and Toshiyuki Matsui

1. Introduction

It is thought that it takes 15–30 years from the appearance of a gastric cancer cell to patient death [1, 2], and in the course of the process, cancers observable to clinicians have already reached their late stages. In some cases, the growth of gastric cancer increases drastically and in others, there is almost no change in the growth of cancer cells for years. Thus, the growth of gastric cancer can take various forms, because various factors such as the degree of differentiation, the presence of an ulcer in the lesion, and differences in immunity among individuals exert influence. In the past, the progress of gastric cancer was estimated by retrospective studies, prospective observations, or assumptions based on the growth curve. However, none of the previous research efforts based on these methods have succeeded in elucidating fully the natural course of gastric cancer [3].

2. Growth Rates and Types of Gastric Cancer

Because gastric cancer is affected by food that passes through the gastric cavity, gastric acid, and peristalsis, its growth is slower than that of cancers originating in parenchymatous organs [1, 2]. It is also well known that ulcers formed in the stomach and fibrous tissues produced by the ulcers inhibit the growth of gastric cancer.

Nishizawa et al. [4] studied how X-ray images of depressed-type early gastric cancer changed with time. In the study they reported that: (1) the duration of intramucosal cancer is more than 10 years when the growth of the cancer is slow, but is assumed to be 2–5 years in most cases; (2) there is not as much variation in the time period cancer remains in the submucosa (after entering the submocosa) as with intramucosal cancer, being from 6 months to 1 year in most cases; and (3) the time period in which cancer spreads from the muscularis propria to the serosa is also assumed to be within 6 months. In 1978, Nakamura et al. [5] tried to estimate the growth curve on the assumption that the growth rate of the area of gastric cancer that was overlooked by endoscopy was on a fixed curve. That is, the growth rate of the tumor area (S in cm^2) could be expressed by a quadratic curve ($S = aT^2 + bT + c$, $a =$ 0.1–0.3) based on the relationship with elapsed time (T) (Fig. 1). There may be cancers that grow exactly as shown in the curve, but many do not coincide with the pattern because the curve was derived from clinical data obtained by retrospective study. Accordingly, it must be difficult to express the growth of all gastric cancers in this curve.

The course of gastric cancer growth varies widely from patient to patient. Some studies have divided patients with gastric cancer into groups. Inokuchi et al. [6] studied the prognoses of gastric cancers including advanced cases. They classified gastric cancers into two types: superficially spreading growth type (super type) and penetrating growth type (pen type), and reported that super-type cancers grow very slowly, while pen-type cancers grow rapidly. Takahashi [7] studied the growth of gastric cancers in patients where lesions could be examined retrospectively by endoscopy, classifying them according to their macroscopic type. The macroscopic type of gastric cancer that was most frequently seen at early stages was type IIc, which made up 54% of all cases. With regard to morphological changes, all of the elevated cancers originated from elevated-type (IIa) early cancers, and all of the depressed cancers originated from depressed-type or flat-type (IIc or IIb) early cancers. They also found that the course of cancer growth could be divided into three types: (1) cancer that begins to invade deeply from its early stages, (2) cancer that remains in its early stages for a long time, and (3) somewhere between the two. Because all of the cancers that remained in the early stages were intramucosal cancers, they assumed that the muscularis mucosae played a role of barrier in the course of cancer growth.

3. Rapid-Growing Gastric Cancer

Among cancers of high malignancy are such examples as scirrhous carcinoma and cancers that invade deeply into the gastric wall while they are still small in size. Yao [8] pointed out that there is a type of gastric cancer that is difficult to detect in its early stages and likely to be found only after it has reached its advanced stages, i.e.,

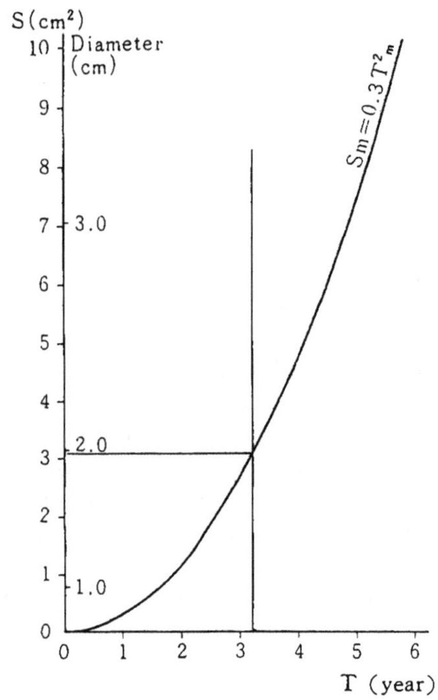

Fig. 1. Growth curve of gastric cancer [5]. *S*, size; *T*, time

a rapid-growing gastric cancer. Inokuchi et al. [6] reported that the pen-type cancers grow rapidly and have a poor prognosis, as described above. According to Inokuchi et al., many pen-type cancers are first detected macroscopically as a combination of elevated and depressed types such as IIa+IIc, and these cancers eventually progress to advanced gastric cancer. In 1979, Yoshida et al. [9] reported that the lesions at the early stages of type-2 or -4 gastric cancers are often detected only as minor changes that do not look abnormal, but grow rapidly [9]. They pointed out the necessity of focusing on nonulcerous, minor changes, rather than ulcerous lesions, to detect lesions that grow rapidly. It seems that the lesions mentioned here are IIb-type lesions. According to Yoshida et al. [10], lesions that show slight abnormalities, such as a pale red area, discoloration, or irregularities of the mucosa, grow rapidly, eventually progressing to type-2, -3, or -4 gastric cancer. They also recommended that the shapes of cancers subject to follow-up should be correlated with the progress of the cancers as follows: "The phases of gastric cancer are classified into two types: The phase in which cancer grows relatively slowly (slow-growing phase) and the phase in which cancer grows rapidly and invades (rapid-growing phase)." Cancer takes the shape of IIc-type or IIa-type early cancer during the slow-growth phase, and takes the shape of IIa+IIc-type, type-2, or type-3 cancer upon reaching the rapid-growth phase because it involves an elevation inside and/or around the lesion. That is, it would be more reasonable to think that the macroscopic type of cancer reflects the course of its growth and progress.

In addition to depressed lesions, the relationship between the initial lesions of elevated lesions and the course of their growth has also been studied. In 1997, Miwa et al. [11] analyzed the growth course of elevated-type early cancers, and divided them into two groups: a group that did not show any abnormality at the first X-ray examination and a group with abnormalities. They reported that cancer grew faster in the former group.

4. Slow-Growing Gastric Cancer

In 1967, Okabe [12] performed a retrospective study and pointed out that the growth of gastric cancers varies widely; some grow very slowly and some grow very rapidly. At the same time, he reported that IIc-type cancer 2 cm or larger in diameter is peculiar because it may develop to advanced cancer similar to IIc-type cancer with a relatively good prognosis. In 1979, Yoshida et al. [10] analyzed the initial lesions of advanced cancers and concluded that many of those similar to IIc-type cancer were ulcerous lesions that grew slowly.

Two major factors that could delay the growth of cancer are exfoliation of tumor caused by peptic ulcer and inhibition of tumor growth by fibrosis. Horinouchi et al. [13] reported that the range of invasion did not spread in patients who had peptic ulcers in cancer lesions. Nakamura et al. [14] also reported that the horizontal growth of cancer was extremely slow in patients in whom cancers were complicated by ulcers. Gastric ulcer as a complication in the course of gastric cancer can be seen as a phase in the so-called malignant cycle. That is, the position of the cancer changes (Fig. 2) in the following cycle: (1) diffuse type (cancer resides in the regenerated mucous membrane surface of the ulcer scar and around this membrane), (2) open type (cancer resides in the margin of the open ulcer, and (3) marginal type (the bottom of the ulcer is mainly covered with noncancerous, regenerated mucous membrane and the cancer resides in the margin of the ulcer). Fibrosis caused by ulcers coexistent with gastric cancer is considered to be the biggest factor in slowing the cancer's growth. With regard to the histological types of cancers, Mai et al. [15] reported that well-differentiated and moderately differentiated cancers tend to grow slowly, and there are some cases of poorly differentiated adenocarcinoma that progress slowly while repeating the above malignant cycle.

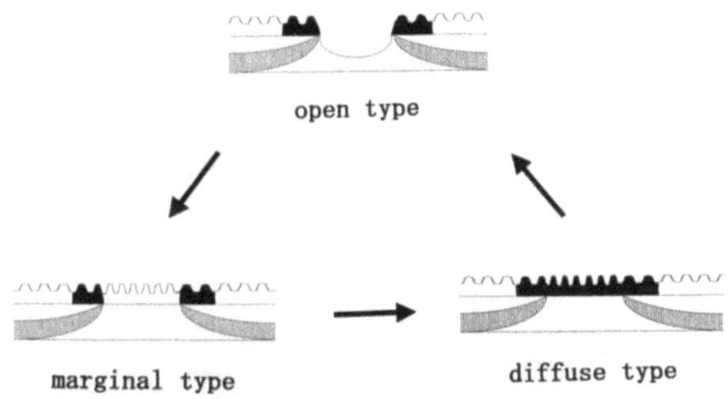

Fig. 2. Malignant cycle. The position of the cancer changes in the cycle. *Diffuse type*: cancer resides in the regenerated mucous membrane surface of the ulcer scar and around this membrane; *open type*: cancer resides in the margin of the open ulcer; *marginal type*: the bottom of the ulcer is mainly covered with noncancerous, regenerated mucous membrane and the cancer resides in the margin of the membrane

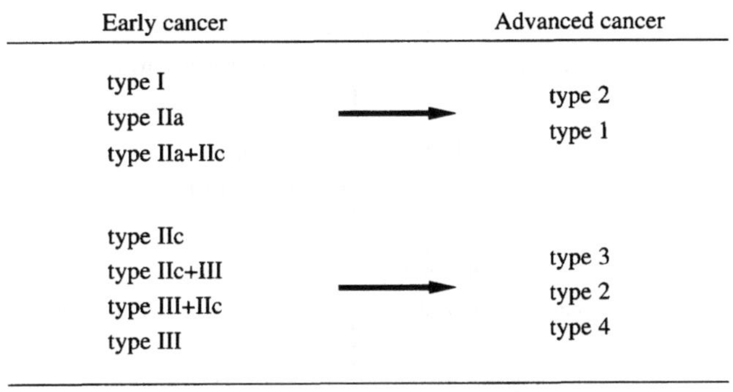

Fig. 3. Development of macroscopic appearances when early cancers progress to advanced cancers

5. Progress from Early to Advanced Cancer

In many of the clinical studies that have been done so far, the actual courses of gastric cancer from the early stages to advanced cancer have not been revealed as yet because the duration of patient follow-up has been too short. Yoshida et al. [16] attempted to deduce the natural history of gastric cancer by examining the clinicopathologic characteristics of removed lesions, on the assumption that the macroscopic type of a removed lesion represents part of the natural history of gastric cancer at a certain time point. The study included 3002 patients who underwent resection of solitary gastric cancer (937 cases of early cancer, 480 cases of muscularis propria-subserosal cancer, and 1585 cases of subserosal or deeper cancer) and whose lesions were imaged satisfactorily by endoscopy. Of the clinicopathologic characteristics, they used factors that do not change over time, namely, sex, site of lesion, and histological type, for determination, and obtained the degree of similarity to macroscopic type for determination by a multivariate analysis. The results of the study showed a close correlation between the following cancers, similar to each other in shape: (1) IIa+IIc-type early cancer and type-2 advanced cancer or localized type-3 cancer, (2) elevated-type early cancer and elevated-type advanced cancer, and (3) depressed-type early cancer and advanced cancer similar to IIc type. Also, (4) type-3 and type-4 cancers that invaded as far as the serosa were very similar to nonulcerous IIc-type early cancers with few converging folds in patients in their thirties to forties. From the above results, they concluded that there was temporal continuity in clinicopathologic characteristics between early cancers and advanced cancers that were similar in macroscopic appearance.

Many cases of elevated type early gastric cancer (types I, IIa and IIa+IIc) grow to advanced cancers type 2 and type 1 macroscopically. One of the reasons why elevated type early cancers develop into type 2 cancers is that the center of the lesions disintegrates and forms an ulceration. These lesions do not pass through the malignant cycle and gradually increase in size. On the other hand, almost all depressed type early gastric cancers (types IIc, IIc+III, III+IIc and III) develop into type 3, 2, or 4 advanced cancer macroscopically. Many cases of depressed type early cancer have ulcerations in cancerous foci. Some cases do not enlarge while going through the malignant cycle and other cases become larger showing a cancerous ulceration (Fig. 3).

Scirrhous gastric cancer is defined as an undifferentiated gastric cancer accompanied by remarkable fibrosis that tends to invade diffusely and widely into the submucosa or deeper, mainly around the fundic glands. It grows rapidly and carries a poor prognosis. Many studies have been performed to find out what the initial lesion of this type of cancer looks like. Nakamura et al. [17] guessed that its primary focus was IIc-type cancer without converging folds, that was 2 cm or smaller in diameter and was to be found in the region of the fundic glands. Linitis plastica cancer, which is used as an almost equivalent term for scirrhous gastric cancer, shows a shape similar to a leather bottle when viewed on X-rays. Nakamura et al. [17] also defined the course of the growth of linitis plastica as follows: (1) pre-linitis plastica: invasion of IIc-like early cancer into the submucosa of the fundic gland area does not exceed one quarter of the circumference of the stomach; (2) latent linitis plastica: invasion exceeds one quarter of the circumference of the stomach but does not cause narrowing of the gastric cavity; (3) typical linitis plastica: invasion spreads widely and causes narrowing of the gastric cavity. They also guessed that it would take approximately 6.3 years

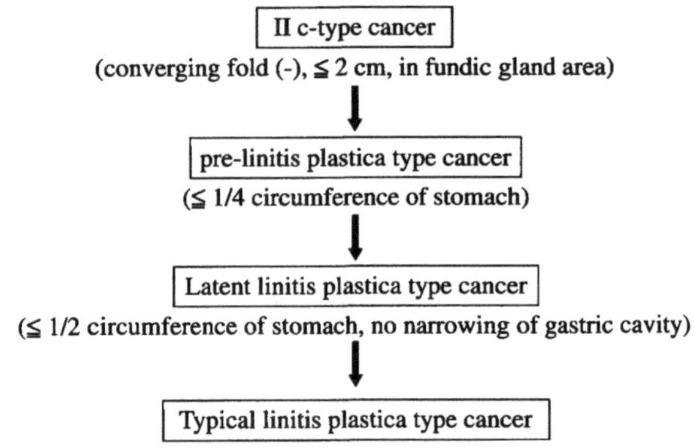

Fig. 4. Development of scirrhous gastric cancer

from carcinogenesis to completion of a linitis plastica cancer (Fig. 4).

However, some researchers think that growth courses are not as uniform as Nakamura et al. pointed out. Ohgushi et al. [18] reported on the characteristics of the initial lesions of scirrhous gastric cancer. Many of the initial lesions were IIc-type lesions that were relatively small in size, but there were also large IIc-type lesions that showed signs of hardening or insufficient extension, suggesting that they had already invaded the submucosa 2 or 3 years previously. Mai et al. [15] reported that it takes at least 3 years, and sometimes 5 or 6 years, from the time that an initial lesion becomes clinically detectable to the time that scirrhous gastric cancer is completed.

5.1 Case 1

A 62-year-old man. The patient visited the hospital to have a medical check-up. Converging folds were found on the posterior wall of the gastric corpus on a barium X-ray examination (Fig. 5). Although this finding was overlooked, X-ray findings were compatible with a IIc-type early cancer. He refused farther examination. When he visited the hospital again 1 year 9 months later, the lesion had become a scirrhous gastric cancer as shown in Fig. 6.

5.2 Case 2

A 52-year-old man. A whitish spot with an uneven surface was found on the lesser curvature of the gastric antrum by endoscopy (Fig. 7). The site was biopsied and the lesion was diagnosed as a poorly differentiated adenocarcinoma. The patient did not visit the hospital thereafter. Two years and 10 months later, endoscopy revealed that the lesion had progressed to a type-3

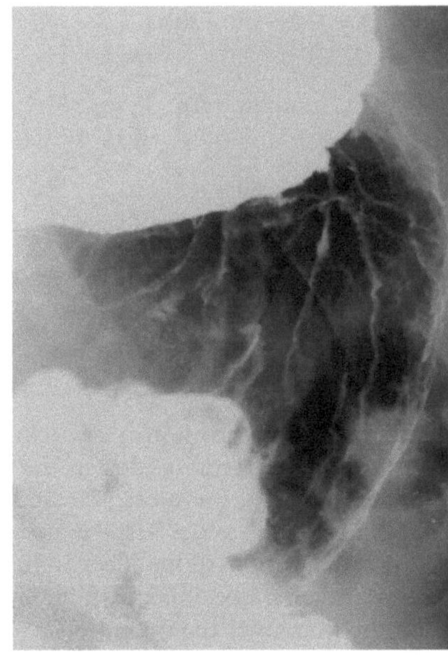

Fig. 5. Case 1. Converging folds were found on the posterior wall of the gastric body on a X-ray examination, and were assumed to be indicative of a IIc-type early gastric cancer

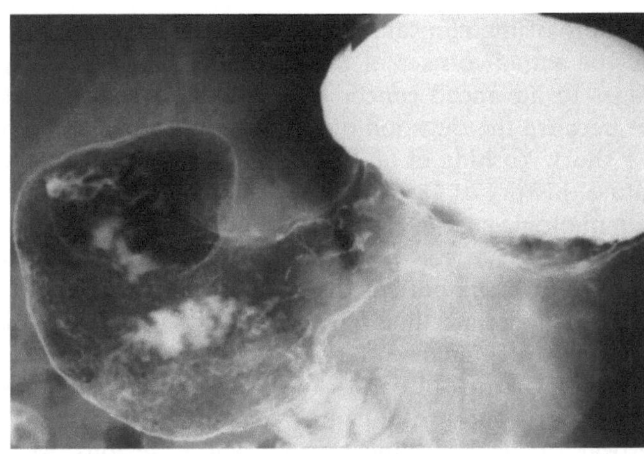

Fig. 6. Case 1. X-ray examination performed 1 year and 9 months later, showed the lesion had become a scirrhous gastric cancer

cancer (Fig. 8). The first endoscopy showed it was a IIb type cancer restricted to the mucosa. When he underwent surgery, the tumor had penetrated the serosa.

5.3 Case 3

A 55-year-old man. Figure 9 shows a IIc-like lesion at the tip of a fold on the posterior wall of the middle of the gastric body. Biopsy was not performed at that time. One year and 9 months later, examination of the same

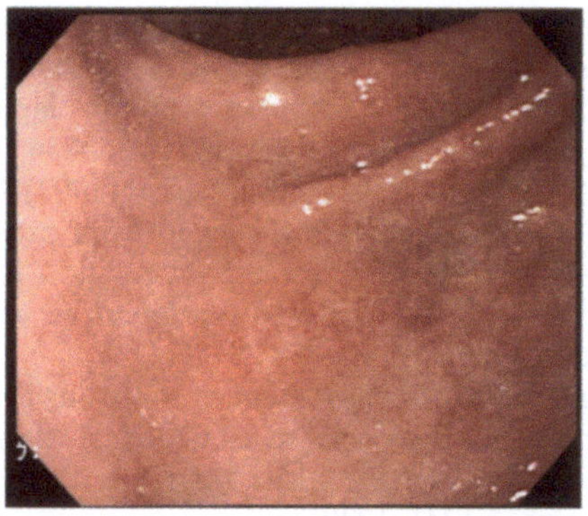

Fig. 7. A whitish spot with an uneven surface was found on the lesser curvature of the gastric antrum by endoscopy. The lesion is considered to be a IIb-type gastric cancer limited to the mucosa

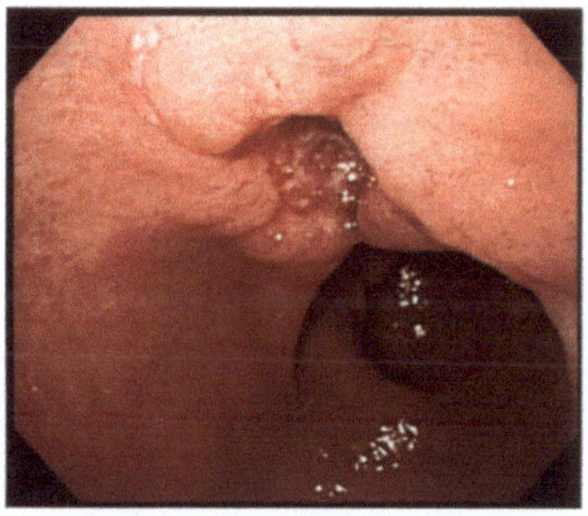

Fig. 8. Case 2. Two years and 10 months later, endoscopy revealed that the lesion was a type 3 advanced cancer, penetrating the serosa

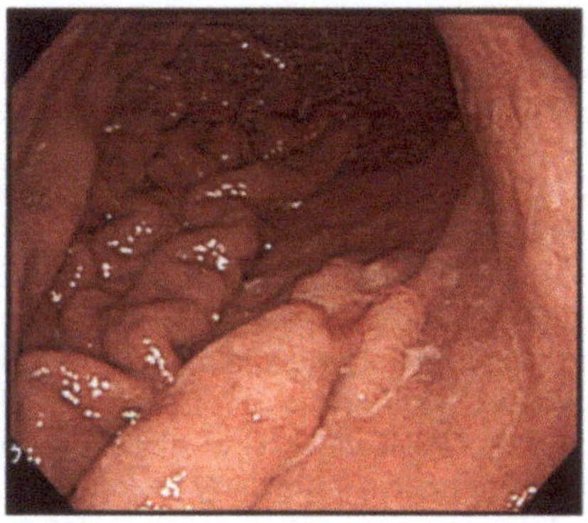

Fig. 9. Case 3. A IIc-like lesion is seen at the tip of a fold on the posterior wall of the middle of the gastric body

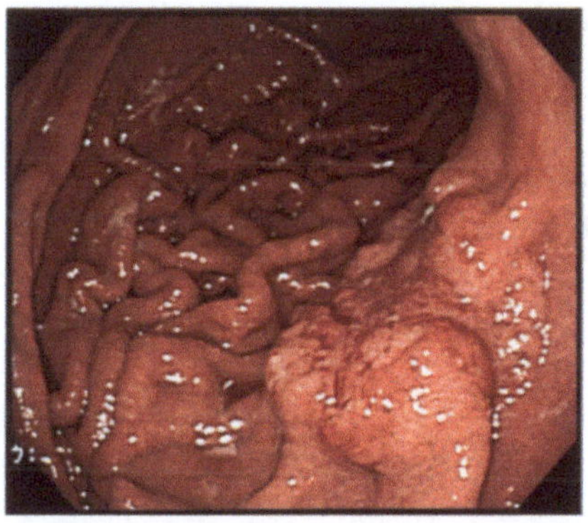

Fig. 10. Case 3. One year and 9 months later, a picture at the same site shows a type-2 cancer. The lesion turned out to be a moderately differentiated tubular adenocarcinoma invading the muscularis propria. It was suggested that this IIc-type gastric cancer developed into a type-2 gastric cancer

site shows a type-2 cancer (Fig. 10). The lesion turned out to be a moderately differentiated tubular adenocarcinoma with invasion into the proper muscle layer. It was suggested that this IIc-type early gastric cancer developed into a type-2 advanced gastric cancer.

6. Conclusion

The relationship between the growth of gastric cancer and its preceding lesions is still controversial, despite all the studies. In the early stages of gastric carcinogenesis, there is a IIb-like lesion, which will develop to IIa-type or IIc-type early cancer. The growth rates of these cancers vary widely. Either way, they are destined to develop into advanced cancers. In future studies, it will be necessary to further analyze the course of the growth of gastric cancer.

References

1. Collins VP, et al (1956) Observation on growth rates of human tumors. Am J Roentgenol 76:988–1000
2. Fujita S (1978) Biology of early gastric carcinoma. Pathol Res Pract 163:297–309
3. Matsui T, Yao T (2001) Natural history of gastric carcinoma (in Japanese). Nippon Rinsho 59:583–588
4. Nishizawa M, Nomoto K, Ueno M, et al (1992) Natural history of gastric cancer in a fixed population—with emphasis on depressed sm cancer (in Japanese with English abstract). Stomach Intest 27:16–24
5. Nakamura K, et al (1978) Relationship between the size of gastric cancer and time-growth curve (in Japanese). Stomach Intest 13:89–93
6. Inokuchi K (1986) Natural history of gastric carcinoma viewed from growth patterns of early carcinoma (in Japanese with English abstract). Jpn J Cancer Chemother 13:1105–1118

7. Takahashi M (1987) Retrospective study on the endoscopic pictures of gastric cancer detected by gastric mass survey (in Japanese with English abstract). Gastroenterol Endosc 29:1956–1970
8. Yao T (1976) Courses of gastric cancer and problems with early gastric cancer viewed from a retrospective study (in Japanese). Jpn J Clin Exp Med 53:2938–2942
9. Yoshida S, Oka Y, Yoshimori M, et al (1979) Endoscopic studies of the growth of gastric cancer (in Japanese). Prog Dig Endosc 15:11–15
10. Yoshida S, Ootu A, Kondo H, et al (1979) Endoscopic approach to progression from early to advanced cancer of the stomach (in Japanese with English abstract). Stomach Intest 32:825–834
11. Miwa H, Iwazaki R, Ohkura R, et al (1977) Radiological retrospective study of gastric cancer in humans: two patterns of development in elevated type gastric cancer. J Gastroenterol Hepatol 12:599–605
12. Okabe H (1967) Courses of early gastric cancer—position of early gastric cancer in the natural history of gastric cancer (in Japanese). Jpn J Clin Med 25:1336–1345
13. Horinouchi K, Yao T, Okabe H (1972) Malignant cycle of advanced cancer (in Japanese with English abstract). Stomach Intest 7:583–592
14. Nakamura K, Kato Y, Misono T, et al (1980) Growing progress to carcinoma of linitis plastica type of the stomach from cancer development (in Japanese with English abstract). Stomach Intest 15:252–234
15. Mai M, Mibayashi Y, Okumura Y, et al (1992) The natural history of gastric carcinoma viewed from prospective or retrospective follow-up studies—in relation to histological type and growth patterns (in Japanese with English abstract). Stomach Intest 17:39–50
16. Yoshida S (1988) Development of scirrhous cancer of the stomach: a speculation from clinical materials obtained. (in Japanese with English abstract). Jpn J Cancer Chemother 15:1241–1249
17. Nakamura K, et al (1975) Histopathological study on primary focus of linitis plastica—Relationship between carcinoma arisen from the fundic gland mucosa and linitis plastica (in Japanese with English abstract). Stomach Intest 10:79–86
18. Ohgushi H, Yao T, Iwashita A (1980) The primary foci of linitis plastica type of gastric cancer and their chronological change (in Japanese with English abstract). Stomach Intest 15:1129–1136

2. Colorectal Cancer: Retrospective, Prospective, and Histologic Observations

Tetsuichiro Muto

1. Introduction

The natural course of colorectal cancers is not well understood because of the difficulties of investigation. It is not allowed ethically to observe the index lesions in situ in order to investigate their natural course.

There are two ways, *direct* and *indirect*, to elucidate the natural course of colorectal neoplasms. The *direct* way is undertaken by collecting cases of colorectal benign or malignant lesions which were not treated initially for some reason, due to either refusal of treatment by patients themselves or misdiagnosis on barium enema (BE) examination. By comparing the index lesions at different periods their natural course can be estimated in terms of the time and shape sequence. Such study is extremely time consuming and only a few studies have been published in the literature [1]. However, the observed data, though small in number, are most reliable and tell us some part of the true aspects concerning the natural course of colorectal neoplasms. These studies were conducted based on the concept that most colorectal cancers arise from preexisting adenomas, known as the adenoma–carcinoma sequence, therefore the index lesions are almost always polypoid in shape. From studies in the past it has been surmised that the adenoma–carcinoma sequence takes more than 10 years and it is a slow-growing process for an adenoma to become a cancer [2].

On the other hand, the *indirect* way is undertaken by histologic examination of either surgically or colonoscopically resected specimens. From meticulous histologic comparisons, particularly morphologic changes, the natural course can be estimated, but only indirectly [3]. By gathering these data from both *direct* and *indirect* ways together, the natural course of colorectal cancers, on the basis of the adenoma–carcinoma sequence concept, has become partially understood. The details of this understanding will be presented in this chapter.

2. Methods of Study

As mentioned above, the study was undertaken by two methods. When a patient with colorectal cancer came to the Surgical Department of the University of Tokyo Hospital and was found to have received a BE examination previously, and the previous films were available to check the presence of initial lesions, the virtual changes of the shape and time sequence could be *directly* measured. The problem with this study was that the pathology of the initial index lesion, mostly polypoid in shape, was not tested because it was missed on BE examination. Therefore, it was not clear whether it was initially a benign adenoma or an early cancer. An early cancer is defined here either as confined to the mucosa (mucosal cancer: m-ca) or invading to the submucosa only (sub-mucosal cancer: sm-ca), which belongs to category 5 in the Vienna classification (Table 1) [4]. As it is hard to distinguish an adenoma from an m-cancer on BE alone and the shape of both lesions looks the same, the index lesions are assumed to be m-cancer for calculating the time sequence in this context. Otherwise, it is extremely difficult to solve this question.

The indirect way was undertaken by histologic observations of collected polypoid adenomas containing a focal cancer in them (m-ca and sm-ca). The observation was particularly focused on the shape of the muscularis mucosae, stressing its relevance to the polyp shape and to the adenoma–carcinoma sequence [3].

Initially only the natural course of polypoid lesions was investigated; however, recently several data have been accumulated for that of nonpolypoid neoplasms. Nonpolypoid neoplasms are defined here as slightly elevated, flat, or even depressed neoplasms, which in Japan are officially classified as superficial elevated (IIa), superficial flat (IIb), and superficial depressed (IIc) [5]. They are novel colorectal neoplasms, either adenomas or early cancers. They are called superficial lesions as well; however, the term nonpolypoid will be used in this context. Superficial elevated adenoma has also been called "flat adenoma," the concept being well accepted worldwide [6]. The role of polypoid and nonpolypoid neoplasms as precursors of colorectal cancers is different and therefore, their natural course will be discussed separately.

3. Natural Course of Polypoid Lesions

The aim of the study of the natural course of colorectal early cancers is to find answers to the questions, how long will it take for an adenoma to become a cancer (time sequence) and how will the morphologic changes (morphologic sequence) occur?

3.1 Time Sequence

This study is only possible under *direct* observation. To understand the problems we have to face, several examples will be presented here.

3.1.1 Case 1 [16]

A broad-based sigmoid polyp, 1 cm in diameter, was followed by BE once a year for 5 years without presenting any size change; however, at the sixth examination it became larger and the resected specimen showed a sm-ca, 1.5 cm in diameter, on the fold (Fig. 1). This case was in the pre-polypectomy period and therefore, the patient was followed up with a BE every year. Of course it is not clear when m-ca developed, and the time sequence from an adenoma to a carcinoma will be either 6 years or 1 year because the size has only changed during the last year of the observation period.

Table 1. Vienna classification of gastrointestinal epithelial neoplasia

1. Negative for neoplasia/dysplasia
2. Indefinite for neoplasia/dysplasia
3. Noninvasive low-grade neoplasia (low-grade adenoma/dysplasia)
4. Noninvasive high-grade neoplasia
4.1 High-grade adenoma/dysplasia
4.2 Noninvasive carcinoma (CIS)
4.3 Suspicious for invasive carcinoma
5. Invasive neoplasia
5.1 Intramucosal carcinoma
5.2 Submucosal carcinoma or beyond

3.1.2 Case 2 [1]

Retrospectively a broad-based rectal polyp, less than 1 cm in diameter, was found to become sm-ca, 1.5 cm across, in 2 years and 3 months (Figs. 2 and 3). However, malignant transformation was assumed to have occurred between 1971 and 1972 in 1 year and 9 months, because there was no sign of sm-ca on BE taken in 1970 and 1971 (Fig. 2). In the early 1970s when colonoscopy was used but the polypectomy technique had not yet been introduced, many polyps were followed by colonoscopy and consequently, information on the natural course was obtained as described in cases 1 and 2.

3.1.3 Case 3 [1]

A semipedunculated sigmoid polyp, 1.5 cm in diameter, was proven to be a benign tubulovillous adenoma with

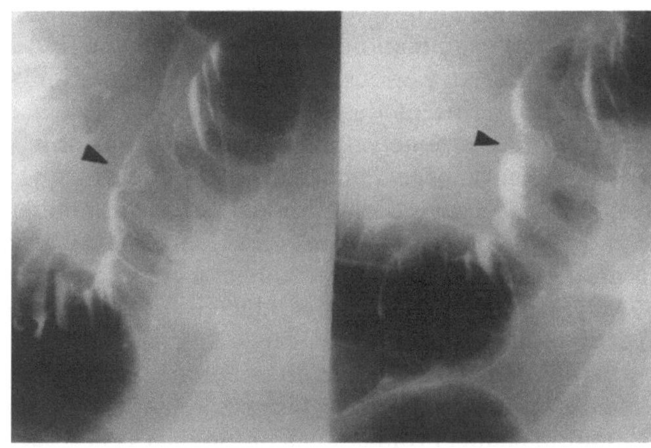

Fig. 1. Barium enema taken in 1965 (*left*) and 1971 (*right*). The change of the size and the shape can be noticed (case 1). The *arrowheads* indicate the index lesion

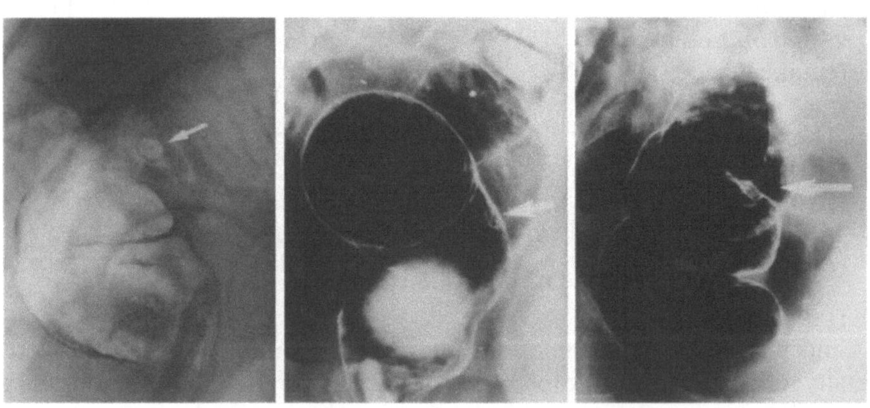

Fig. 2. Barium enema taken in July 1970 (*left*), January 1971 (*middle*), and October 1972 (*right*). The marked change of the size and the shape can be noticed between 1971 and 1972 (case 2). The *arrows* indicate the index lesion

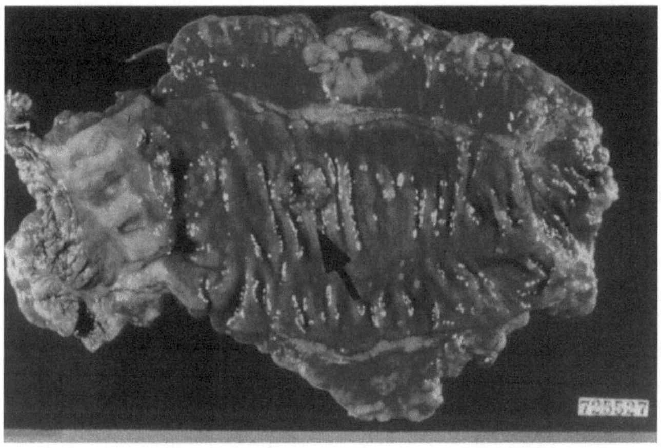

Fig. 3. An ulcerating cancer of the rectum (*arrow*), 1.5 cm in diameter invading to the submucosa only (case 2)

forceps biopsy and followed up in a conventional manner (Fig. 4, top). Only 9 months later the patient complained of marked anal bleeding and colonoscopy revealed an ulcerating sigmoid cancer, 3 cm in diameter, at the same site of the previous adenoma, and sigmoidectomy was performed. Histologically it was a well-differentiated adenocarcinoma invading into the proper muscle (Fig. 4, bottom). To our knowledge, this is an example of the most rapid malignant transformation from an adenoma (probably m-ca) to an adenocarcinoma.

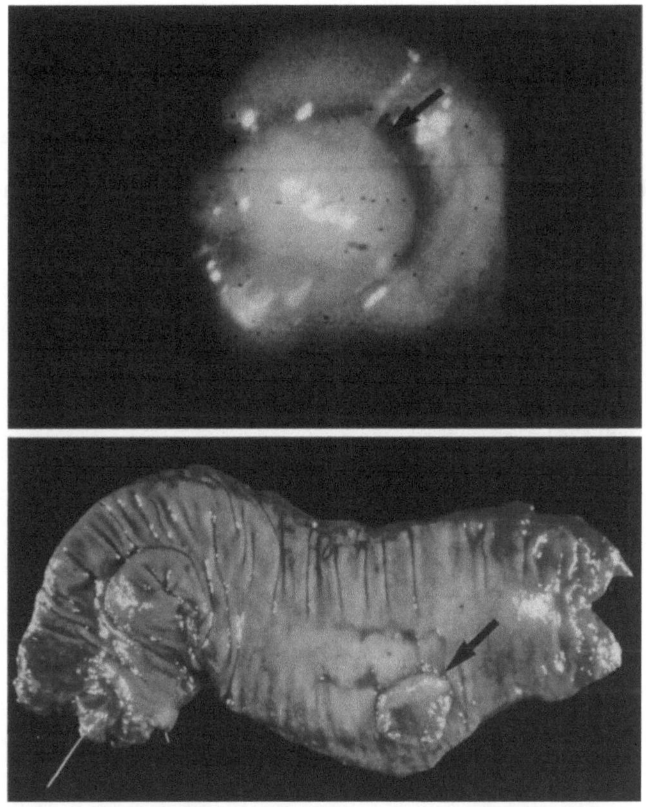

Fig. 4. Colonoscopic findings of the sigmoid polyp (*top, arrow*) 1.5 cm in diameter showing no sign of malignancy and a resected ulcerating cancer of the sigmoid colon (*bottom, arrow*), 3 cm in diameter, invading to the proper muscle (case 3). The time interval was only 9 months

3.1.4 Case 4 [17]

A semipedunculated rectal adenoma, 7 mm in diameter, in a patient with adenomatosis coli was found to become a sm-ca, 2.5 cm in diameter, in 2 years and 2 months (Fig. 5). Considering the low risk of containing mucosal cancer in an adenoma less than 1 cm in diameter (less than 10%), the actual progression from m-ca to sm-ca was assumed to have occurred in less than 2 years. There are only a few reports in the literature describing the time sequence from a polypoid lesion to a carcinoma [1]. It was estimated to be 2–18 years by Scarborough et al. [7] and 5–28 years by Muto et al. [2], showing quite a large disparity of time sequence.

The difference in the time sequence could well be explained by the different point of recognition of the index polyps, as shown in Fig. 6. When the recognized index polyp is an entirely benign adenoma, malignant transformation may well take many years, i.e., $t_1 + t_2 + t_3 + t_4 + t_5 + t_6$. On the other hand, when it is mucosal cancer (m-ca) which cannot be diagnosed on BE examination, it needs only a short period of time, e.g., $t_5 + t_6$. Each interval from t_1 to t_6 is not precisely known, and the intervals are most likely to differ in individual cases. The

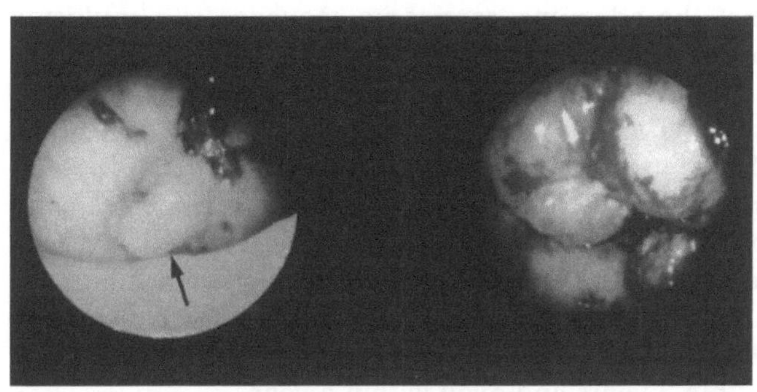

Fig. 5. A semipedunculated rectal adenoma, 7 mm in diameter, in a patient with adenomatosis coli (*left, arrow*) and an ulcerating rectal cancer 2.5 cm in diameter (case 4). The time interval was 2 years and 2 months

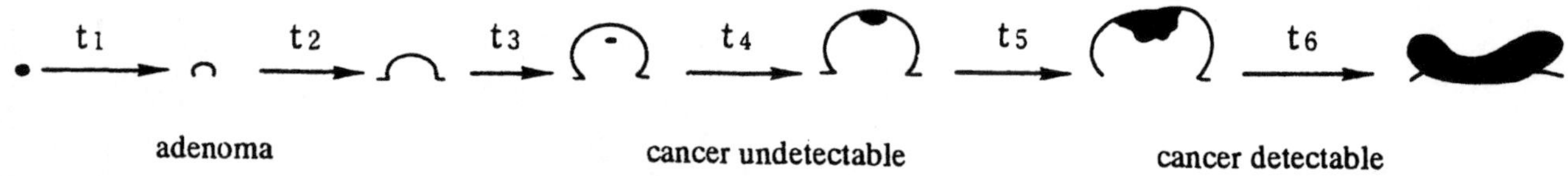

Fig. 6. A schema showing sequential time interval from an adenoma to a cancer

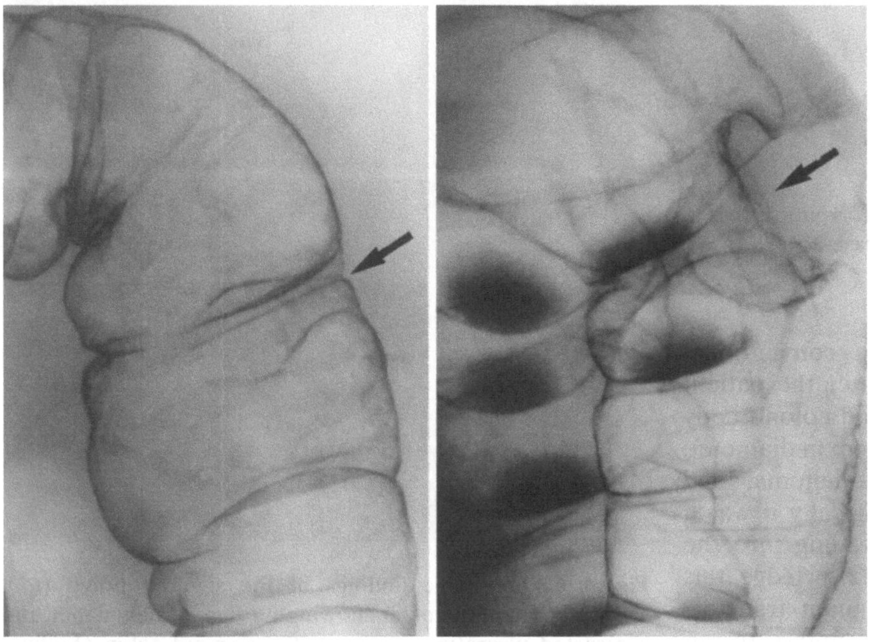

Fig. 7. A sessile lesion missed on the previous barium enema examination (*left*, *arrow*) became an ulcerating cancer of the ordinary type (*right*, *arrow*). It took only 1 year (case 5)

long interval of Σtn does not necessarily mean a slow progression of the adenoma–carcinoma sequence; however, the short interval as seen in case 3 indicates that the progression from m-ca to advanced cancer ($t_5 + t_6$) can occur even within a year. It has been believed that the adenoma–carcinoma sequence is a multistep phenomenon, from a small adenoma to a larger adenoma with a higher grade of atypia, and from a larger adenoma with severe atypia to an invasive cancer thence to an advanced cancer. Although there is no definite proof yet, the last step of this sequence seems to be more rapid than previously anticipated, as seen in case 3. The cases presented here, though limited in number, clearly show that a colorectal cancer can develop from a pre-existing neoplasm, mostly adenoma, within 3 years and even within a year.

3.2 Morphologic Sequence

When talking about the shape of colorectal polyps, there are several categories such as (a) pedunculated (long stalk), (b) semipedunculated (short stalk), (c) broad-based, and (d) sessile. One tended to assume that colorectal cancers develop from adenomas with a long stalk; however, the observed examples did not support this view. All precursor lesions presented here were either semipedunculated or broad-based (cases 1–4) but not pedunculated. Spratt et al. erroneously described a schema showing a polyp with a long stalk to become an advanced cancer [8]. Case 5 clearly shows the transformation from a sessile lesion to an advanced cancer (Fig. 7). It is interesting to note that this phenomenon took place within a year, indicating the possibility of rapid progression [17].

Mucosal cancers were collected from the resected and polypectomized specimens in order to study the proportion of early cancers with each shape [3]. As seen in Table 2, the majority were either semipedunculated (short stalk), broad-based, or sessile, and there was no pedunculated sm-ca in the series (Table 2). The histologic observation of the resected adenomas revealed the different features of the muscularis mucosae according to the different polyp shapes. Pedunculated polyps have thick and dense muscularis mucosae with an inverted V shape which can be a strong barrier against cancer inva-

Table 2. Relationship of size and shape in colorectal early cancer (polypectomy series)

Size	Long stalk	Short stalk	Broad-based	Sessile	Total	
<1 cm	1	4	8 (3)	1	14 (3)	24%
1–2 cm	8	11 (2)	6 (2)	4 (1)	29 (5)	51%
≧2 cm	3	6 (2)	4 (2)	1 (1)	14 (5)	24%
Total	12	21 (4)	18 (7)	6 (2)	57 (13)	24%
	21%	37%	31%	11%		

Numbers in parentheses are for submucosal cancer

sion. On the other hand, broad-based or sessile polyps have loose muscularis mucosae with a Greek omega or flat shape which seems to be a weak barrier against cancer invasion. These histologic differences may reflect the significance of the polyp shape as a precursor of colorectal cancer [3]. Ushio et al. retrospectively investigated 18 cases of colorectal cancers which showed the natural course of colorectal neoplasms [9]. It is interesting to note that the time sequences were variable from 2 to 10 years and the shapes of the index lesions were all nonpedunculated except one. The general trend of the time and the morphologic sequence mentioned above was also confirmed by Ushio's large number of experiences.

It has been believed that the malignancy rate is higher with increasing size, based on the study of surgically resected colorectal neoplams [2]. However, after introduction of the polypectomy technique it was found that even small adenomas, around 1 cm in diameter, have a much higher malignancy rate than previously appreciated [10]. It should be kept in mind that the adenoma–carcinoma sequence operates not only in large adenomas but also on smaller adenomas around 1 cm in diameter. Our experiences (cases 1, 2, 4) together with Ushio's data, showing the smallest initial size to be 7 mm in diameter, clearly confirmed these new findings.

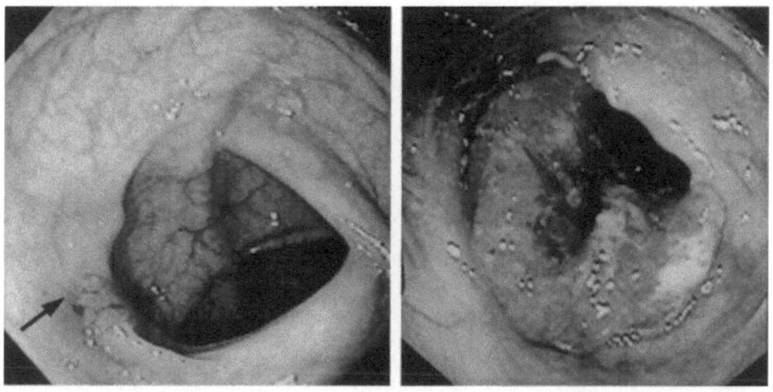

Fig. 8. An ulcerating early cancer of IIc type (*left, arrow*) grew to a protuberant advanced cancer 1 year later (*right*) (case 6)

4. Natural Course of Nonpolypoid Lesions

4.1 Time Sequence

As mentioned previously, very few data on the natural course of nonpolypoid lesions were collected because of the difficulties in detecting the index superficial lesions retrospectively. The data are only available when patients refuse treatment. As seen in case 6, the initial index lesion was diagnosed as sm-ca of IIc type on colonoscopy, and colectomy was recommended; however, the patient refused the surgical treatment. Fifteen months later the index lesion had grown to a protuberant advanced carcinoma (Fig. 8). As there are only a few cases reported in the literature, the time interval of the nonpolypoid adenoma–carcinoma sequence is still an enigma [11, 12]. Because the muscularis mucosae of nonpolypoid lesions is very thin and loose, it is assumed that cancerous invasion into the submucosa through the weak barrier could occur easily and rapidly. However, this is not the case in the report by Matsui et al [12]. According to their observations the doubling times of nonpolypoid early cancers were longer than those of polypoid cancers, without any significant difference.

4.2 Morphologic Sequence

As seen in cases 5 and 6, it is clear that ordinary ulcerating carcinomas develop from nonpolypoid lesions as well. By collecting as many small m-ca and sm-ca as possible, one can speculate on the sequential morphologic changes (Fig. 9). From the histologic observations particularly of the similar features of the muscularis mucosae, the origin of these three lesions shown in Fig. 9 are assumed to be superficial elevated adenomas. It is shown that in the first step a focal carcinoma arising in a superficial elevated adenoma becomes polypoid due to cancerous invasion associated with surrounding fibrous reaction (Fig. 9, middle) and in the next step, it becomes a much more elevated polypoid lesion (Fig. 9, bottom). It is not well known whether this polypoid sm-ca will grow to an advanced polypoid cancer, which is

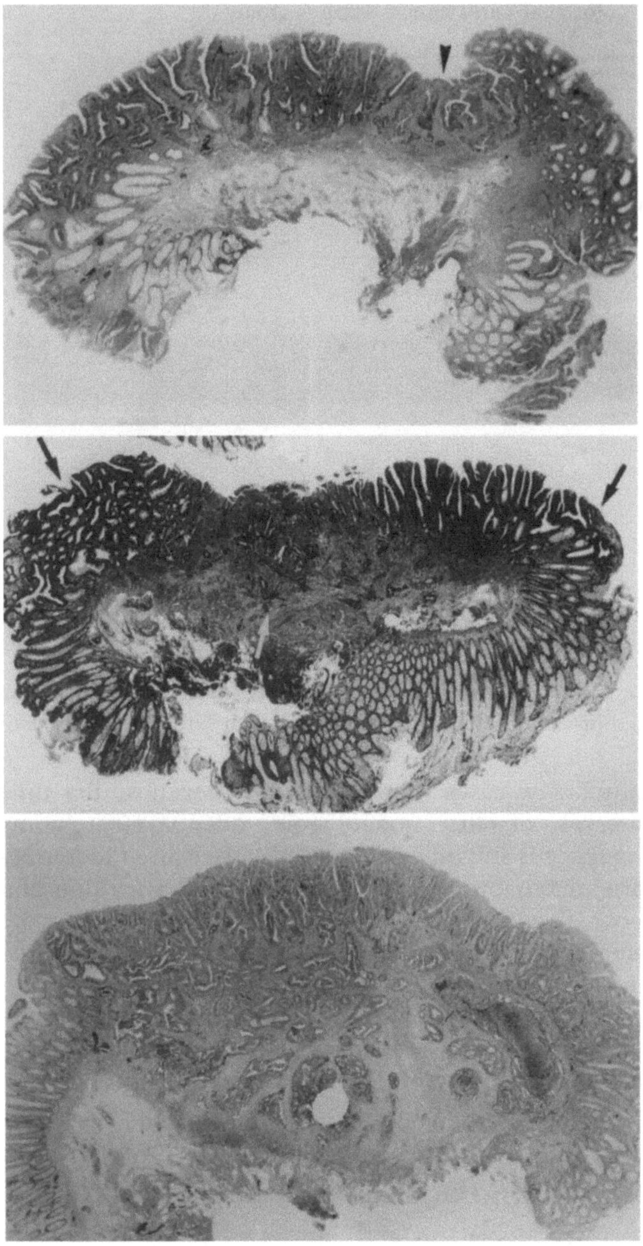

Fig. 9. Three polypectomized cancers presenting probable morphologic changes from top to bottom. Focal cancer in a superficial elevated adenoma (*top*, *arrowhead*) becomes polypoid by cancerous invasion and fibrous reaction of the surrounding tissue (*middle*, *arrows* indicating residual adenomatous tissue). It becomes much more elevated with increasing cancer invasion (*bottom*). The configuration of the muscularis mucosae is similar to that of superficial elevated adenomas

rather rarely seen in everyday practice, or to an ulcerating cancer after continuous ulceration. On the other hand, there are a few examples suggesting a superficial elevated adenoma to progress to a small ulcerating carcinoma without an intermediate phase of a polypoid lesion. There is a report suggesting that some depressed-type lesions may undergo a polypoid shape [11, 13]. More details will be described in Chapter 4 by Kashida et al. in this Part.

Table 3. Growth type and rate of K-ras mutation

Adenoma	%		Invasive cancer (sm-ca)	%
Polypoid	80	48 (Polypoid + Type IIa)	Polypoid	56
			Ulcerating	
Nonpolypoid (Type IIa)	33		PG	50
Nonpolypoid (Type IIc)	9		NPG	6

sm-ca, submucosal cancer; PG, polypoid growth; NPG, nonpolypoid growth

Because of the small number of cases available for the study and the limited incomplete data, it is immature to draw any concrete conclusions on the natural course of nonpolypoid neoplasms for the present. Shimoda et al. reported two types of ulcerating early colorectal cancers: polypoid growth type (PG) and nonpolypoid growth type (NPG) [14]. Put simply, the edge of PG consists of cancer itself whereas that of NPG is covered by the normal mucosa (Fig. 10). It is interesting to note that the prevalence of K-ras mutation, usually present in the adenoma–carcinoma sequence, was found to be present in 50%–80% of both polypoid adenomas and PG cancers, whereas it was in less than 10% in both depressed adenomas and NPG cancers (Table 3) [15]. From these data the origin of NPG and PG cancers may well be depressed adenomas and polypoid adenomas, respectively. Gathering all data together it can be assumed that there are at least two or possibly three pathways of colorectal carcinogenesis, from polypoid, nonpolypoid neoplasms, and de novo origin [15]. It is expected that the novel knowledge of molecular biology may shed more light on the study of the natural course of colorectal cancer in the future.

5. Conclusions

From accumulated observations, though limited, the natural course of (early) colorectal cancer was clarified to some extent as follows.

1. The time sequence of the polypoid adenoma–carcinoma sequence is variable depending on the time of recognition of the index lesions. However, the last step of progression from a mucosal cancer to an advanced cancer could be as rapid as less than 1 year.
2. The time sequence of the nonpolypoid adenoma–carcinoma sequence is not well known but could be more rapid than that of polypoid lesions.

Fig. 10. The edge of a polypoid growth type cancer consists of cancer itself (*left*) and that of a nonpolypoid growth type is covered with the normal mucosa (*right*)

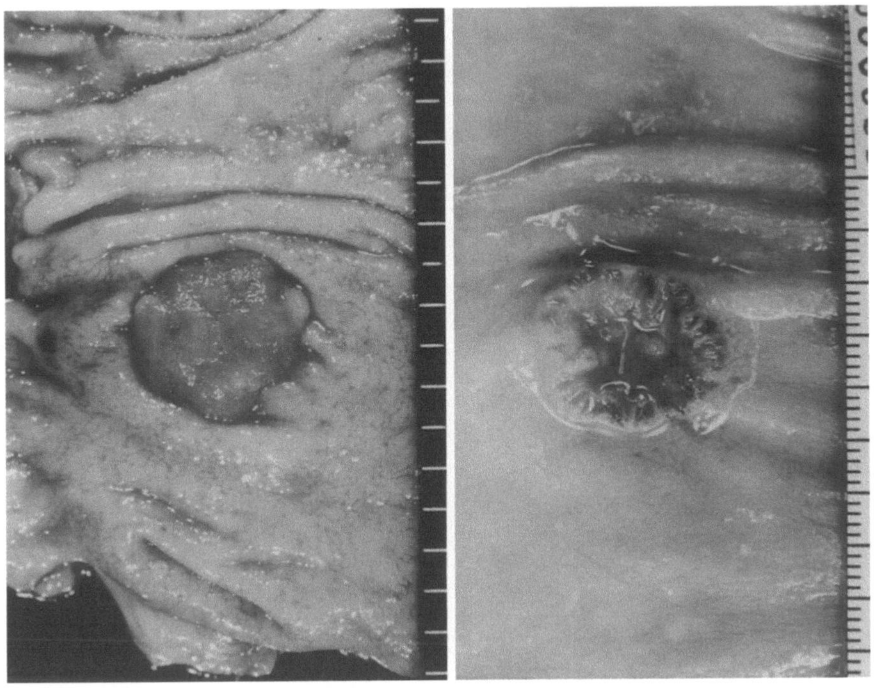

3. Polypoid adenoma can develop into ulcerating cancers. Adenomas around 1 cm in diameter, broad-based or sessile in shape, play a greater role in the polypoid adenoma–carcinoma sequence.

4. Nonpolypoid adenomas are new precursors of colorectal cancers; however, the proportion of this origin in ordinary cancers is not yet clarified because of a lack of enough proven examples.

5. The knowledge of molecular biology should be used for further understanding of the natural course of early colorectal cancers.

References

1. Muto T, Kamiya J, Kusama S, et al (1982) Rapid evolution of colon cancer from a polyp: report of two cases. Am J Proctol Gastroenterol Colon Rectal Surg 33:15–24
2. Muto T, Busssey HJ, Morson BC (1975) The evolution of cancer of the colon and rectum. Cancer 36:2251–2270
3. Muto T, Kamiya J, Sawada T, et al (1983) Morphogenesis of human colon cancer. Dis Colon Rectum 26:257–262
4. Schlemper RJ, Riddell RH, Kato Y, et al (2000) The Vienna classification of gastrointestinal epithelial neoplasia. Gut 47:251–255
5. Japanese Society for Cancer of the Colon and Rectum (1997) Japanese classification of colorectal carcinoma. 1st edn. Kanehara, Tokyo, pp 70–74
6. Muto T, Kamiya J, Sawada T, et al (1985) Small "flat adenoma" of the large bowel with special reference to its clinicopathologic features. Dis Colon Rectum 28:847–851
7. Scarborough RA (1960) The relationship between polyps and carcinoma of the colon and rectum. Dis Colon Rectum 3:336–342
8. Spratt JS Jr, Ackerman LV, Moyer CA (1958) Relationshop of polyps of colon to colonic cancer. Ann Surg 148: 682–698
9. Ushio K, Shima Y, Goto Y, et al (1985) Growth and progression of colorecal cancer: retrospective study based on roentgenologic findings (in Japanese). Stomach Intest 20: 843–858
10. Muto T, Kamiya J, Sawada T, et al (1980) Colonoscopic polypectomy in diagnosis and treatment of early carcinoma of the large intestines. Dis Colon Rectum 23:68–75
11. Umetani N, Muto T, Kawamura Y, et al (2001) Superficial depressed early carcinoma that developed into protuberant advanced carcinoma in the transverse colon. J Gastroenterol 36:48–51
12. Matsui T, Tsuda S, Yao K, et al (2000) Natural history of early colorectal cancer. Dis Colon Rectum 43(suppl):S18–S22
13. Watari J, Saito Y, Orii Y, et al (1996) Prospective observation of superficial colorectal neoplasms (in Japanese). Stomach Intest 13:1599–1606
14. Shimoda T, Ikegami M, Fujisawa J, et al (1989) Early colorectal carcinoma with special reference to its development de novo. Cancer 64:1138–1146
15. Muto T, Nagawa H, Watanabe T, et al (1997) Colorectal carcinogenesis: historical review. Dis Colon Rectum 40(suppl):S80–S85
16. Muto T, Williams C (1972) Diagnosis of early carcinoma of the colon with fibreoptic colonoscope (in Japanese). Stomach Intest 7:101–106
17. Muto T, Saito Y, Adachi M, et al (1990) Morphogenesis of colorectal carcinoma (in Japanese). Jpn J Clin Radiol 35:1277–1288

3. Colorectal Cancer: Ulcerative Colitis-Associated Neoplasia

Kazuaki Kitajima, Shigehiko Fujii, Takahiro Fujimori, Tsutomu Chiba, and Akira Terano

1. Introduction

The incidence of colorectal neoplasia is increased in patients with long-standing and extensive ulcerative colitis (UC), and death from colorectal neoplasia is the most important factor for long-term mortality in patients with UC. To improve the prognosis of patients with UC-associated neoplasia, it is very important to diagnose it at an early or precancerous state in patients with long-standing UC. However, UC-associated neoplasia is often difficult to detect endoscopically and difficult to discriminate from inflammatory regenerative epithelium pathologically. There are three important problems in diagnosing UC-associated neoplasia: the first is how to detect UC-associated dysplasia and early cancer endoscopically; the second is how to discriminate UC-associated dysplasia from inflammatory regenerative epithelium pathologically; and the third is how to identify individuals at increased risk of neoplasia, especially dysplasia, in patients with long-standing and extensive UC. We reviewed the clinicopathological and genetic characteristics of UC-associated neoplasia focusing on these three problems.

2. How to Detect UC-Associated Dysplasia and Early Cancer Endoscopically

For the purpose of detecting UC-associated dysplasia and the early stage of cancer, surveillance colonoscopy has been recommended for patients with long-standing and extensive UC. Several long-term prospective studies have been undertaken to evaluate the benefit of surveillance colonoscopy, and most of these results suggested that this modality contributed to the early detection of UC-associated neoplasia [1–8]. However, some of these reports also showed that the cancer was detected at a late stage in an appreciable number of patients, despite surveillance colonoscopy [2, 3, 7]. Furthermore, there were other reports that the effectiveness of surveillance colonoscopy would be doubtful [9–11]. Thus, it is still a matter of debate whether or not surveillance colonoscopy with random biopsies is effective for the early detection of UC-associated neoplasia.

According to the World Health Organization classification, the pit pattern of the mucosal surface of sporadic colorectal tumors is thought to predict the histology of the tumors [12]. However, the usefulness of the magnifying endoscope and the pit pattern classification for detecting UC-associated neoplasia is still unclear. In our study [13, 14], the pit pattern of UC-associated neoplasias (UC-III and -IV) differed from that of UC-I and -II lesions (Table 1). UC-III and -IV lesions showed a packed distribution of oval and/or club-shaped and/or branch-shaped pits, whereas UC-I lesions showed circular and/or oval pits that were distributed regularly and UC-II lesions showed circular and/or oval pits that were scattered throughout the area. Recently, Kiesslich et al. [16] reported the usefulness of chromoendoscopy for detecting UC-associated neoplasia. A randomized controlled trial was performed to examine whether chromoendoscopy using the pit pattern classification can facilitate early detection of UC-associated neoplasia. They showed that both the sensitivity and the specificity for differentiation between non-neoplastic and neoplastic lesions was 93% using the pit pattern classification. These findings suggest that observation of the pit pattern using a magnifying endoscope might make it possible to diagnose UC-associated neoplasia more accurately and to practice surveillance colonoscopy more efficiently. However, unlike sporadic neoplasia, more than a few non-neoplastic lesions display club- and/or branch-shaped pits; therefore, it remains unclear whether this method is practical for surveillance colonoscopy. Further studies are needed to determine the potential utility of the observation of the pit pattern as an adjunctive technique for endoscopically identifying neoplasia in non-neoplastic inflamed epithelium.

3. How to Discriminate UC-Associated Dysplasia from Inflammatory Regenerative Epithelium Pathologically

Although UC-associated dysplasia is not only a precursor of colitic cancer but may also be a marker for existence of colitic cancer in other areas of the colorectum, there are differences in the diagnostic criteria that

Table 1. Histological classification of the neoplastic epithelium arising in ulcerative colitis (UC)

UC-I	Inflammatory change
UC-II	Indefinite
UC-IIa	Probably inflammatory
UC-IIb	Probably neoplastic
UC-III	Neoplastic but not carcinoma
UC-IV	Carcinoma

Source: Research Committee of Inflammatory Bowel Disease at the Ministry if Health and Welfare of Japan, 1993 [15].

Table 2. Biopsy classification of dysplasia in inflammatory bowel disease

Negative
Normal mucosa
Inactive (quiescent) colitis
Active colitis
Indefinite
Probably negative (probably inflammatory)
Unknown
Probably positive (probably dysplasia)
Positive
Low-grade dysplasia
High-grade dysplasia

Source: Inflammatory Bowel Disease Morphology Study Group, 1983 [17].

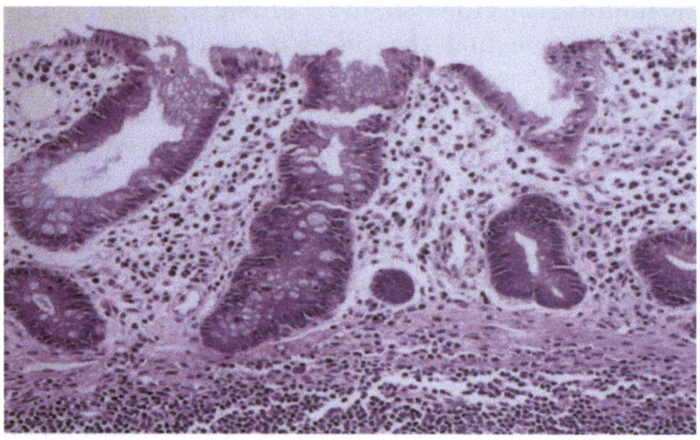

Fig. 1. Histological findings of "UC-IIa," probably inflammation, lesion. This epithelium shows a relative loss of tubular glands, and there are irregular or distorted glands accompanied by goblet cell depletion and dispolarity of goblet formation. However, there is only minor nuclear stratification and no significant loss of nuclear polarity. So this epithelium could be interpreted as UC-IIa

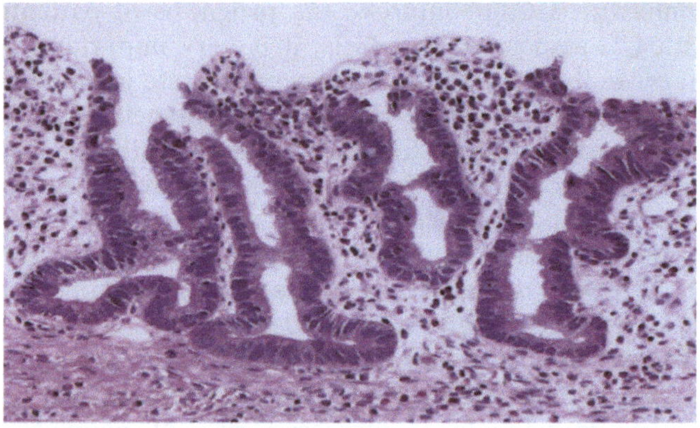

Fig. 2. Histological findings of "UC-IIb," probably neoplasia, lesion. Tubular glands show distortion and branching. Epithelial cells show cuboidal or low columnar shapes and goblet cells are almost absent. Basal polarity of the nuclei is almost maintained, but nuclear hyperchromasia, pleomorphism and enlargement are apparent. This epithelium thus could be interpreted as UC-IIb

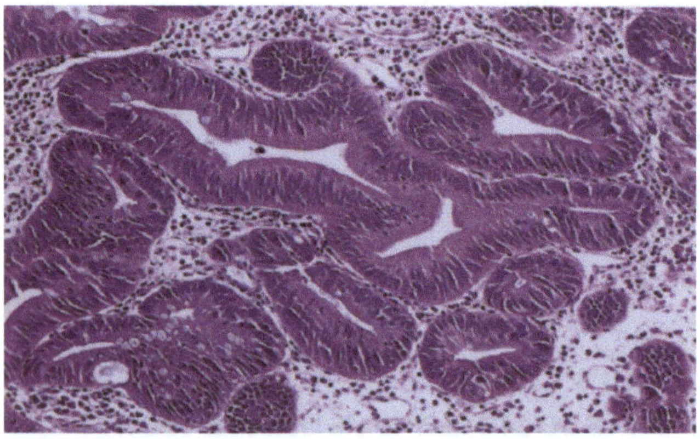

Fig. 3. Histological findings of "UC-III," neoplastic lesion but not carcinoma. The features of cytological atypia in UC-III closely resembles those of adenoma in noncolitic patients. Thus, there is nuclear stratification that extends beyond the mid portion of the cell, hyperchromasia and pleomorphism of the nuclei. Crypt architecture shows back-to-back configuration

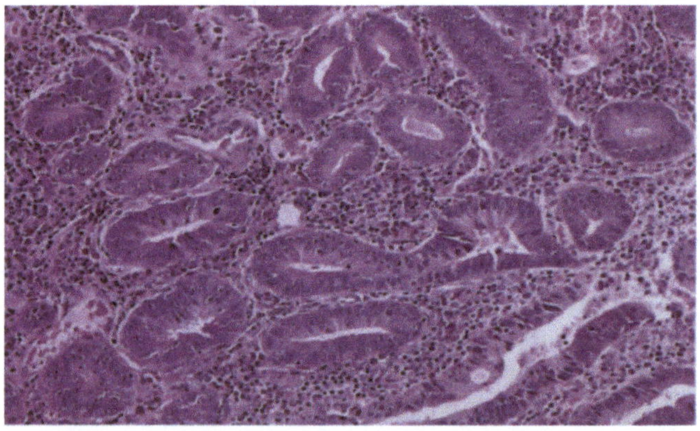

Fig. 4. Histological findings of "UC-IV," carcinoma. There is irregular proliferation of glands, partly marked budding, or gland-in-gland configuration. Nuclear hyperchromasia and pleomorphism as well as enlargement are apparent and the polarity of the nuclei is lost

Table 3. Nuclear accumulation of p53 protein by histological diagnosis

Histological diagnosis	*n*	Positive staining (%)
Inflammatory change (UC-I)	5	0 (0)
Indefinite, probably inflammatory (UC-IIa)	38	0 (0)
Indefinite, probably neoplastic (UC-IIb)	35	14 (40.0)
Neoplastic but not carcinoma (UC-III)	24	14 (58.3)
Carcinoma (UC-IV)	18	11 (61.1)

different pathologists use for dysplasia. In 1983, the Inflammatory Bowel Disease Morphology Study Group attempted to verify a standardized terminology and classification for the assessment of dysplasia in UC. In Western countries, this is now the standard classification for dysplasia (Table 2) [17]. Also in Japan the interpretation of "dysplasia" in UC varied from one pathologist to another. To solve this problem, in 1993 the Research Committee on Inflammatory Bowel Disease of the Ministry of Health and Welfare of Japan proposed a new classification for UC-associated neoplasia (Table 1) [15]. This classification is used for clinical and research purposes and applies to both colectomy and biopsy specimens. Figures 1–4 show the histological characteristics of each stage of UC-associated neoplasia. However, it is not easy to discriminate between UC-associated dysplasia and regenerative epithelium by the hematoxylin and eosin (H&E)-stained biopsy specimen. Furthermore, there are still differences in the diagnostic criteria that different pathologists use for dysplasia.

To improve the accuracy of pathological diagnosis, it may be necessary to use modalities other than those that are currently available using conventional techniques. It is generally agreed that the genetic alterations (p53, K-ras, APC, etc.) that occur in tumor progression in UC-associated neoplasia, called the dysplasia–carcinoma sequence, would be different from that occurring in sporadic colorectal cancer [14, 18, 19]. Several reports have shown that the rate of *p53* alterations was high in UC-associated neoplasia and suggested that *p53* alteration would be an early event in the development of UC-associated neoplasia [14, 20–23].

We investigated alteration of the *p53* gene using immunohistochemistry in 120 colectomy specimens from eight patients with UC who had undergone total colectomy for UC-associated neoplasia [13]. The nuclear accumulation of p53 protein was 0% (0 of 5 specimens) in UC-I, 0% (0 of 38 specimens) in UC-IIa, 40.0% (14 of 35 specimens) in UC-IIb, 58.3% (14 of 24 specimens) in UC-III, and 61.1% (11 of 18 specimens) in UC-IV (Table 3). However, in UC patients where there was no dysplasia or cancer, there was no demonstrable abnormal nuclear accumulation of the p53 protein [24]. Thus, *p53* alteration seems to be an early event in the development of dysplasia in the dysplasia–carcinoma sequence. If we were not able to discriminate dysplasia from regenerative epithelium in pathological specimens, this molecular analysis would contribute to an accurate pathological diagnosis of UC-associated dysplasia.

Table 4. Mutation of the *p53* gene (exons 5–8) by histological diagnosis

Histological diagnosis	*n*	*p53* exons 5–8 mutation (%)
Inflammatory change (UC-I)	2	0 (0)
Indefinite, probably inflammatory (UC-IIa)	10	2 (20.0)
Indefinite, probably neoplastic (UC-IIb)	10	8 (80.0)
Neoplastic but not carcinoma (UC-III)	13	12 (92.3)
Carcinoma (UC-IV)	8	8 (100)

Table 5. Mutation of the *p53* gene (exons 5–8) in lesions that showed negative staining for immunohistochemistry

Histological diagnosis	*n*	*p53* exons 5–8 mutation (%)
Inflammatory change (UC-I)	2	0 (0)
Indefinite, probably inflammatory (UC-IIa)	10	2 (20.0)
Indefinite, probably neoplastic (UC-IIb)	7	5 (71.4)
Neoplastic but not carcinoma (UC-III)	8	7 (85.7)
Carcinoma (UC-IV)	6	6 (100)

However, negative staining for p53 protein does not always indicate normality of the *p53* gene. When the *p53* gene has a nonsense mutation or frame shift, p53 protein does not accumulate in the nucleus in spite of the gene abnormality. Therefore, we investigated alternation of the *p53* gene in 43 specimens by using polymerase chain reaction–single-strand conformation polymorphism (PCR–SSCP) analysis within exons 5–8 [13]. The proportion of samples with a mutation of the *p53* gene was 0% (0 of 2 specimens) of UC-I, 20.0% (2 of 10 specimens) of UC-IIa, 80.0% (8 of 10 specimens) of UC-IIb, 92.3% (12 of 13 specimens) of UC-III, and 100% (8 of 8 specimens) of UC-IV (Table 4). In 81 specimens that showed negative immunohistochemical staining of p53, 33 specimens were included in the PCR-SSCP analysis. The proportion that was shown to be positive for the mutation was 0% (0 of 2 specimens) of UC-I, 20.0% (2 of 10 specimens) of UC-IIa, 71.4% (5 of 7 specimens) of UC-IIb, 85.7% (7 of 8 specimens) of UC-III, and 100% (6 of 6 specimens) of UC-IV (Table 5). This result suggests that analysis of the *p53* mutation using PCR–SSCP is more accurate than immunohistochemistry for discrimination between UC-associated neoplasia and regenerative epithelium. This technique should be adopted for an accurate pathological diagnosis of UC-associated neoplasia.

4. How to Identify Individuals at Increased Risk of Neoplasia, Especially Dysplasia, in Patients with Long-Standing and Extensive UC

As mentioned in the Introduction, it is still controversial as to whether surveillance colonoscopy is effective in the early detection of neoplasia. There is a great need for sensitive markers to identify individuals at increased risk of neoplasia among patients with long-standing and extensive UC. Several reports revealed some molecular alterations (e.g., p53, DNA aneuploidy, chromosomal instability, Sialyl-Tn antigen, K-ras, p16 hypermethylation, microsatellite instability) of non-neoplastic epithelium in UC patients with neoplasia, and suggested the possibility that these molecular alterations would be candidates for new markers.

Recently, some noteworthy studies were published. Issa et al. [25] reported that UC patients with neoplasia have age-related methylation in non-neoplastic epithelium, whereas UC patients without neoplasia do not. In a study to clarify whether analysis of age-related methylation in non-neoplastic epithelium can predict increased neoplastic risk, we also analyzed methylation of the estrogen receptor (ER) gene in non-neoplastic epithelium throughout the entire colorectum from patients with long-standing and extensive UC, with and without colorectal neoplasia. As a result, methylation of the ER gene was significantly more frequent in non-neoplastic epithelium from UC patients with neoplasia compared with chronic colitic epithelium from UC patients without neoplasia, and the ER gene was extensively methylated in non-neoplastic colorectal epithelium throughout the entire colorectum of UC patients with neoplasia [26]. O'Sullivan et al. [27] reported that telomere lengths were shorter in non-neoplastic samples from UC patients with neoplasia than in those from UC patients without neoplasia. These reports suggest that analysis of age-related methylation and telomere length would be useful markers for identifying individuals at increased risk of neoplasia among patients with long-standing and extensive UC. Furthermore, it is anticipated that analysis of a single biopsy sample, e.g. a rectal biopsy, may have the possibility of helping to identify UC patients at particularly high risk of developing neoplasia, in contrast to the large number of biopsy samples needed for surveillance colonoscopy at present. The determination of the predictive power of these molecular alterations as markers in the surveillance of UC patients awaits further studies.

In this chapter, we demonstrated three critical problems concerning the diagnosis of UC-associated dysplasia and colitic cancer, and discussed the possibility of solving these problems. Only by tackling the problems discussed can we obtain a more accurate diagnosis and make an appropriate treatment plan for patients with UC.

References

1. Rozen P, Baratz M, Fefer F, et al (1995) Low incidence of significant dysplasia in a successful endoscopic surveillance program of patients with ulcerative colitis. Gastroenterology 108:1361–1370
2. Lindberg B, Persson B, Veress B, et al (1996) Twenty years' colonoscopic surveillance of patients with ulcerative colitis. Detection of dysplastic and malignant transformation. Scand J Gastroenterol 53:1195–1204
3. Lashner BA (1992) Recommendations for colorectal cancer screening in ulcerative colitis: a review of research from a single university-based surveillance program. Am J Gastroenterol 87:168–175
4. Suzuki K, Muto T, Shinozaki M, et al (1995) Results of cancer surveillance in ulcerative colitis. J Gastroenterol 30 suppl:40–42
5. Karlen P, Kornfeld D, Broström O, et al (1998) Is colonoscopic surveillance reducing colorectal cancer mortality in ulcerative colitis? A population based case control study. Gut 42:711–714
6. Lennard-Jones JE, Melville DM, Morson BC, et al (1990) Precancer and cancer in extensive ulcerative colitis: findings among 401 patients over 22 years. Gut 31: 800–806
7. Nugent FW, Haggitt RC, Gilpin PA (1991) Cancer surveillance in ulcerative colitis. Gastroenterology 100:1241–1248
8. Choi PM, Nugent FW, Schoetz DJ (1993) Colonoscopic surveillance reduces mortality from colorectal cancer in ulcerative colitis. Gastroenterology 105:418–424
9. Taylor BA, Pemberton JH, Carpenter HA, et al (1992) Dysplasia in chronic ulcerative colitis: implications for colonoscopic surveillance. Dis Colon Rectum 35: 950–956
10. Axon ATR (1991) Surveillance in ulcerative colitis does not work and cannot work. In: Riddell RH (ed) Dysplasia and cancer in colitis. Elsevier, New York, pp 43–48
11. Axon ATR (1994) Cancer surveillance in ulcerative colitis—a time for reappraisal. Gut 35:587–589
12. Hamilton SR, Vogelstein B, Kudo S, et al (2000) Carcinoma of the colon and rectum. In: Hamilton SR, Aaltonen LA (eds) Pathology and genetics of tumours of the digestive system. World Health Organization classification of tumours. IARC Press, Lyon, pp 105–119

13. Fujii S, Fujimori T, Chiba T (2003) Usefulness of analysis of p53 alteration and observation of surface microstructure for diagnosis of ulcerative colitis-associated colorectal neoplasia. J Exp Clin Cancer Res 22: 107–115
14. Fujii S, Fujimori T, Kashida H (2002) Ulcerative colitis-associated neoplasma. Pathol Int 52:195–203
15. Konishi F, Wakasa H, Kino I, et al (1993) Histological classification of the neoplastic epithelium arising in ulcerative colitis. Annual report (for 1992) of the Research Committee of Inflammatory Bowel Disease (in Japanese with English abstract). The Ministry of Health and Welfare of Japan, Tokyo, pp 153–156
16. Kiesslich R, Fritsch J, Holtmann M, et al (2003) Methylene blue-aided chromoendoscopy for the detection of intraepithelial neoplasia and colon cancer in ulcerative colitis. Gastroenterology 124:880–888
17. Riddell RH, Goldman H, Ransohoff DF, et al (1983) Dysplasia in inflammatory bowel disease: standardized classification with provisional clinical applications. Hum Pathol 14:931–968
18. Fujimori T, Kawamata H, Kashida H (2001) Precancerous lesions of the colorectum. J Gastroenterol 36: 587–594
19. Fujimori T, Satonaka K, Yamamura-Idei Y, et al (1994) Non-involvement of ras mutations on flat colorectal adenomas and carcinomas. Int J Cancer 57:51–55
20. Holzmann K, Klump B, Borchard F, et al (1998) Comparative analysis of histology, DNA content, p53 and Ki-ras mutations in colectomy specimens with long-standing ulcerative colitis. Int J Cancer 76:1–6
21. Yin J, Harpez N, Tong Y, et al (1993) p53 point mutations in dysplastic and cancerous ulcerative colitis lesions. Gastroenterology 104:1633–1639
22. Harpaz N, Peck AL, Yin J, et al (1994) p53 protein expression in ulcerative colitis-associated colorectal dysplasia and carcinoma. Hum Pathol 25:1069–1074
23. Brentnall TA, Crispin DA, Rabinovitsch PS, et al (1994) Mutations in the p53 gene: an early marker of neoplastic progression in ulcerative colitis. Gastroenterology 107: 369–378
24. Toda J, Nagasako K, Fujimori T, et al (1998) The study of genetic changes in colorectal cancer with ulcerative colitis (in Japanese with English abstract). Nippon Shokakibyo Gakkai Zasshi (Jpn J Gastroenterol) 95:123–132
25. Issa JP, Ahuja N, Toyota M, et al (2001) Related articles, links accelerated age-related CpG island methylation in ulcerative colitis. Cancer Res 61 (9):3573–3577
26. Fujii S, Tominaga K, Kitajima K, et al (2005) Methylation of the estrogen receptor gene in non-neoplastic epithelium as a marker of colorectal neoplasia risk in long-standing and extensive ulcerative colitis. Gut (in press)
27. O'Sullivan JN, Bronner MP, Brentnall TA, et al (2002) Chromosomal instability in ulcerative colitis is related to telomere shortening. Nat Genet 32 (2):280–284

4. Colorectal Cancer: The Importance of Depressed Lesions in the Development of Colorectal Cancer

Hiroshi Kashida, Shin-ei Kudo, Tsukasa Takeuchi, and Kazuo Ohtsuka

1. Introduction

Concerning the development of colorectal carcinoma, two main doctrines have been advocated: the one called "adenoma–carcinoma sequence" theory [1] maintains that a cancer develops from normal mucosa through a stage of adenoma, and the other, called "*de novo*" theory [2], claims that a carcinoma emerges directly from normal epithelium without going through a process of adenoma. It is now believed and widely accepted that a sporadic colorectal cancer evolves through either of these two pathways. In carcinogenesis, a single cell transforms into a cancer cell, proliferates through frequent mitoses, and gradually forms a mass. It takes a certain time for a cancer to be diagnosed as such after its birth. According to the Japanese rule [3], early colorectal cancer is defined as being limited to the mucosa or invading only as far as the submucosa, regardless of the presence or absence of lymph node metastases. The term "early" does not always imply that the lesion exists right after its birth, but means only that it is early enough for the tumor to be completely cured. Thus, the term "early" does not reflect the time course of the tumor, nor does it fully represent its biological nature.

2. Gross Appearance of Early Colorectal Neoplasm

Several kinds of classification have been advocated for early colorectal cancer. According to the Japanese rules [4], early colorectal cancers are divided into: type I, protruded (Ip, Isp, Is); type II, superficial (IIa, IIb, IIc); and type III, excavated. Shimoda et al. [5] classified them into carcinomas with polypoid growth (type PG) and carcinomas with nonpolypoid growth (type NPG), from a pathological point of view. The Paris classification of superficial gastrointestinal neoplastic lesions [6] is largely based on the Japanese classification.

Colorectal adenomas and early carcinomas can be grossly divided into three groups: protruded or polypoid, slightly elevated, and slightly depressed (Fig. 1) [7]. The slightly depressed-type colorectal cancers can be absolutely depressed or can be accompanied by a slightly elevated margin. The periphery is usually covered with normal mucosa and is elevated because of the compression by the carcinoma or because of submucosal proliferation of tumor cells. It is worth noting that the elevated margin does not usually consist of adenomatous tissue. The transition from the carcinoma to the adjacent normal colonic mucosa is abrupt and often there is no evidence of "residual" adenoma.

The terminology "flat adenoma" was put forward by Muto et al. [8] in 1985. It referred to a type of neoplastic lesion that is slightly elevated and plateau-like, with a reddish surface and sometimes a central depression. The thickness of the adenomatous component was defined as no more than twice that of the adjacent non-neoplastic mucosa. In addition to the flat-surfaced lesion, a depressed variety of flat adenoma was described, which marked the beginning of the confusion about the depressed lesions and flat adenomas [9]. It is true that some adenomas appear to have a depression and resemble depressed-type early cancers. The depression in a slightly depressed-type colorectal cancer is rather extensive and clearly demarcated. In contrast, the "depression" in flat adenomas is actually an ill-defined pseudodepression with only a thorny or groove-like appearance. Adenomas with a pseudodepression should be differentiated from truly depressed lesions, because the former are almost invariably benign. In other words, depressed lesions are not part of flat adenomas but should rather be regarded as a different entity [10].

As Kobayashi and Sivak [11] pointed out, the terminology "flat" is often confusing. What are called "flat" adenomas are not absolutely flat but are slightly elevated. Likewise, some depressed cancers are somewhat elevated as a whole although they definitely contain a discrete depression. Comprehensive terms such as "nonpolypoid" or "superficial" are also misleading so should be used with care.

Some slightly elevated adenomas spread extensively and circumferentially along the colonic wall although being very short in height. These large, slightly elevated adenomas are sometimes malignant, but not so advanced in spite of their large diameter. We [12] advocated a category "laterally spreading tumor," which is defined as lesions larger than 10 mm in diameter but extending circumferentially rather than vertically. This is further divided into a granular type that is composed of fine granules and a nongranular type that is devoid of apparent nodules or granules.

3. Differences Between Depressed Lesions and Slightly Elevated Adenomas

Kariya et al. [13] reported the first case of slightly depressed early colon carcinoma in the Japanese language in 1977. Kudo et al. published their own cases in Japanese in 1986 [14], and in English in 1993 [15]. Rates of submucosal invasion in slightly depressed-type lesions (Table 1) are 8.0% in lesions not exceeding 5 mm, 45.0% in those of 6–10 mm, and 68.7% in those of 11–15 mm. Depressed lesions show submucosal invasion even when they are very small, strongly suggesting that they grow rather rapidly to become advanced cancer at an early stage [16, 17].

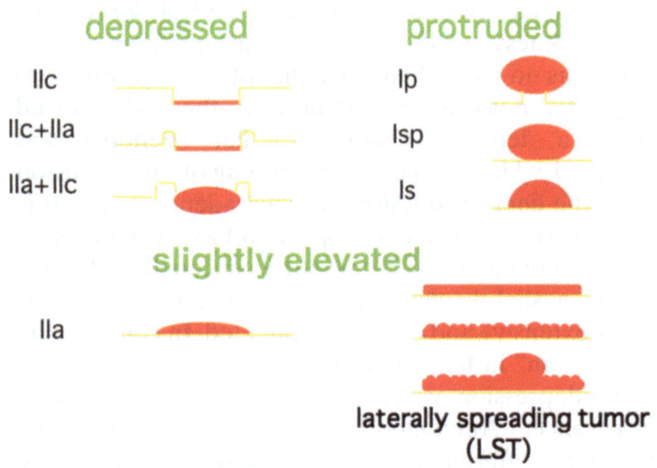

Fig. 1. Gross appearances of early colorectal cancers and adenomas

Slightly depressed-type early colorectal cancers, as well as slightly elevated adenomas, were first thought to be unique to a localized area in Japan or the East, but recently an increasing number of similar lesions has been witnessed also in Western countries [18–21]. Although depressed early colorectal cancers are still only rarely found, taking into account the difficulty of endoscopic detection of such tumors and their rapid growth, there should still be far more being overlooked than detected. It would be easy to regard these as rare exceptions, but it is necessary to question whether this is really the case.

According to the initial series of "flat adenomas" [8, 22], about 40% of them contained focal carcinomas or severely dysplastic tubules, which was one of the reasons why the authors regarded slightly elevated adenomas as precursors of invasive cancers. These studies dealt with only about 30 cases of such lesions. We have encountered more than 8500 cases of slightly elevated adenomas. Rates of submucosal invasion in slightly elevated lesions (Table 1) are 0.03% for those not exceeding 5 mm, 0.18% for those of 6–10 mm, and 1.9% for those of 11–15 mm, which are even lower than those in protruded polyps. Therefore, slightly elevated lesions are usually benign or only focally malignant and grow very slowly, not becoming invasive until they are rather large.

Muto et al. [8] described that "flat adenomas with a central depression" were more malignant than others. We suppose that they were rather true slightly depressed lesions with marginal elevation than what are now called adenomas with a pseudodepression. It is re-emphasized that depressed lesions and slightly elevated adenomas should be regarded as different entities and that the malignant potential of slightly elevated lesions should not be overrated.

Table 1. Rate of submucosal (T1) cancer in colorectal neoplasms excluding advanced cancers

Gross appearance	Size (mm) 0–5	6–10	11–15	16–20	≥21	Total
Depressed	20/249	63/140	46/67	18/20	14/16	161/492
	8.0%	45.0%	68.7%	90.0%	86.7%	32.7%
Slightly elevated	2/6479	2/1095	10/521	17/178	59/266	90/8539
	0.03%	0.18%	1.9%	9.6%	22.1%	1.1%
Protruded	0/5807	56/4376	85/1071	62/375	65/215	268/11844
	0%	1.3%	7.9%	16.5%	30.2%	2.3%
Total	22/12535	121/5611	141/1659	97/573	138/497	519/20875
	0.18%	2.2%	8.5%	16.9%	27.8%	2.5%

Apr 1985–May 2004

4. Adenoma–Carcinoma Sequence Theory and De Novo Theory

For over four decades two opposing theories have been argued regarding the pathogenesis of colorectal cancers: the so-called polyp-cancer sequence [1] and the *de novo* carcinogenesis [2]. The former claims that almost all colorectal cancers arise from adenomatous polyps. On the other hand, small colorectal cancers without any adenomatous remnant have been reported [23–25]. After the initial reports [13, 14, 26], depressed lesions are drawing many colonoscopists' attention as candidates for proving *de novo* carcinogenesis.

It has long been believed that colorectal cancers evolve from polyps. Does every colorectal cancer evolve from an adenomatous polyp [27, 28]? The majority of advanced colorectal cancers are ulcerated rather than protruded. Few researchers have witnessed an intermediate-stage colorectal cancer between a benign polyp and an advanced depressed carcinoma, a significant number of small colonic cancers without any adenomatous remnant have been reported [23–25], and benign adenomatous tissue is seen only in about 20% of advanced colorectal carcinomas [5, 29].

The supporters of the adenoma–carcinoma theory assert that the adenomatous polyp has been ulcerated or sloughed away during the development. But this may not be the case because most small early cancers without an adenomatous remnant are not ulcerated.

Perhaps a carcinoma may have overgrown the polyp, destroying the evidence of precursor adenomatous polyp? Shimoda et al. [5] described that in early colorectal cancers that showed polypoid growth, about 90% contained an adenomatous element; while in those that showed nonpolypoid growth, none contained any adenomatous remnants although they were significantly smaller (average diameter 8.7 mm) than those with polypoid growth (average diameter 16.8 mm). If the adenomatous precursor is to be gradually replaced by the carcinoma, a higher incidence of adenomatous remnants should be recognized in smaller lesions. Such a tendency is observed in polypoid carcinomas but is not seen in slightly depressed carcinomas [30]. Thus the existence of small, submucosally invasive carcinomas without identifiable residual adenomatous tissue seems to give evidence to the theory of *de novo* development of colorectal carcinoma [31–34].

Meanwhile, there is no evidence either that colorectal cancers without an adenomatous component really arise de novo from absolutely normal mucosa. An alternative explanation may be that these lesions arise from very small microadenomas which are rapidly replaced by the expanding carcinoma. It is difficult to prove which is true—whether a cancer arises from a microadenoma that is replaced rapidly by carcinomatous tissue, or strictly *de novo* from an isolated dysplastic cell that degenerates readily without going through an adenomatous step. In any case such a rapid development of cancer looks quite different from the conventional polyp–cancer concept. It would be natural to believe that there is also a *de novo* pathway in colorectal cancer development.

De novo carcinogenesis from flat mucosa without going through an adenomatous stage is not rare in the gastrointestinal tract other than the colorectum. The studies of chemically induced colorectal carcinomas in experimental animals [35, 36] have shown evidence in support of *de novo* carcinogenesis. It is only in the human colorectum that the adenoma-carcinoma sequence is regarded as the main pathway of carcinogenesis. The genetic studies also seem to support there being at least two pathways in colorectal cancer development.

5. Development of Colorectal Cancer: From Polypoid to Ulcerated, or from Depressed to Elevated?

Concerning the natural history of small adenomas, some studies [37, 38] suggested that many small adenomas either do not grow or sometimes diminish in size if followed. As mentioned above, the malignant potential of slightly elevated adenomas is not so different from that of protruded polyps. It can be speculated that slightly elevated adenomas follow the adenoma–carcinoma pathway, which is a very slow event.

Does a colorectal neoplasm always grow in a manner from a polyp to a depressed advanced cancer? There is enough evidence to believe that some lesions evolve from a slightly depressed lesion to an elevated cancer. A small invasive cancer half depressed and half elevated was reported [38]. If a polypoid neoplasm had invaded the submucosa and became ulcerated, the depressed part should have been more deeply invasive than the elevated part. Actually, in this study the elevated part was submucosally invasive but the depressed part was confined to the mucosal layer. There was no ulceration or adenomatous remnant, and the rim of the lesion was covered with normal mucosa. It was speculated that a depressed lesion partly invaded the submucosa, the cancer cells proliferated in the submucosa, and as a result the lesion became half elevated.

We have encountered many lesions that are somewhat elevated as a whole but can be considered to have evolved from slightly depressed lesions [38]. The

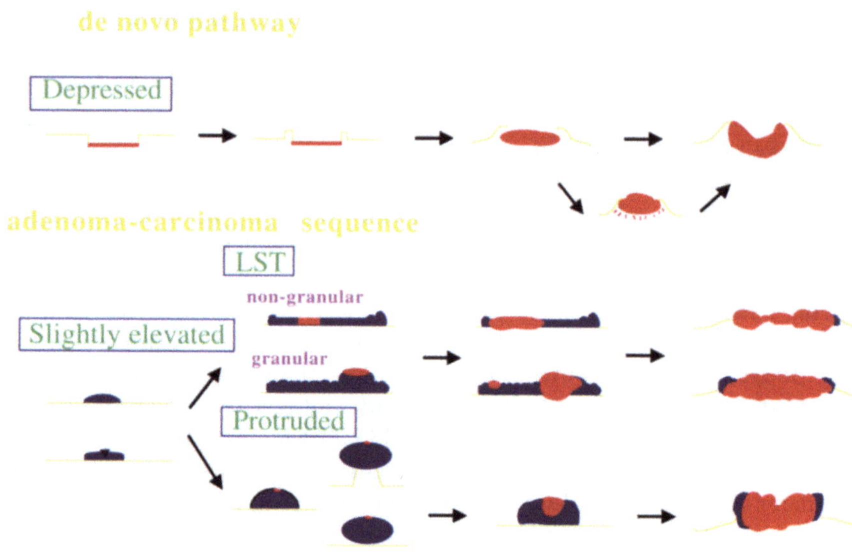

Fig. 2. Schematic demonstration of speculated natural courses of colorectal cancer development. *orange part*: cancer; *blue part*: adenoma. *LST*, laterally spreading tumor

lesions were elevated as a result of cancer proliferation in the submucosa. In such cases, the lesions looked like simple polypoid lesions at first sight, but after spraying of dye the depression was recognized. These polyp-mimicking cancers with slight depression may represent the transient and intermediate stage of the "depressed lesion-advanced carcinoma" sequence. Our theory about the natural course of early colorectal neoplasm is schematically summarized in Fig. 2.

6. Genetic Alterations in Colorectal Tumorigenesis

The adenoma–carcinoma sequence theory in the colorectum was supported by Vogelstein et al. [39] Multistep carcinogenesis had been assumed in other organs as well, but the study by Vogelstein's group was epoch-making in that they connected the genetic alterations to morphological changes in colorectal tumors. The first genetic alteration recognized in colorectal tumorigenesis is that of the *APC* (adenomatous polyposis coli) gene. Mutational activation of the K-*ras* oncogene is considered to play a role in the progression of size and grade of atypia in the adenoma–carcinoma sequence. In studies comparing the K-*ras* mutation and the configuration of the colorectal tumors, K-*ras* mutations were detected in as many as 70% of protruded adenomas, whereas they were rare in superficial adenomas [40]. Superficial colorectal tumors are regarded as candidates for de novo carcinogenesis and seem to be associated with specific genetic alterations different from those in the adenoma–carcinoma sequence. It is speculated that once becoming overt carcinoma, the consecutive changes are similar regardless of the lesion's initial form or whichever pathway it has followed. *p53* alteration is not only frequently witnessed in the development of carcinoma through the adenoma–carcinoma sequence, but is also shown to be a frequent event in de novo carcinogenesis [38]. It would be important to determine the genetic profiles of early colorectal cancers and precancerous lesions classified by their configuration.

References

1. Morson BC (1974) The polyp cancer sequence in the large bowel. Proc R Soc Med 67:451–457
2. Helwig EB (1947) The evolution of adenomas of the large intestine and their relation to carcinoma. Surg Gynecol Obstet 84:36–49
3. Japanese Society for Cancer of the Colon and Rectum (1997) Japanese classification of colorectal carcinoma. Kanehara, Tokyo, p 20
4. Japanese Society for Cancer of the Colon and Rectum (1997) Japanese classification of colorectal carcinoma. Kanehara, Tokyo, p 6
5. Shimoda T, Ikegami M, Fujisaki J, et al (1989) Early colorectal carcinoma with special reference to its development de novo. Cancer 64:1138–1146
6. The Paris endoscopic classification of superficial neoplastic lesions: esophagus, stomach, and colon (2003) Gastrointest Endosc 58(Suppl 6):S3–S43
7. Kashida H, Kudo S (2003) Magnifying colonoscopy, early colorectal cancer, and flat adenomas. In: Waye JD, Rex DX, Williams CB (eds) Colonoscopy: principles and practice. Blackwell, Malden, pp 478–486
8. Muto T, Kamiya J, Sawada T, et al (1985) Small "flat adenoma" of the large bowel with special reference

to its clinicopathologic features. Dis Colon Rectum 28: 847–851
9. Kudo S, Kashida H, Tamura S, et al (1997) The problem of "flat" colonic adenoma. Gastrointest Endosc Clin North Am 7:87–98
10. Sakashita M, Aoyama N, Maekawa S, et al (2000) Flat-elevated and depressed, subtypes of flat early colorectal cancers, should be distinguished by their pathological features. Int J Colorect Dis 15:275–281
11. Kobayashi K, Sivak Jr MV (1998) Flat adenoma: are Western colonoscopists careful enough? Endoscopy 30: 487–489
12. Kudo S, Kashida H, Nakajima T, et al (1997) Endoscopic diagnosis and treatment of early colorectal cancer. World J Surg 21:694–701
13. Kariya J, Mizuno K, Mayama M (1977) A case of early colonic cancer type IIc associated with familial polyposis coli (in Japanese with English abstract). Stomach Intest 12:1359–1364
14. Kudo S, Muto T (1986) Superficial depressed type (IIc) of colorectal carcinoma (in Japanese with English abstract). Gastroenterol Endosc 28:2811–2813
15. Kudo S (1993) Endoscopic mucosal resection of flat and depressed types of early colorectal cancer. Endoscopy 25:455–461
16. Hirata I, Tanaka M, Sugimoto K, et al (1991) Clinicopathological study on flat and depressed minute colorectal carcinomas. Dig Endosc 3:526–535
17. Iishi H, Tatsuta M, Tsutsui S, et al (1992) Early depressed adenocarcinomas of the large intestine. Cancer 69: 2406–2410
18. Stolte M, Bethke B (1995) Colorectal mini-de novo carcinoma: a reality in Germany too. Endoscopy 27: 286–290
19. Fujii T, Rembacken BJ, Dixon MF, et al (1998) Flat adenomas in the United Kingdom: are treatable cancers being missed? Endoscopy 30:437–443
20. Hart AR, Kudo S, Mackay EH, et al (1998) Flat adenomas exist in asymptomatic people: important implications for colorectal cancer screening programs. Gut 43:229–231
21. Saitoh Y, Waxman I, West AB, et al (2001) Prevalence and distinctive biologic features of flat colorectal adenoma in a North American population. Gastroenterology 120: 1657–1665
22. Wolber RA, Owen DA (1991) Flat adenomas of the colon. Hum Pathol 22:70–74
23. Spjut HJ, Frankel NB, Appel MF, et al (1979) The small carcinoma of the large bowel. Am J Surg Pathol 3: 39–46
24. Crawford BE, Stromeyer FW (1983) Small nonpolypoid carcinomas of the large intestine. Cancer 51:1760–1763
25. Kuramoto S, Oohara T (1988) Minute cancers arising de novo in the human large intestine. Cancer 61:829–834
26. Kudo S, Tamura S, Hitota S, et al (1995) The problem of de novo colorectal carcinoma. Eur J Cancer 31A: 1118–1120
27. Castlemann B, Krickstein HI (1962) Do adenomatous polyps of the colon become malignant? N Engl J Med 267:469–475
28. Ackerman LV, Spratt JS (1963) Do adenomatous polyps become cancer? Gastroenterology 44:905–908
29. Hermanek P, Crall FP (1986) Early (microinvasive) colorectal carcinoma. Int J Colorect Dis 1:79–84
30. Tada S, Yao T, Iida M, et al (1993) A clinicopathologic study of small flat colorectal carcinoma. Cancer 74: 2430–2435
31. Vas W, Somers S, Stevenson G (1982) Rapid growth of carcinoma of the colon. Gastrointest Endosc 28:19–21
32. Jelinek GP, Nava HR, Nime F (1983) Small primary de novo adenocarcinoma of the colon with mesenteric lymphatic metastasis. J Surg Oncol 23:185–188
33. Herrera L, Hanna S, Castillo N, et al (1991) Primary de novo adenocarcinoma of the colon measuring 8 mm in diameter with lymph node metastases: report of a case. Dis Colon Rectum 34:275–279
34. Minamoto T, Mai M, Ogino T, et al (1993) Early invasive colorectal carcinomas metastatic to the lymph node with attention to their nonpolypoid development. Am J Gastroenterol 88:1035–1039
35. Maskens AP, Dujardin-Loits RM (1981) Experimental adenomas and carcinomas of the large intestine behave as distinct entities: most carcinomas arise de novo in flat mucosa. Cancer 47:81–87
36. Chang WW (1984) Histogenesis of colon cancer in experimental animals. Scand J Gastroenterol 104:27–43
37. Hoff G, Foerster A, Vatn MH, et al (1986) Epidemiology of polyps of the rectum and colon; recovery and evaluation of unresected polyps two years after detection. Scand J Gastroenterol 21:853–862
38. Kudo S, Kashida H, Tamura T, et al (1999) Colonoscopic diagnosis and management of non-polypoid ECC (early colorectal cancer). World J Surg 23:694–701
39. Vogelstein B, Fearon ER, Hamilton SR, et al (1988) Genetic alterations during colorectal-tumor development. N Engl J Med 319:525–532
40. Fujimori T, Satonaka K, Yamamura-Idei Y, et al (1994) Non-involvement of ras mutations on flat colorectal adenomas and carcinomas. Int J Cancer 57:51–55

5. Natural Course of Squamous Cell Carcinoma of the Esophagus

Misao Yoshida

The process of growth and development of carcinoma of the esophagus is an interesting theme of study. Recent progress in early detection of squamous cell carcinoma of the esophagus has allowed us to know features of esophageal carcinoma at every stage of growth and development. In this chapter, such growth and development is estimated through clinical and pathological analyses of 435 superficial esophageal cancer lesions conducted at the Tokyo Metropolitan Komagome General Hospital, Tokyo, Japan.

1. Overview of Growth and Development of Esophageal Cancer

Regarding squamous cell carcinoma of the esophagus, a close relationship is apparent between size of lesions, number of lesions, and depth of invasion. The number of patients with superficial esophageal cancers increases until the size of the lesion reaches 20mm. Thereafter, the number of superficial cancers decreases as the size of the lesion increases. Submucosal invasion appears when the size of the lesion exceeds 5mm, and the incidence of submucosal cancer increases as the size of the lesion increases. The total number of superficial esophageal cancers decreases as the ratio of submucosal cancer (sm2 and sm3) increases (Figs. 1–3). These facts suggest that esophageal mucosal cancers can increase in size until reaching 20mm. At the same time, some cancers begin to invade the submucosa when the size of lesion exceeds 5mm. A considerable number of superficial esophageal cancers probably grow over sm3 rapidly and the number of superficial esophageal cancers decreases as the size of the lesion increases to over 20mm.

2. Gross Findings of Superficial Esophageal Cancer

According to the guidelines for treatment of esophageal cancer, superficial esophageal cancer can be classified into three basic types [1]. Cancer lesions of the protruding type (type I) and the distinctly depressed type (type III) are highly likely to have moderate (sm2) or severe (sm3) invasion into the submucosa, while cancer lesions of the slightly elevated, flat and slightly depressed types (type II) have a high probability of being mucosal cancers (Tables 1–3).

3. Minute Cancers as Initial Cancer of the Esophagus

Nowadays in Japan, the size of minute cancers of the esophagus is defined as 5mm or less. The majority of minute cancers (84% of 26 minute cancers) is confined to the epithelium (EP) and is flat (type IIb). Others are slightly elevated (type IIa) 4%, slightly depressed (type IIc) 8%, and distinctly depressed (type III) 4%. Submucosal invasion was found only in type III minute cancer (4% of all minute cancers) (Fig. 4), strongly suggesting that the initial cancer lesion is a very small and flat cancer (type IIb) confined to the epithelium. At the same time, a small number of minute cancers probably differentiates into other types such as type IIc, IIa, and so on, from the minute type IIb lesion before they grow to a size of 5mm. Considering these facts, the true initial cancer lesion may be a type IIb lesion smaller than 5 mm. Among all type IIb lesions, the number of type IIb cancers less than 5mm in size is relatively large. They decrease in number as they increase in size, and type IIb cancers larger than 20mm in size are rare (Fig. 5).

4. Development from Minute Cancers

Type IIc cancers are most frequent among superficial esophageal cancers, followed by type IIb and type IIa (Fig. 6). A minute type IIc cancer is rare, but there is a large number of type IIc cancers over 10mm while the number of type IIc cancers gradually decreases as they increase in size to over 20mm (Fig. 7). The same phenomenon has been found in cases of type IIa cancers (Fig. 8). Type IIc and IIa cancers with a size of less than 10mm showed simple endoscopic findings such as only a slight depression or a slight elevation. In some lesions

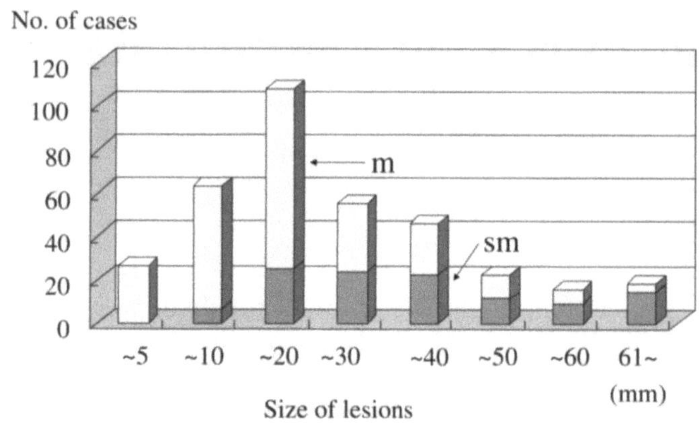

Fig. 1. Size and depth of invasion

Table 1. Gross classification of superficial esophageal cancer

I	Ip	Ipl	Isep
II	IIa	IIb	IIc
III	III		

Source: Japanese Society for Esophageal Diseases, March 1992.

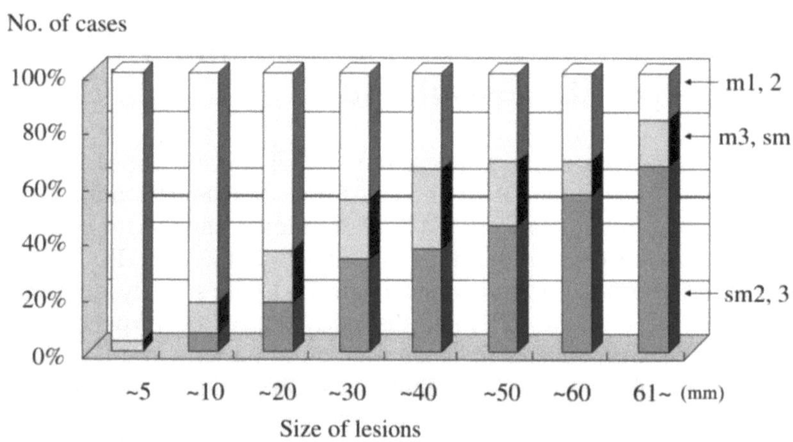

Fig. 2. Size and depth of invasion: percentages

Table 2. Gross findings of mucosal cancer

Type	No. of lesions	sm	m
I	62	92%	10%
II	349	14%	86%
III	24	96%	4%

n = 435.

Table 3. Gross findings of mucosal cancer

Type	No. of lesions	sm	m
IIa	45	4%	96%
IIb	66		100%
IIc	238	19%	81%

n = 349.

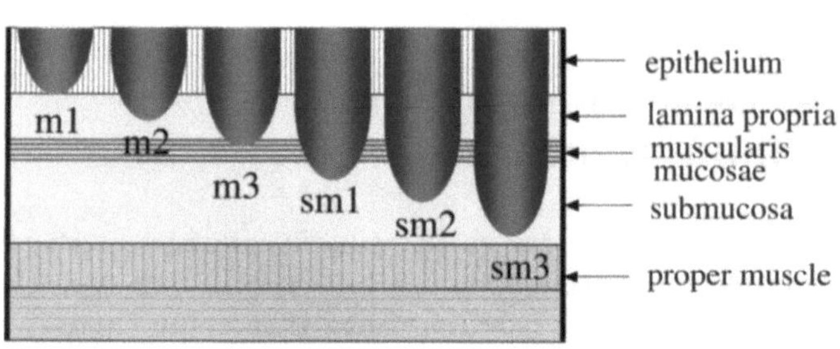

Fig. 3. Subclassification of the depth of invasion

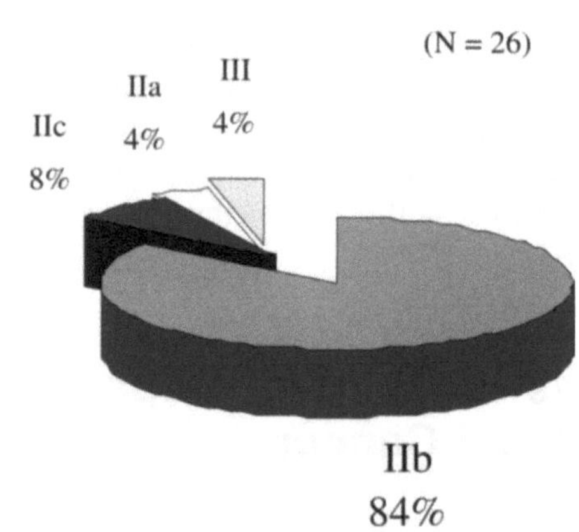

Fig. 4. Minute cancers of the esophagus

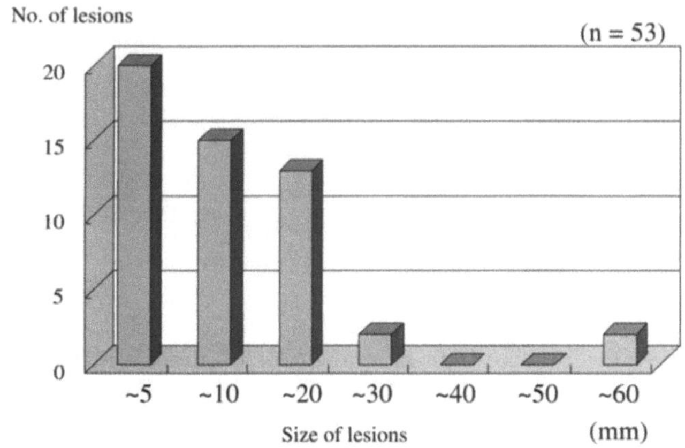

Fig. 5. Type IIb esophageal cancers

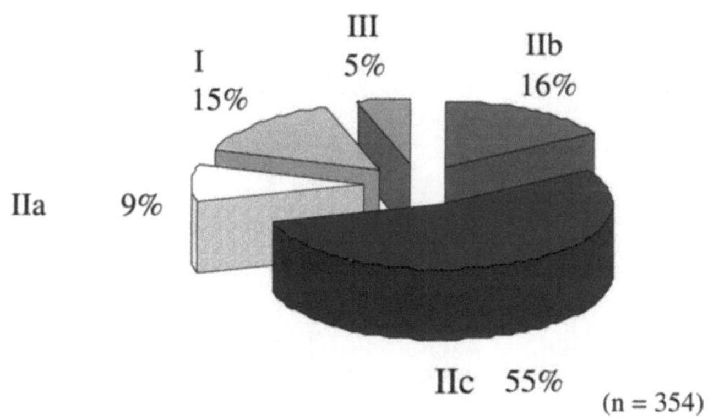

Fig. 6. Endoscopic findings of superficial esophageal cancer

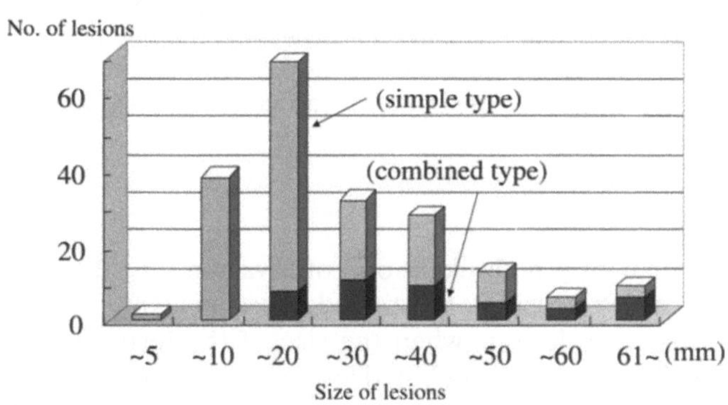

Fig. 7. Type IIc esophageal cancers: simple type and combined type

different appearances are combined, such as a slight depression with a slight elevation (IIc+IIa) or a slight depression within a slightly elevated cancer lesion (IIa+IIc). This suggests that some small initial cancers (type IIb) probably grow and develop into small and simple type IIc or type IIa cancers and begin to lose the type IIb character before they have reached a size of 10 mm. Type IIc cancers then develop a partial elevation or a limited and deeper depression, and type IIa cancers

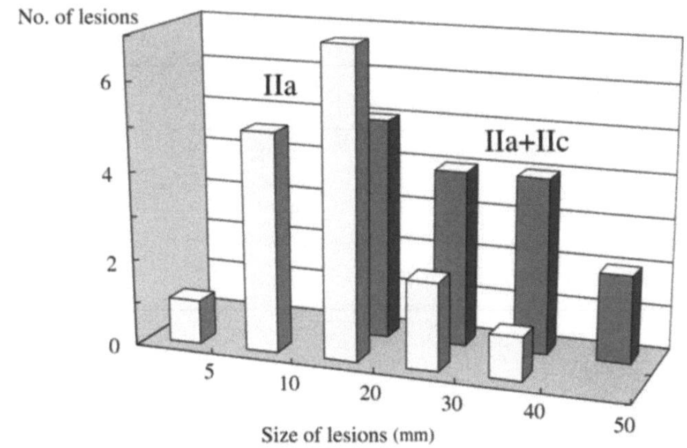

Fig. 8. Type IIa esophageal cancers

then develop a partial depression (combined types), as they increase in size. The proportion of combined cancers among type IIc and IIa cancers increases as the size of the lesions increases (Figs. 7 and 8).

5. Growth and Development from Mucosal Cancer to Submucosal Cancer

5.1 Cancer Invasion and Lymph Node Metastases

Subclassification of depth of cancer invasion was carried out in studies on depth of cancer invasion and pathological features of superficial esophageal cancers. Mucosal cancers are classified into three groups, namely, m1 (intraepithelial cancer), m2 (invasion into the lamina propria mucosae), and m3 (invasion reaching the muscularis mucosae). Submucosal cancers are also classified into three groups, namely, sm1 (slight invasion into the submucosa), sm2 (invasion reaching the middle third of the submucosa), and sm3 (invasion into the deeper third of the submucosa) (Fig. 3). Lymph node metastasis is very rare among m1 and m2 cancers while it is frequent among sm2 and sm3 cancers (47%). The incidence of lymph node metastasis is 6% in m3 cancers and 11% in sm1 cancers. Clinical differentiation of superficial esophageal cancers into three categories such as m1 plus m2, m3 plus sm1, and sm2 plus sm3 is important in the selection of treatment (Table 4).

5.2 m3 and sm1 Cancers

The mode of cancer invasion in superficial esophageal cancer is not uniform because a deeper invasion is

Table 4. Lymph node metastasis in superficial esophageal cancer

Depth of invasion	No. of cases	Vascular invasion	Lymph node metastasis
m1,2	22	4.5%	0%
m3	16	56%	6%
sm1	9	78%	11%
sm2,3	96	97%	47%
Total	143	77%	33%

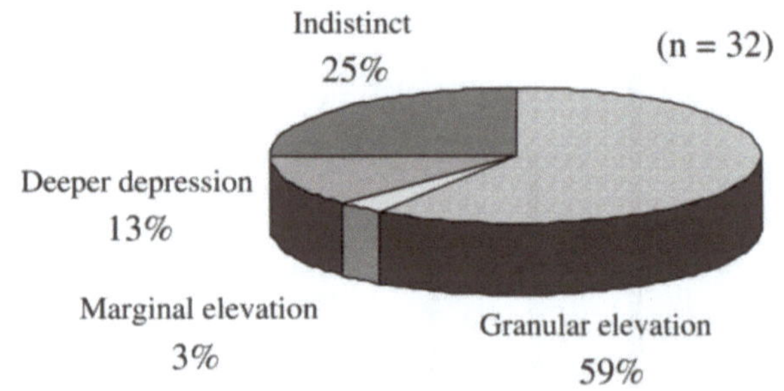

Fig. 9. Endoscopic findings at the site of m3 invasion in type IIc

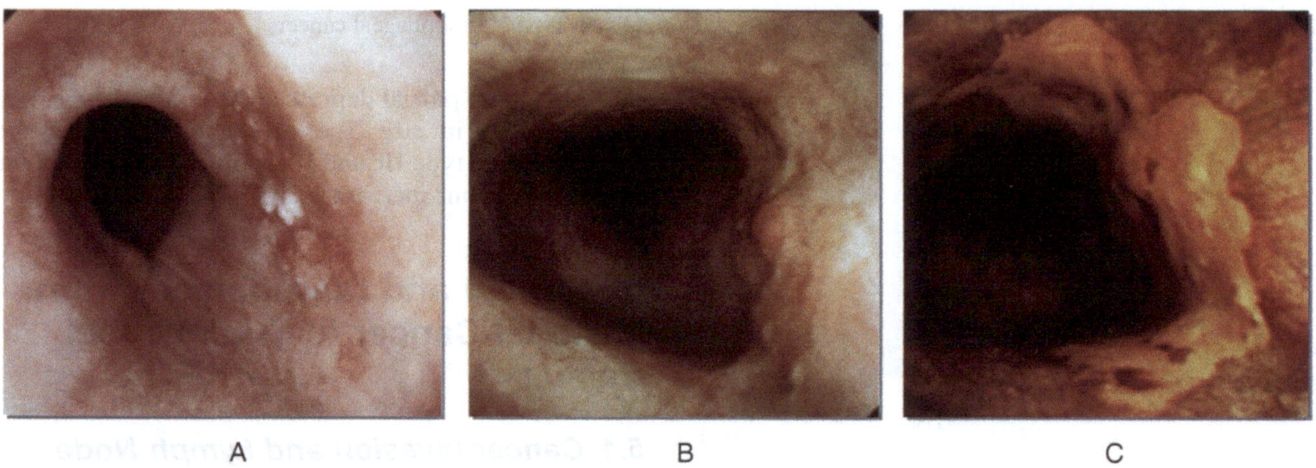

Fig. 10A–C. Endoscopic pictures of type IIc cancer lesions. Cancer invasion into the deeper layer is probably partial and present in only a narrow area. Invasion must be detected on endoscopic observation. Granular elevations in the depressed area suggest deeper invasion. **A** A few coarse granular elevations in the depressed area suggest deeper invasion over a narrow area reaching the muscularis mucosae (m3). **B** A type IIc cancer is noted with a slight depression and reddening. **C** The irregular shape and size are delineated by the unstained area after iodine staining. A nodular elevation in the depressed area suggests cancer invasion reaching the submucosa (sm)

usually limited to a small part of a cancer lesion. Clinical signs of the development toward a submucosal cancer from a mucosal cancer begin when cancer invasion reaches the muscularis mucosae (m3). The site of deeper invasion in a mucosal cancer can be detected by endoscopic observation in 75% of all m3 cancer cases. Small, granular elevations or a partially deeper depression in a type IIc cancer strongly suggest deeper invasion, while a type IIc cancer with a very narrow area of invasion does not allow us to find any clinical abnormalities (Figs. 9–11).

5.3 Growth into Submucosal Cancers

Protruding cancer (type I) and distinctly depressed cancer (type III) are types of superficial esophageal cancer with a high likelihood of invasion into the submucosa. Protrusion or distinct depression is observed as simple type lesions when the size of the lesion is less than 20mm, while combined lesions are frequent among type I and type III cancers when they are over 20mm. These facts probably suggest that small mucosal cancers may develop into small submucosal cancers such as type I or type III with simple gross findings, and may increase in size up to 20mm. In addition, type IIc mucosal cancers may begin to invade into deeper layers presenting with a partial elevation or a deeper depression, and may finally develop into type I or type III submucosal cancers (Figs. 12–15). Most advanced esophageal cancers reaching the proper muscular layer can be classified into protruding type or ulcerative type. Most of them are combined with mucosal cancer (IIc: 70% and IIb: 7%). Cancers with simple protrusion or simple

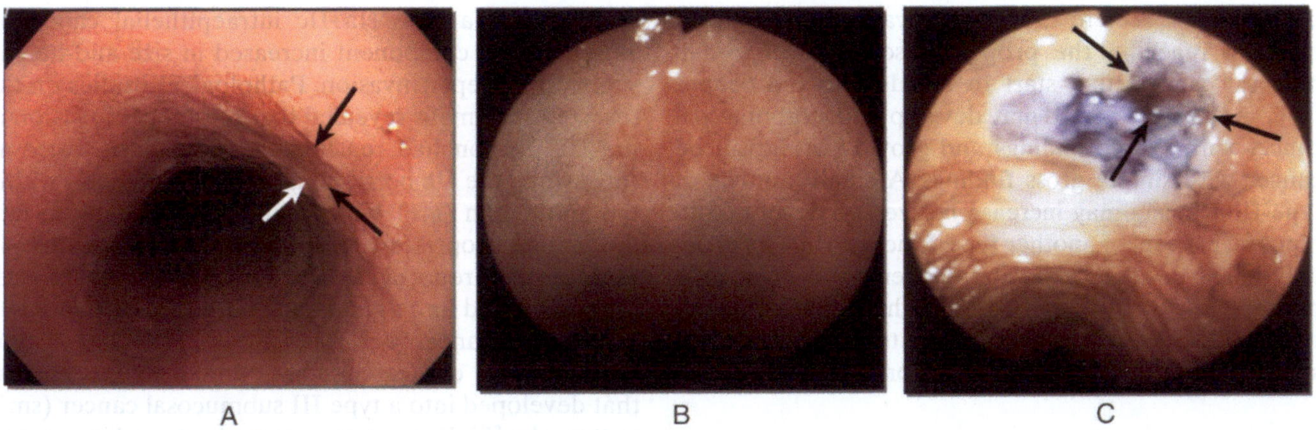

Fig. 11A–C. Endoscopic pictures of partially deeper depressions in type IIc cancers. Localized deeper depression in a type IIc lesion suggests deeper invasion. **A** There is a small deeper depression with distinct redness noted in a type IIc cancer, which suggests invasion over a narrow area reaching the muscularis mucosae (m3). **B** A small type IIc cancer with irregular shape. **C** Endoscopic toluidine blue–iodine (TB-I) double staining of **B** revealed a small blue-stained area with a deeper depression and irregular surface at the proximal part of the slightly depressed area, which suggests cancer invasion over a narrow area into the muscularis mucosae (m3)

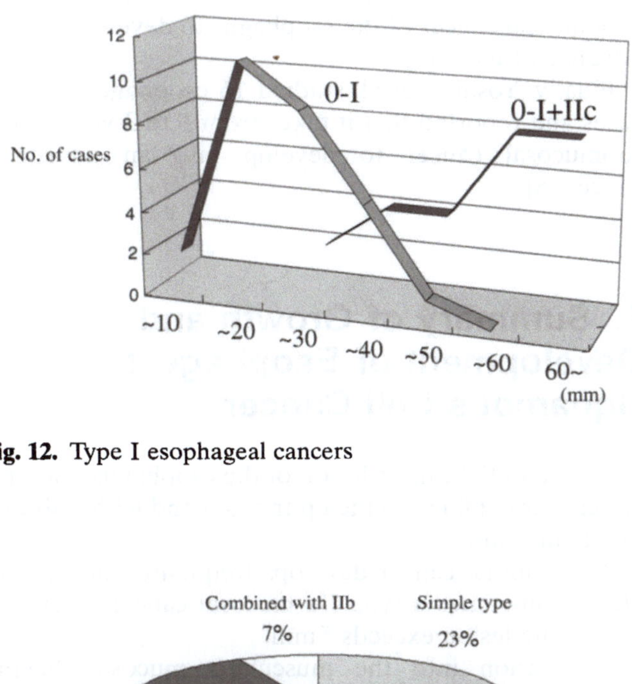

Fig. 12. Type I esophageal cancers

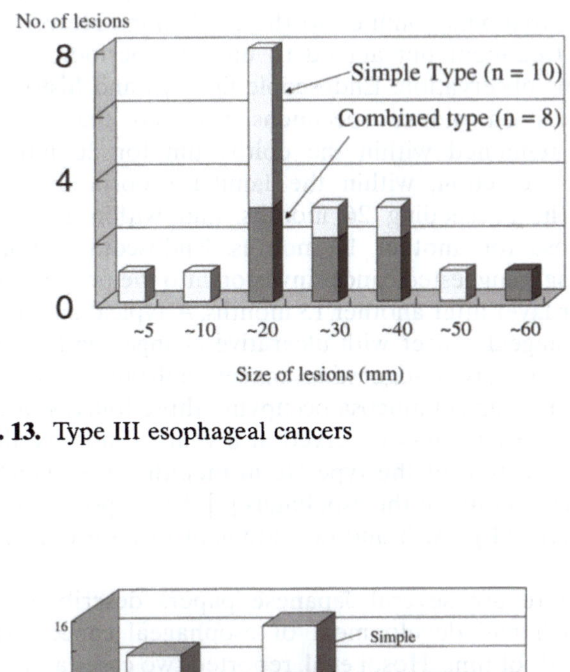

Fig. 13. Type III esophageal cancers

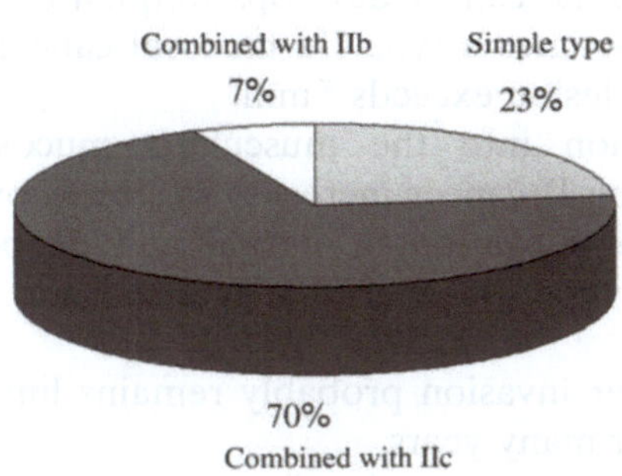

Fig. 14. Esophageal cancer that reaches the proper muscle, classified into simple versus combined types

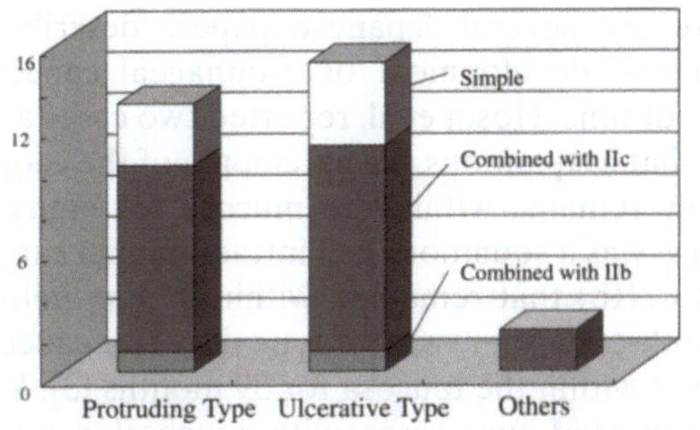

Fig. 15. Esophageal cancer that reaches the proper muscle, classified into protruding versus ulcerative types

ulceration are seen in 23% of all advanced cancers with invasion reaching the proper muscular layer. Small mucosal cancers that start to invade into the deeper layer in the early period may develop into a submucosal cancer with simple findings and grow to an advanced cancer with simple gross findings. A small number of type IIb cancers may increase in size and develop into mucosal cancers of another type. Mucosal cancers probably begin to invade into the deeper layer, presenting partial elevation or depression, which may grow to become distinct protrusion or ulceration when the invasion reaches the submucosa or beyond.

6. Natural Course of Esophageal Cancer

We seldom have a chance to observe the natural course of esophageal cancer from mucosal cancer to advanced cancer. Hayashi reported on an elderly man who had a type IIc esophageal cancer. Pathological studies on biopsy specimens strongly suggested squamous cell carcinoma confined to the epithelium. He refused any treatment but agreed to undergo periodic endoscopic observation. Endoscopic findings and histologic studies on biopsy specimens revealed that cancer had remained within the epithelium for 26 months after detection, within the lamina propria mucosae for the succeeding 26 months, and within the submucosa for another 11 months. Endoscopic findings strongly suggested cancer invasion into the proper muscular layer after another 13 months. A typical advanced esophageal cancer with ulcerative changes with an ill-defined margin suggesting cancer infiltration into the surrounding submucosa occupying three fourths of the circumference was observed at 8 years 4 months after the detection of the type IIc intraepithelial squamous cell carcinoma of the esophagus [2]. This report showed the typical growth and development of an esophageal cancer.

There are several Japanese papers describing the growth and development of esophageal cancer over periods of time. Hosoi et al. reported two cases and suggested that a squamous cell carcinoma of the esophagus probably remains within the mucosa for many years. One case was a squamous cell intraepithelial carcinoma (type IIc+IIb) that remained within the epithelium for 56 months; another was a type IIc+IIb cancer that remained within the mucosa for 59 months [3]. Yamada et al. reported two cases with mucosal cancer that showed deeper invasion over the course of a few years. One case was a type IIc mucosal cancer that developed into a type I protruding submucosal cancer after 3 years; another was a type IIa+IIc intraepithelial cancer in which the IIa component increased in size and height, suggesting deeper invasion. Pathological studies on the resected specimens revealed that the cancer invasion in the IIa portion had reached the muscularis mucosae (m3) while the IIc portion had mostly remained within the epithelium (m1), with small areas of invasion into the lamina propria mucosae (m2) after 18 months [4]. Momma et al. reported a case of type IIc mucosal cancer that developed into a small type III distinctly depressed submucosal cancer (sm1) in 4 weeks, as well as a type IIc squamous cell carcinoma confined to the mucosa that developed into a type III submucosal cancer (sm1) in 9 weeks [5]. Kato et al. reported a type IIc mucosal cancer with a partial elevation suggesting invasion reaching the muscularis mucosae (m3) or slight invasion into the submucosa (sm1). The slight elevation in the type IIc lesion developed into a type I protrusion with moderate histological invasion into the submucosa (sm2) [6].

Yamada et al. carried out a retrospective study on the growth and extension of esophageal carcinoma in 13 cases. They estimated that it takes about 1 year for a submucosal cancer of the esophagus to develop into an advanced cancer [7].

Finally, Yoshida et al. studied 16 esophageal cancer cases and reported that it takes from 1 to 3 years for a submucosal cancer to develop into an advanced cancer [8].

7. Summary of Growth and Development of Esophageal Squamous Cell Cancer

1. The initial cancer lesion of the esophagus is a type IIb cancer confined to the epithelium and with a size of less than 5 mm.
2. An initial cancer develops frequently into a type IIc or sometimes a type IIa mucosal cancer when the size of the lesion exceeds 5 mm.
3. Invasion into the muscularis mucosae begins when a type II cancer increases in size to over 10 mm. A granular elevation or partial and deeper depression in a type IIc cancer suggests a site of deeper invasion.
4. Cancer invasion probably remains limited to the mucosa for many years.
5. Mucosal cancers develop protrusions or distinct depressions, and grow into submucosal cancers of the protruding type (type I) or the distinctly depressed type (type III).

6. A small number of submucosal cancers is noted when the size of the lesion exceeds 5 mm, and the proportion of submucosal cancers is increased among superficial cancers over 20 mm in size.

7. Cancer invasion probably remains within the submucosa at least for 1 year before developing into advanced cancer, resulting in a decreased number of superficial esophageal cancers that are over 20 mm in size.

References

1. Japanese society for esophageal diseases (1999) Guidelines for the clinical and pathological studies on carcinoma of the esophagus (9th edn). Kanehara, Tokyo
2. Hayashi T (1995) Superficial esophageal carcinoma (type 0–IIc) followed up endoscopically for eight years and four months, report of a case. Stomach Intestine 30: 1357–1363
3. Hosoi T, et al (1995) Retrospective study of superficial esophageal carcinoma, report of two cases. Stomach Intestine 30:1372–1378
4. Yamada Y, et al (1995) Type 0-I superficial esophageal cancer in which the course of development was observed, report of two cases. Stomach Intestine 30:1391–1396
5. Momma K, et al (1995) Type 0–IIc esophageal cancer lesions developing into type 0–III, report of two cases. Stomach Intestine 30:1397–1402
6. Kato H, et al (1995) Esophageal cancer of superficial and slightly depressed type rapidly developing into superficial and protruding type. Stomach Intestine 30:1403–1407
7. Yamada A, et al (1988) Retrospective study of growth and extension of esophageal carcinoma with reference to its X-ray findings. Stomach Intestine 23:1199–1207
8. Yoshida T, et al (1988) Growth and progression of esophageal cancer. Stomach Intestine 23:1222–1228

VII. Surgical Treatment and Survival Rate of Early Cancer

1. Surgical Treatment and Survival Rate of Early Cancer

Michio Kaminishi, Shoji Shimoyama, Hirokazu Yamaguchi, Fumio Aoki, Nobuyuki Shimizu, Sachiyo Nomura, Toshiki Mimura, Naoki Hiki, Masaki Kawahara, Yasuyuki Seto, and Ken-ichi Mafune

1. Early Gastric Cancer

1.1 Introduction

Subtotal gastrectomy with lymphadenectomy including Group 2 lymph nodes, D2 lymphadenectomy, has been performed in Japan as a standard surgical treatment for gastric cancer regardless of its stage, and good survival rates have been obtained. However, retrospective analysis of the results revealed that about 80% of early cancers have no lymph node involvement, suggesting curative treatment of these early cancers without the standard D2 lymphadenectomy; they may be curative with limited surgery. Limited surgery includes two limitations, the scope of the gastrectomy and lymphadenectomy. In terms of quality of life (QOL) after gastric surgery, preservation of the gastric function and less invasive surgery are desirable. In this section, we discuss indications and results of limited surgery for early gastric cancer. Furthermore, application of a newly developed surgical treatment will be proposed.

1.2 Lymph Node Involvement

We analyzed 624 cases of solitary early gastric cancer resected at our institution over the last years from 1976 to 1997. There were 352 cases of mucosal and 272 cases of submucosal cancer. According to the Rules of the Japanese Gastric Cancer Association [1], clinicopathological features were investigated. In regard to macroscopic type, cancers were divided into elevated, i.e. protruded and superficial elevated (I and IIa), depressed (IIc), and combined (IIa+IIc) types. Furthermore, the depressed type was classified as with or without an ulcer or ulcer scar (see Table 1, ul(−) vs ul(+)). According to Lauren's classification [2], the histological type of cancer was divided into intestinal (pap, tub) and diffuse (por, sig, muc) types.

Table 1 shows the relationship between the macrosopic type and depth of cancer invasion. The depressed type occupied 75% of all cancers and three quarters of the depressed type were associated with an ulcer or ulcer scar [3]. Regarding the depth of cancer invasion, the incidence of submucosal cancer was higher in the combined type compared with the other types. There was no close relationship between histological type and depth of cancer invasion, nor between association of ulcer or ulcer scar and depth of invasion. However, the depth of invasion showed a close relationship with the size of the cancer (Table 2).

The incidence of lymph node involvement was 3.7% in mucosal cancer (13/352) and 18.4% in submucosal cancer (50/272). The results are quite similar to other reports [3–6]. In mucosal cancer, the involved lymph nodes were mostly located in the perigastric region (11/13), the Group 1 lymph nodes, and all lymph node-positive cases were of the depressed type with ulceration or ulcer scar in the cancerous lesion. Histologically, 12 of 13 cases were of the undifferentiated type (por, sig). In submucosal cancer, 6% of the cases showed involvement of distant lymph nodes, the Group 2 (N2) or the Group 3 (N3) lymph nodes, irrespective of macroscopic type (Table 3).

The incidence of lymph node involvement increased according to not only the depth of cancer invasion, but also the size of the cancer. Tables 4 and 5 show the relationship between size of cancer, histological type, and lymph node involvement reported by the Cancer Institute Hospital in Japan. In differentiated type cancer, only 3 of 784 mucosal cancers (0.4%) showed lymph node involvement without evident relation to cancer size. In contrast, mucosal cancer of the undifferentiated type and submucosal cancers, both of the differentiated and undifferentiated types, showed a positive relationship between lymph node metastasis and the size of the cancer. As stated later, multivariate analysis revealed a strong correlation between lymph node involvement and cancer recurrence, even if the cancer was limited to the mucosa [7–10].

1.3 Survival Rate of, and Mode of Recurrence in Early Gastric Cancer

The Japanese Society for Gastric Cancer and Japanese Gastric Cancer Association have been carrying out

Table 1. Macroscopic type and depth of cancer invasion in early gastric cancer

Macroscopic type	Depth	
	m	sm
Elevated (n = 80)	54 (68%)	26 (32%)
Combined (n = 76)	20 (26%)	56 (74%)
Depressed (n = 468)		
ul(−) (n = 117)	71 (61%)	46 (39%)
ul(+) (n = 351)	207 (59%)	144 (41%)

Source: Department of Gastrointestinal Surgery, University of Tokyo, 1976–1997.
Combined, elevated + depressed; ul, ulceration or ulcer scar within the lesion; m, mucosal; sm, submucosal.

Table 2. Depth of invasion and size in early gastric cancer

Size (mm)	Depth	
	m	sm
0–5 (n = 13)	11 (85%)	2 (15)
6–10 (n = 51)	40 (78%)	11 (22%)
11–15 (n = 74)	43 (58%)	31 (42%)
16–20 (n = 96)	57 (59%)	39 (41%)
21–25 (n = 74)	39 (53%)	35 (47%)
26–30 (n = 83)	51 (61%)	32 (39%)
31–40 (n = 87)	46 (53%)	41 (47%)
41–50 (n = 61)	27 (44%)	34 (56%)
≥51 (n = 85)	38 (45%)	47 (55%)

Source: Department of Gastrointestinal Surgery, University of Tokyo, 1976–1997.

Table 3. Incidence and site of lymph node involvement in early gastric cancer

Depth	n0	n1	n2	n2
M (n = 352)	399 (96%)	11 (3%) dif 1 undif 10	2 (1%) dif 0 undif 2	0 (0%)
SM (n = 272)	222 (82%)	34 (12%) dif 21 undif 13	13 (5%) dif 10 undif 3	3 (1%) dif 1 undif 2

Source: Department of Gastrointestinal Surgery, University of Tokyo, 1976–1997.
dif, differentiated adenocarcinoma; undif, undifferentiated adenocarcinoma.

nationwide registration of gastric cancer cases and annually analyze more than 10000 cases. Table 6 shows the cumulative 5-year survival rates in each stage after standard D2 lymph-adenectomy. This was 93.4% in Stage IA, which includes mucosal and submucosal cancer without lymph node involvement, and 87% in Stage IB, which includes mucosal and submucosal cancer with perigastric lymph node metastasis and cancer invading the muscular or subserosal layer without lymph node metastasis. Sasako et al. of the National Cancer Center Hospital in Japan reported that cumulative 5-year survival rates of mucosal and submucosal cancer were 94.3% and 91.0%, respectively. Excluding other causes of death, the rates increased to 99.3% and 98.2% in mucosal and submucosal cancer, respectively [11].

In our series, we have had 43 deaths in early gastric cancer within 5 years of gastrectomy. Among these, only four cases manifested cancer recurrence, or 0.6% of early gastric cancer. One of them was mucosal and three were submucosal cancers, but all cases were preoperatively diagnosed as advanced. Macroscopically, two cases were of the depressed and two were of the mixed type. No cases manifested peritoneal dissemination. These results are quite similar to many other reports. Furthermore, we had six cases of cancer recurrence more than 5 years after curative surgery [12], all of which manifested hematogenous metastasis. Therefore in early gastric cancer, especially in mucosal cancer, standard radical dissection, in which dissection of the Group 2 lymph nodes (D2), wider resection of the stomach, and burso-omentectomy are performed, is not necessary.

1.4 Limited Surgery

Based on the numerous results of lymph node involvement in early gastric cancer, mucosal cancer is most likely to be a good candidate for limited surgery [13, 14]. Limited surgery consists of the following procedures:

Table 4. Correlation between lymph node involvement, tumor size, and histological type in mucosal cancer

Size (cm)	Differentiated type			Incidence	Undifferentiated type			Incidence
	n0	n1	n2		n0	n1	n2	
≤0.5	46 (100.0)	0 (0)	0 (0)	0/46 (0)	16 (100.0)	0 (0)	0 (0)	0/16 (0)
0.6–1.0	114 (100.0)	0 (0)	0 (0)	0/114 (0)	68 (98.6)	1 (1.4)	0 (0)	1/69 (1.4)
1.1–2.0	306 (100.0)	0 (0)	0 (0)	0/306 (0)	272 (98.6)	4 (1.4)	0 (0)	4/276 (1.4)
2.1–3.0	164 (99.4)	1 (0.6)	0 (0)	1/165 (0.6)	177 (97.8)	4 (2.2)	0 (0)	4/181 (2.2)
3.1–4.0	82 (98.8)	0 (0)	1 (1.2)	1/83 (1.2)	98 (91.6)	8 (7.5)	1 (0.9)	9/107 (8.4)
4.1–5.0	36 (100.0)	0 (0)	0 (0)	0/36 (0)	58 (89.2)	2 (3.1)	5 (7.7)	7/65 (10.8)
≥5.1	33 (97.1)	1 (2.9)	0 (0)	1/34 (2.9)	64 (92.8)	4 (5.8)	1 (1.4)	5/69 (7.2)
Total	781 (99.6)	2 (0.3)	1 (0.1)	3/784 (0.4)	753 (96.2)	23 (2.9)	7 (0.9)	30/783 (3.8)

Source: Department of Surgery, Cancer Institute Hospital, 1952–1999.
Percentages are given in parentheses.

Table 5. Correlation between lymph node involvement, tumor size, and histological type in submucosal cancer

Size (cm)	Differentiated type				Undifferentiated type			
	n0	n1	n2	n3 and/or n4	n0	n1	n2	n3 and/or n4
≤0.5	8 (100.0)	0 (0)	0 (0)	0/8 (0)	6 (100.0)	0 (0)	0 (0)	0/6 (0)
0.6–1.0	35 (97.2)	1 (2.8)	0 (0)	0/36 (0)	25 (78.1)	6 (18.8)	1 (3.1)	1/32 (3.1)
1.1–2.0	98 (88.3)	12 (10.8)	1 (0.9)	1/111 (0.9)	78 (89.7)	8 (9.2)	1 (1.2)	1/87 (1.1)
2.1–3.0	93 (80.9)	14 (12.2)	8 (7.0)	8/115 (7.0)	102 (80.3)	20 (15.8)	5 (3.9)	5/127 (3.9)
3.1–4.0	134 (79.3)	25 (14.8)	10 (5.9)	10/169 (5.9)	145 (81.9)	25 (14.1)	7 (4.0)	7/177 (5.5)
4.1–5.0	112 (70.4)	34 (21.4)	13 (8.2)	13/159 (8.2)	106 (70.2)	32 (21.2)	13 (8.6)	13/151 (8.6)
≥5.1	48 (64.0)	18 (24.0)	9 (12.0)	9/75 (12.0)	62 (70.5)	16 (18.2)	10 (11.3)	10/88 (11.4)
Total	528 (78.5)	104 (15.5)	38 (5.6)	38/673 (5.6)	524 (78.4)	107 (16.0)	37 (5.6)	37/668 (5.5)

Source: Department of Surgery, Cancer Institute Hospital, 1952–1999.
Percentages are given in parentheses.

Table 6. Cumulative 5-year survival rate of patients with standard D2 surgery

Stage	+E	U	M	L	Whole	Total
IA	71.4	88.0	95.1	93.0	100.0	93.4
	(7)	(225)	(910)	(854)	(8)	(2030)
IB	68.8	82.5	91.0	86.6	57.1	87.0
	(21)	(163)	(300)	(243)	(7)	(725)
II	44.9	63.7	72.7	66.1	66.6	68.3
	(28)	(117)	(200)	(198)	(19)	(541)
IIIA	33.7	44.6	57.0	53.0	17.0	50.1
	(30)	(137)	(150)	(167)	(25)	(485)
IIIB	21.7	26.2	35.4	35.2	10.1	30.8
	(24)	(73)	(71)	(98)	(28)	(273)
IV	16.1	17.1	23.2	13.6	11.0	16.6
	(40)	(120)	(92)	(152)	(67)	(440)
Total	35.9	61.3	82.6	74.8	25.6	73.7
	(150)	(835)	(1723)	(1712)	(154)	(4494)

Source: Japanese Gastric Cancer Association, registered cases in 1991.
Percentages are given in parentheses.
+E, positive for esophageal invasion; Whole, whole stomach; U, M, L, upper, middle, and lower third of the stomach.

Table 7. Macroscopic type and depth of cancer invasion in our series of limited surgery

Macroscopic type	Depth	
	m	sm
Elevated ($n = 38$)	31 (81.6%)	7 (18.4%)
Depressed ($n = 142$)	110 (77.5%)	32 (22.2%)
Combined ($n = 8$)	3 (37.5%)	5 (62.5%)
Total	144	44

Table 8. Data of patients with lymph node involvement in our series of limited surgery

Depth	m	5/144 (3.5%)
	sm	5/44 (11.4%)
LN group	1	10
	2	0
Macroscopic type	Elevated	0
	Depressed	10
	Combined	0
Ulceration	(+)	9
	(−)	1
Histological type	Intestinal	2
	Diffuse	8
Tumor size (cm)		3.8 ± 2.6[a]

LN, lymph node.
[a] Mean ± SD.

dissection of the Group 1 and no. 7 lymph nodes (at the root of the left gastric artery), limited resection of the stomach, and omission of burso-omentectomy. In mucosal cancer, the site of lymph node metastasis in the N2 group was the no. 7 lymph node, if present, and peritoneal recurrence was quite rare [15, 16], leading to limited lymph node dissection and preservation of the greater omentum for curative treatment.

From 1980 to 1993, we performed limited surgery on 188 patients with early cancer preoperatively diagnosed with mucosal cancer and Stage Ia. The depth of cancer invasion was evaluated by a barium meal examination, endoscopy, and endoscopic ultrasonography (EUS). Intraoperatively, the stage of cancer was confirmed as Stage Ia and the lesion was palpated from the serosal side. When it was palpable, the patient was excluded from limited surgery and underwent D2 lymphadenectomy. Cancer invading the deep submucosal layer or the muscle layer is easily palpable. Furthermore, as mentioned above, peptic ulceration within the lesion predisposes to cancer invasion and lymph node involvement. Fibrous tissue due to ulcer formation is frequently palpated as an induration. Accordingly, palpation of the lesion is a simple and effective method for the diagnosis of not only cancer invasion, but also the presence of an ulcer or ulcer scar.

The results of limited surgery are shown in Tables 7 and 8. There was cancer invasion to the mucosal and submucosal layers in 144 patients (76.6%) and 44 patients (23.4%), respectively, and there was no case of advanced cancer. Cancer invasion was correctly diagnosed in approximately 80% of the elevated and of the depressed types. Since the adoption of EUS in 1987, only two cases have been misdiagnosed in terms of depth of cancer invasion in the elevated type. However, in the combined type, more than half of the cases were submucosal cancer and the preoperative diagnosis of cancer invasion was unsatisfactory (Table 7). Clinically, it is well known that this type of cancer mimics type 2 cancer and frequently invades the lymphatic and vascular systems, even when it is small. After this experience, the combined type was fundamentally excluded from limited surgery.

In our series of limited surgery, lymph node involvement was observed in 10 patients (5.3%); 5 were mucosal and 5 were submucosal cancers. They were all of the depressed type and 9 of them (90%) were accompanied by an ulcer or ulcer scar within the lesion. The mean size of the lesion was 3.8 cm in diameter. Only one lesion was without ulceration and measured 9 cm in diameter (Table 8). Therefore, one should be cautious of performing limited surgery if a lesion is large or is accompanied by an ulcer or ulcer scar.

In comparison with standard radical surgery, limited surgery resulted in a significantly shorter operating time, less blood loss, and lower incidence of blood transfusion (Table 9). Conclusively, we have had no cases of cancer recurrence after limited surgery.

1.5 Japanese Guidelines for the Treatment of Early Gastric Cancer

The Japanese Gastric Cancer Association proposed clinical guidelines for the treatment of early gastric cancer in 2001, mainly based on obvious evidence and numerous clinical results, including those of limited surgery. Strategies for the treatment of early gastric cancer are postulated in detail according to the status of cancer invasion and lymph node involvement as follows: endoscopic mucosal resection (EMR) for cancers limited to the mucosa, pathologically intestinal type, measuring less than 2 cm in diameter and showing no ulceration; limited surgery A (gastrectomy with D1 + no.7 lymph node dissection, and additionally no. 8a lymph node dissection if the tumor is located in the antrum) for other mucosal cancers and for those with pathologically intestinal type invading the submucosa and measuring less than 1.5 cm in diameter; limited surgery B (gastrectomy with D1 + no. 7, 8a, 9 lymph node dissection) for cancers limited to the mucosa, macroscopically N1-positive but N2-negative, and measuring less than 2 cm in diameter, or for those not adaptable to limited surgery A and invading the submucosa but macroscopically node negative. Cases of early gastric cancer not fulfilling the above-mentioned criteria should undergo standard radical surgery with D2 lymph node dissection (Fig. 1).

Table 9. Operating time, blood loss, and blood transfusion in limited surgery compared with standard surgery

	Limited surgery	Conventional surgery	*P* value
Operating time (h)	3.8 ± 1.0	4.6 ± 1.0	<0.05
Blood loss (g)	311 ± 194	502 ± 485	<0.01
Incidence of transfusion	6/188 (3.2%)	14/136 (10.3%)	<0.05

Values are expressed as mean ± SD.

	NO	N1	N2
T1 (M)	IA EMR (en bloc resection) (differentiated type, ≤2.0 cm, without ulceration) limited surgery A (cases not fulfilling the above conditions)	IB limited surgery B (≤ 2.0 cm) standard surgery (> 2.0 cm)	II standard surgery
T1 (SM)	IA limited surgery A (differentiated type, ≤ 1.5 cm) limited surgery B (cases not fulfilling the above conditions)		

Fig. 1. Clinical guidelines for the treatment of early gastric cancer. *N0*, no lymph node metastasis, *N1*, lymph node metastasis in the group 1 station; *N2*, lymph node metastasis in the group 2 station; *EMR*, endoscopic mucosal resection. *Limited surgery A*, gastrectomy with no. 7 lymph node dissection (additionally no. 8a lymph node is dissected when cancer is located at the antrum); *limited surgery B*, gastrectomy with no. 7, 8a, and 9 lymph node dissection; *standard surgery*, resection of more than two thirds of the stomach and D2 lymphadenectomy proposed by the Japanese Gastric Cancer Association

1.6 Reconstruction After Gastrectomy

Results of surgical treatment for early gastric cancer have shown excellent survival rates and most of the patients are likely to live for a long time after surgery. Accordingly, attention has been paid to QOL after gastrectomy. It is well known that many patients suffer from post-gastrectomy disorders, such as dumping syndrome, malnutrition, diarrhea, anemia, reflux diseases, and so on. The dumping syndrome is caused by emptying of hyperosmolar gastric contents into the small intestine. Reduced gastric acid secretion and prompt emptying inhibit the mixing of acid and gastric contents, predisposing to anemia and disorders of bone metabolism. Reflux diseases are caused by regurgitation of the duodenal contents including bile and pancreatic juice, resulting in reflux esophagitis, reflux gastritis and eventually, gastric remnant cancer. The development of gastric remnant cancer is the worst disorder after gastrectomy. Recently, several reports have claimed an increasing incidence of gastric remnant cancer after gastrectomy for gastric cancer. We clearly demonstrated the effects of gastrectomy and denervation on gastric remnant carcinogenesis [17, 18]. These procedures are inevitably performed with lymphadenectomy. Loss of gastric function, especially loss of pyloric function, is the most critical factor in terms of postgastrectomy disorders. The pylorus, or pyloric antrum, plays an important role in the control of gastric emptying and prevention of duodenogastric reflux. Therefore, preservation of pyloric function may contribute to minimizing post-gastrectomy disorders.

Based on these considerations, Maki et al. performed pylorus-preserving gastrectomy (PPG) about 50 years ago for patients with gastric ulcer and obtained remarkable results [20]. In the PPG procedure, the stomach is dissected 1.5–2 cm proximal to the pyloric ring. Simultaneously, the right gastric and right gastroepiploic vessels are preserved to maintain blood flow and innervation to the pyloric region. However, from the viewpoint of surgery for malignancy, preservation of these vessels may predispose to cancer recurrence as it leaves the lymph nodes at the peripyloric region. In contrast, complete dissection of both the vessels and peripyloric lymph nodes may give rise to ischemia of the pylorus and loss of its function. These considerations have led to a rejection of the application of PPG in gastric cancer surgery. However, in early cancer the incidence of lymph node involvement is very low and most of the involved lymph nodes are adjacent to the cancer lesion. On the other hand, blood flow to the pyloric region is maintained by preservation of the inferior pyloric artery, which branches off from the right gastroepiploic or the gastroduodenal artery when the right gastric artery is severed. These facts have made it possible to apply PPG for early gastric cancer located in the gastric body [21].

We have performed PPG since 1991, in which the right gastric and gastroepiploic arteries are divided with confirmation and preservation of the inferior pyloric branches, and the stomach is dissected 2 cm proximal to the pyloric ring. Figures 2 and 3 show a barium meal study and endoscopic views of a patient with PPG. The ingested barium meal was smoothly emptied from the gastric remnant. Endoscopically, the pyloric ring was open, but no bile staining of the gastric remnant was observed.

Table 10 shows the results of our series of PPG compared with the Billroth I procedure that was performed in cases of gastric cancer mainly located in the antrum

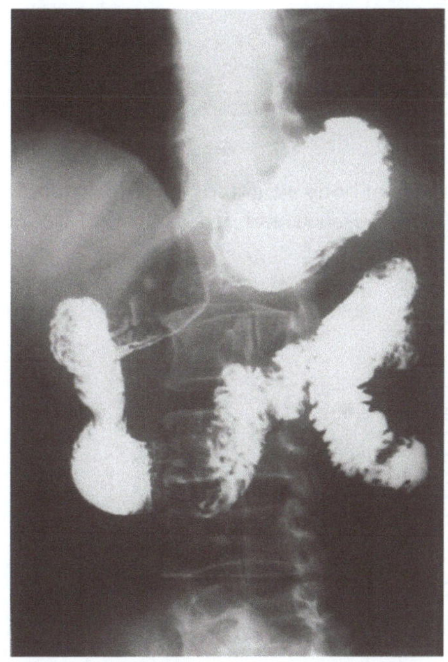

Fig. 2. Barium meal study of a patient with pylorus-preserving gastrectomy (PPG)

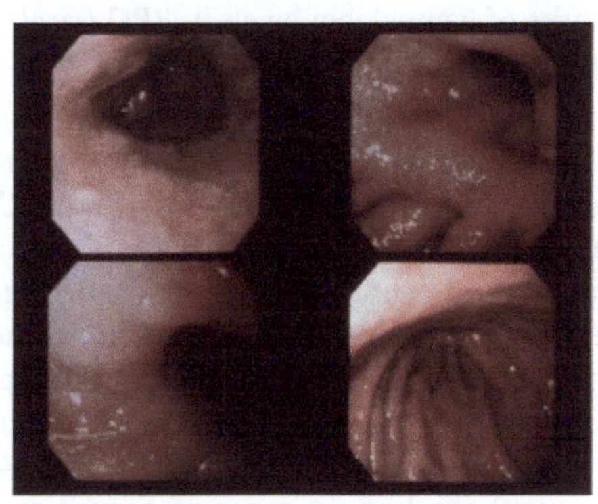

Fig. 3. Endoscopic view of a patient with PPG

Table 10. Results of our series of PPG compared with B-I

	PPG (n = 15)	B-I (n = 28)	P
Early dumping symdrome	6 (40%)	21 (75%)	0.03
Vasomotor symptoms	2 (13%)	13 (46%)	0.02
Late dumping syndrome	7 (47%)	12 (43%)	0.29
Mean total protein concentration (g/dl)	7.3 ± 0.3	7.1 ± 0.4	0.09
Mean serum albumin (g/dl)	4.2 ± 0.2	4.2 ± 0.3	0.47

PPG, pylorus-preserving gastrectomy; B-I, Billroth I procedure.

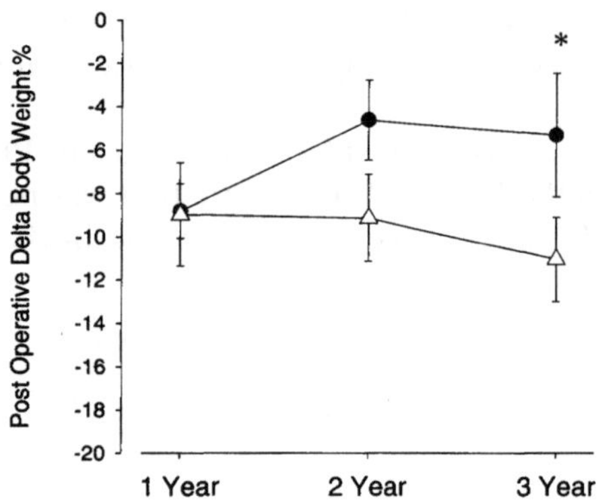

Fig. 4. Changes of body weight loss in pylorus-preserving gastrectomy (*PPG*; *circles*) and B-I Billroth I (*B-I*; *triangles*) groups. *$P < 0.05$ vs B-I

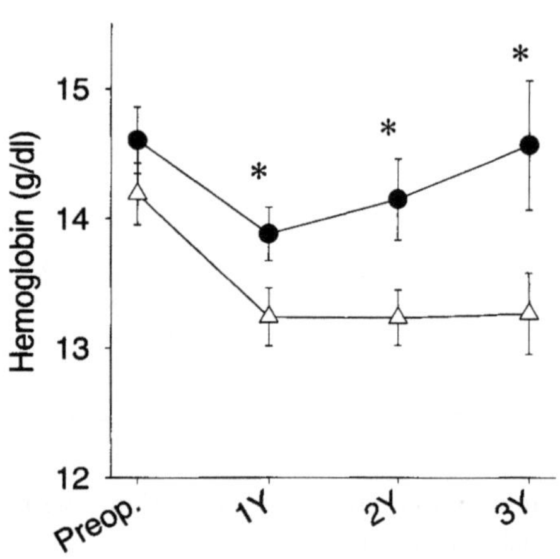

Fig. 5. Changes of hemoglobin levels in PPG (*circle*) and B-I (*triangles*) groups. *$P < 0.05$ vs B-I

in the same period. Pylorus-preserving gastrectomy patients manifested a significantly lower incidence of early dumping syndrome and related vasomotor symptoms. Some patients showed delayed gastric emptying, but related symptoms such as gastric fullness and vomiting after meals subsided 6 months after operation. Consequently, we obtained a significantly lower degree of body weight loss and anemia in PPG (Figs. 4 and 5). In addition, we have had no cases of cancer recurrence [22].

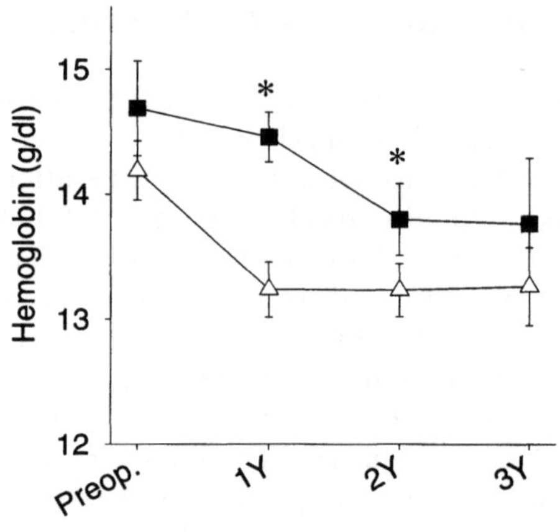

Fig. 6. Changes of blood hemoglobin levels in jejunal interposition (*JIP*; *squares*) and B-I (*triangles*) groups. *$P < 0.05$ vs JIP

The application of PPG is restricted to patients in whom cancer is located in the gastric body, in order to maintain a safe distal margin from the cancerous lesion [23]. When cancer is located in the antrum, a conventional procedure such as Billroth I, Billroth II, or Roux-en-Y is performed as a standard procedure. The Roux-en-Y method can prevent reflux disorders, but cannot minimize dumping syndrome and may promote gallstone formation. To achieve better QOL, we have adopted the jejunal interposition (JIP) since 1996 as a substitute for such procedures when cancer is located in the antrum. In JIP, a 10-cm segment of the upper jejunum is interposed between the gastric remnant and the duodenum. An important technical point in this procedure is to sacrifice a segment of the jejunum in order to maintain blood flow and innervation to the interposed jejunum. The jejunal mesenterium is divided at the proximal side of the interposed jejunum with a jejunal transection, but at the distal side the marginal small vessels of the jejunum are severed 5–10 cm to maintain the mesenterium intact. The preserved innervation to the mesenterium provides a to-and-fro movement of the jejunum as a substitute for the pylorus. Nutritional status is satisfactory and hemoglobin levels are significantly higher than in patients with Billroth I procedure (Fig. 6). Figure 7 demonstrates barium meal studies. Gastric emptying is adequate. Endoscopically, bile staining of the gastric remnant is observed less frequent. In the JIP procedure, all peripyloric lymph nodes are completely dissected, indicating the feasibility of this procedure for patients with Stage I and II advanced gastric cancer without serosal exposure.

Recently, the laparoscopic technique has been applied in gastric surgery. This provides less invasiveness and faster recovery from surgery. On the other hand, open laparotomy is required to perform reconstruction after gastrectomy. Considering these points, we have adopted laparoscopy-assisted gastrectomy (LAG) in which perigastric lymph node dissection is performed under laparoscopy, and subsequent gastric reconstruction is performed through a 6-cm minilaparotomy.

1.7 Laparoscopic Local Resection with Lymph Node Dissection

In terms of QOL, there is a big difference between endoscopic mucosal resection (EMR) and gastrectomy, even if limited surgery combined with PPG or JIP is performed. In the former, the stomach is preserved as it is but in the latter, two thirds of the stomach is resected. Furthermore, the gastrectomy is performed via a laparotomy, and is much more invasive for the patient. To minimize such a big difference, we have adopted local resection of the lesion with lymph node dissection and have done the procedure under laparoscopy since 1998.

The most important point in this treatment is selection of appropriate candidates. The best candidates are patients in whom EMR is not feasible but in whom mucosal cancer without lymph node involvement is preoperatively and correctly diagnosed. However, the accuracy of the preoperative diagnosis of cancer invasion depth is controversial [24]. To select candidates, we analyzed the cases of our series of limited surgery in which cancer was prospectively diagnosed as mucosal cancer and was not palpable intraoperatively. Since 1987, when EUS was first applied for the diagnosis of cancer invasion, 128 cases underwent limited surgery (gastrectomy with no. 7 lymph node dissection). One hundred and seven cases were pathologically mucosal and 21 were submucosal cancer, with an 83.6% accuracy of preoperative diagnosis. Four cases had positive lymph nodes that were limited to the perigastric region, Group 1 lymph nodes, and all of these had ulcers or scars in the lesion. The perigastric lymph node region is divided into six stations in the definition of the Japanese Gastric Cancer Association. In most cases of mucosal cancer, positive lymph nodes were observed only in one station. However, cases in which the cancer was larger than 4 cm in diameter showed positive lymph nodes in two stations, even if ulcers or scars were absent in the lesion. Considering these results, patients in whom cancer is preoperatively diagnosed as mucosal by means of endoscopy and EUS, smaller than 4 cm in diameter, and cancer-negative in the resected lymph node by frozen-section examination are considered to be the best candidates for local resection with perigastric lymph node dissection. Moreover, our series of limited surgery showed no lymph node metastasis in cases of less than 1 cm in diameter with or without ulcers or scars. A similar result was reported in which only one out of 183 cases of less than 1 cm in diameter manifested lymph node metastasis in the perigastric region, even if ulcers or scars were present (Table 4). These results suggest that about 40% of cases of limited surgery can be managed by the new procedure. If the specimen is

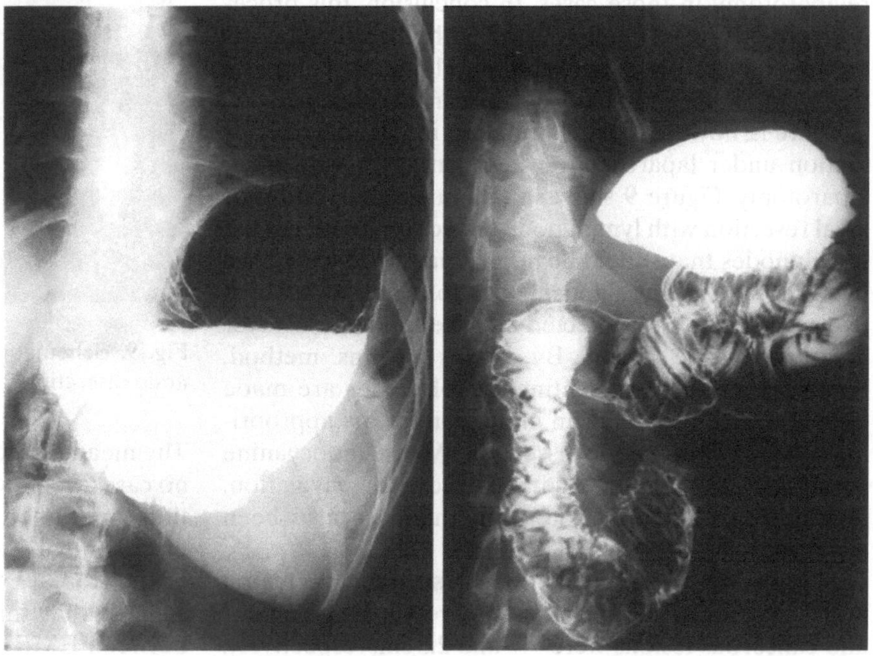

Fig. 7. Barium meal study of patients with JIP

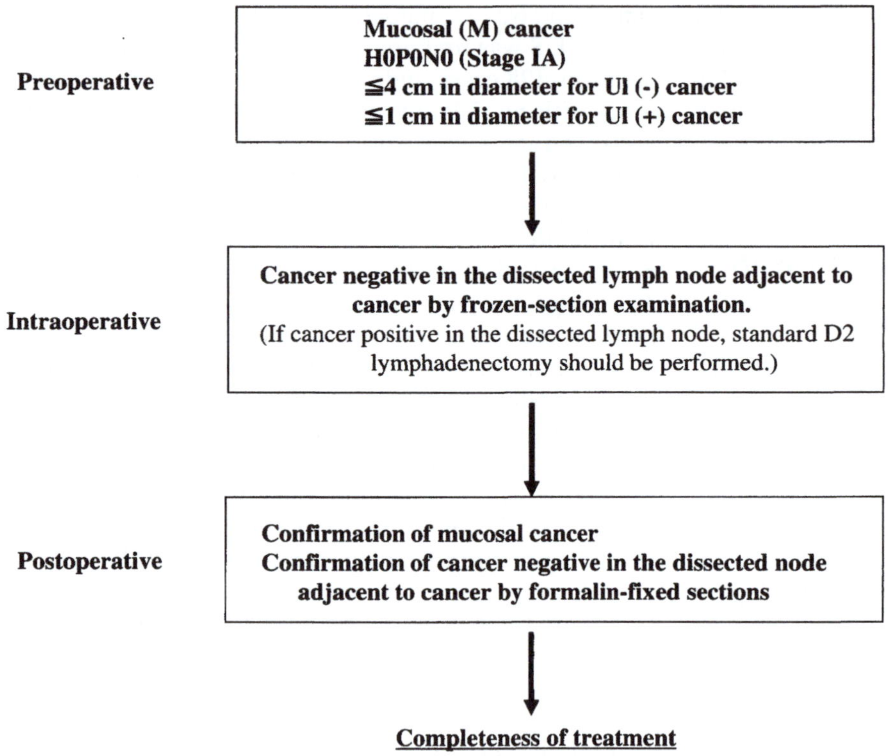

Fig. 8. Flow chart of local resection with lymphadenectomy adjacent to cancer

revealed to be submucosal cancer, or positive for lymph node involvement by intraoperative or postoperative histological examination, standard gastrectomy with D2 lymph node dissection is highly recommended under open laparotomy. Therefore, local resection with lymphadenectomy adjacent to the cancer should be performed under laparoscopy in order to avoid relaparotomy in those cases. In conclusion, this procedure provides confirmation of the pathological diagnosis of the resected specimen and simultaneous complete treatment of the given early gastric cancer (Fig. 8).

There is, however, some limitation in lymph node dissection under laparoscopy when compared with open laparotomy. Figure 9 shows a schematic illustration of local resection with lymph node dissection. To detect the lymph nodes that should be appropriately dissected, we have adopted a lymph node navigation method in which dye is endoscopically injected into the submucosal layer adjacent to the lesion. By means of this method, lymphatic vessels and sentinel lymph nodes are made clearly visible, providing an indication for the appropriate scope of lymph node dissection. We use indocyanine green (ICG) or patent-blue as a tracer for navigation. Application of a radioisotope method has also been reported.

In our series of 24 cases of local resection with lymph node dissection, the mean sizes of resected specimens and cancerous lesions were 7.7 and 2.3 cm, respectively.

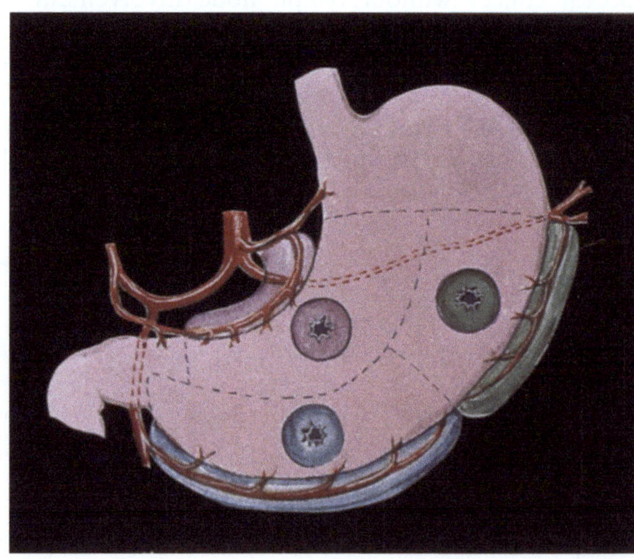

Fig. 9. Schematic illustration of local resection with lymph node dissection

The mean dissected number of lymph nodes was 7.6 and no cases were positive for lymph node metastasis. Nutritional parameters showed no change after surgery. A barium meal study is shown in Fig. 10 and no deformity of the stomach was observed. These preliminary results suggest that this procedure is the best to fill the gap between EMR and gastrectomy [25].

1.8 Summary

A flow chart of our strategy for the surgical treatment of early gastric cancer is shown in Fig. 11. From the viewpoint of QOL, a tailor-made treatment should be promoted in cases of early gastric cancer according to cancer status such as depth of invasion, presence or absence of ulcers or ulcer scars, location, and size.

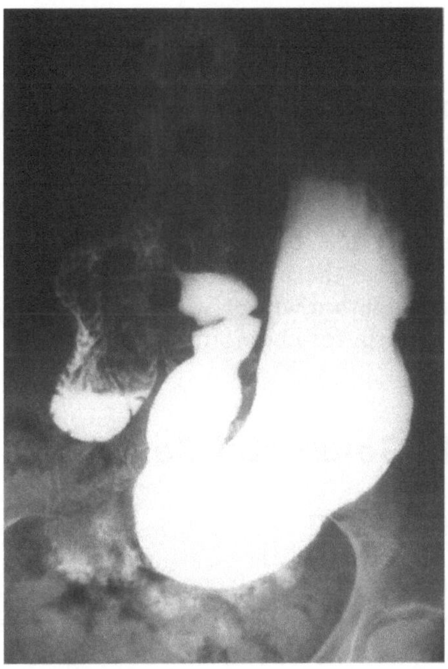

Fig. 10. Barium meal study of a patient with local resection

2. Early Esophageal Cancer

2.1 Introduction

It is well known that the prognosis of esophageal cancer is quite poor and surgical treatment is very invasive for the patients. However, recent advances in the diagnosis of esophageal cancer have yielded an increasing number in the early stage of cancer, and an improvement of the 5-year survival rates from 30% to more than 40% in Japan over the last 10 years.

According to the definition of the Japanese Society for Esophageal Diseases [26], early esophageal cancer is a tumor in which the tumor invasion is restricted in the epithelial or mucosal layer without lymph node metastasis. Therefore, diagnosis of early esophageal cancer is confirmed finally after pathological examination of resected specimens. On the other hand, superficial esophageal cancer is defined as a tumor in which the invasion is restricted in the epithelial, mucosal, or submucosal layer regardless of lymph node metastasis (Fig. 12). The depth of cancer invasion can be diagnosed by means of diagnostic imaging such as endoscopy, endoscopic ultrasonography, or a barium meal study.

Surgical Treatment and Survival Rates of Early and Superficial Esophageal Cancers

With regard to lymph node metastasis, m1 and m2 squamous cell cancers in which the invasion has not reached

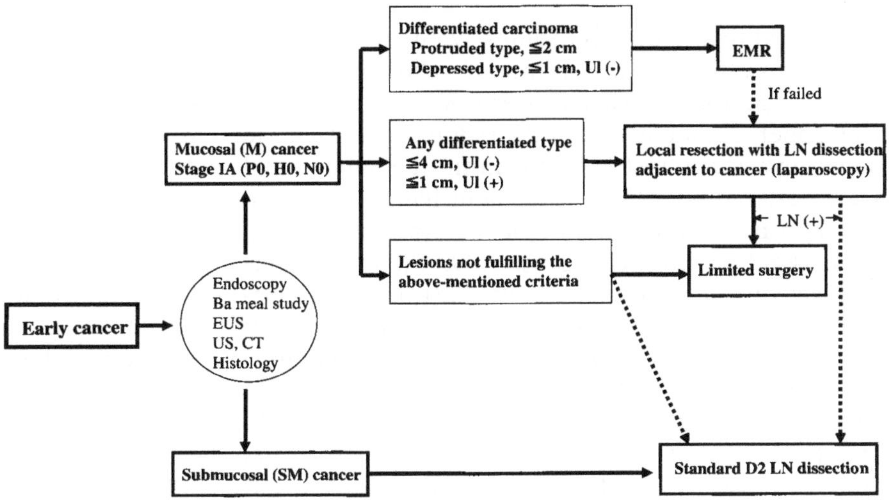

Fig. 11. Flow chart of the treatment of early gastric cancer. *Ba*, barium; *EUS*, endoscopic ultrasonography; *US*, ultrasonography; *CT*, computed tomography; *EMR*, endoscopic mucosal resection; *LN*, lymph node

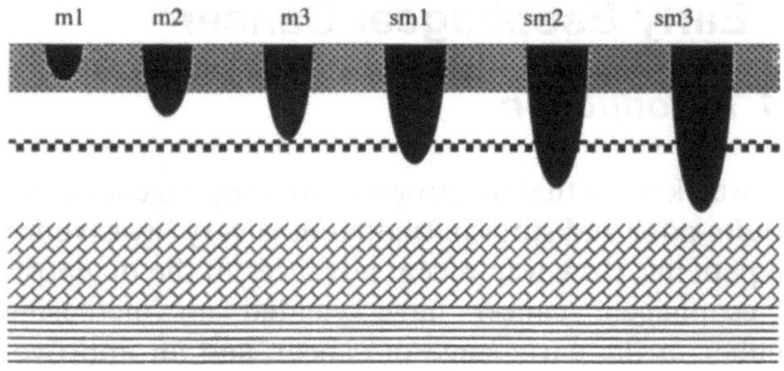

Fig. 12. Subclassification of the depth of cancer invasion in superficial esophageal cancer (Japanese Society for Esophageal Diseases)

the muscularis mucosae have no lymph node metastasis. In m3 and sm1 cancers, the lymph node metastasis rate is 10 to 15%, whereas in sm2 and sm3 cancers it is more than 50%. Furthermore, involvement of lymphatic vessels, one of the important factors related to lymph node metastasis, is observed in about 60% of submucosal cancers.

Based on these facts, EMR of squamous cell carcinoma is indicated for cases in which the depth of cancer invasion is diagnosed as m2 or less. An excellent 5-year survival rate of 80% has been achieved by EMR. If the number of early esophageal cancers is more than 5, or the cancer occupies more than two thirds of the esophageal lumen, EMR may induce severe stenosis of the esophagus, and blunt dissection of the esophagus without thoracotomy is recommended. However, superficial cancer that invades massively into the muscularis mucosae (m3) or into the submucosal layer is an indication for esophagectomy with lymph node dissection. The prognosis after esophagectomy of superficial cancer depends on the status of lymph node metastasis [27, 28]. The data from the registry of the Japanese Society for Esophageal Diseases showed that survival rates of Stage 0 (Tis, N0, M0), I (T1, N0, M0), and II B (T1, N1, M0) according to the UICC classification are 80%, 70%, and 40%, respectively.

In regard to surgical procedures, lymph node dissection of three fields (cervical-thoracic-abdominal field) should be performed when cancer is located in the cervical, upper, or middle part of the esophagus, even if the cancer invasion is restricted to within the submucosal layer. Better prognosis of three-field lymph node dissection compared with two-field (thoracic-abdominal field) dissection has been reported [29, 30]. When superficial cancer is located in the lower part of the esophagus, two-field lymph node dissection through left thoracotomy and laparotomy is sufficient as curative surgery. In cases of early cancer of Barrett's esophagus, lymph node metastasis to the upper and middle mediastinal parts is quite rare. Accordingly, paracardiac and lower mediastinal lymph node dissection via the left thoraco-abdominal approach is recommended [30]. A flow chart of the surgical treatment of superficial esophageal cancer is shown in Fig. 13.

Recently, radiation or chemoradiation therapy for Stage I and II has been challenged and equivalent results to surgical therapy have been reported [31, 32]. Further investigation will be warranted to establish the feasibility criteria for chemoradiation therapy.

3. Early Colorectal Cancer

3.1 Introduction

Early colorectal cancer limited to the mucosa does not have lymph node involvement or distant metastasis. It is, therefore, not life-threatening as long as it is diagnosed and treated properly before invading beyond the muscularis mucosa. This is probably one reason why Western clinicians and pathologists are prone to regard this pathology as adenoma with severe dysplasia rather than carcinoma, although the diagnosis of any disease should be made on its underlying nature, rather than its clinical outcomes.

3.2 Treatment and Survival Rate of Mucosal Cancer

Mucosal colorectal cancer is treated with endoscopic polypectomy or EMR. If some technical difficulties due to the size or location of the lesion hamper its endoscopic removal, segmental resection of the colon by laparoscopic surgery or local resection of the rectum by transanal endoscopic microsurgery (TEM) [33], minimally invasive transanal surgery (MITAS) [34], or a trans-sacral approach [35] could be employed. With these appropriate therapies, the survival rate of mucosal early colorectal cancer should be 100%.

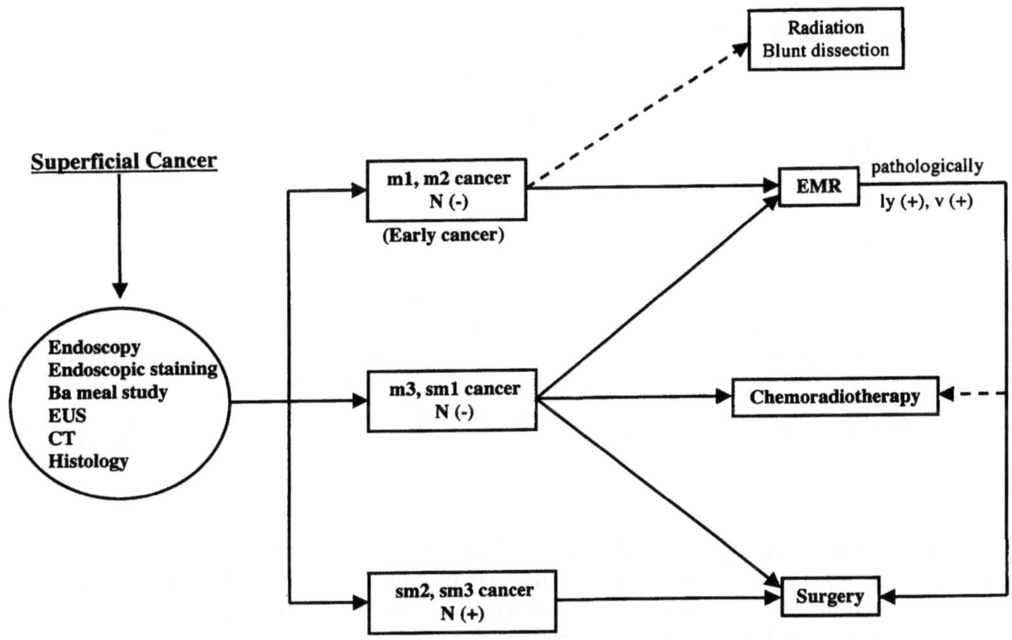

Fig. 13. Flow chart of the treatment of superficial esophageal cancer. *Ba*, barium; *EUS*, endoscopic ultrasonography; *CT*, computed tomography; *EMR*, endoscopic mucosal resection; *ly*, lymphatic vessels permeation; *v*, venous vessels permeation

3.3 Lymph Node Metastasis and Survival Rate of Submucosal Cancer

Colorectal cancer invading into the submucosal layer also has a good prognosis with a 5-year survival rate after surgery of about 90%–97% [36, 37]. A complete cure can be achieved by endoscopic or local resection in most submucosal cancers that are not complicated with lymph node involvement or distant metastasis. It is, therefore, essential to identify lesions that have lymph node metastasis and require surgery with lymph node dissection.

Some 10% of submucosal cancers involve lymph node metastasis, which is one of the strongest prognostic determinants. The cumulative 5-year survival rate is 70%–80% in node-positive patients, compared with 90%–97% in node-negative patients [36, 38, 39]. In our series of 74 patients with submucosally invasive early colorectal cancer, 6 (8%) had lymph node metastasis, and distant metastases to the liver were found in 3 (4%). The 5-year survival rate was 97%, with 83.3% in node-positive and 98.5% in node-negative patients.

Reported risk factors for lymph node metastasis include (i) depth of invasion, (ii) histopathological type of differentiation, (iii) lymphovascular invasion, (iv) configuration of the tumor, and (iv) small clusters of undiffentiated cancer cells called "tumor budding" [39–41]. The simplest, most robust, and useful risk factor is the depth of cancer invasion. The submucosal layer is divided into three portions: upper (sm1); middle (sm2); and lower (sm3) third. In most cases, an accurate diagnosis of depth of invasion can be made comprehensively with endoscopic appearances including "pit patterns [42]," endoscopic ultrasonographic findings [43], and radiological evaluation [44]. As the invasion deepens, the rate of lymph node metastasis increases: sm1, 0%–3%; sm2, 5%–10%; and sm3, 10%–15% [41, 45], as does the rate of distant metastasis: sm1, 0.3%; sm2, 3%; and sm3, 4% [45]. In all three patients with liver metastasis from our series, the depth of invasion was sm3.

3.4 Treatment of Submucosal Cancer

If the lesion is sm1 in depth without other risk factors, endoscopic or local resection would suffice for a complete cure. As for lesions with sm2 invasion that are pedunculated or subpedunculated in configuration, endoscopic or local resection should be performed initially. If the histological examination of the resected specimen reveals further risk factors such as deeper invasion, poor differentiation, or lymphovascular invasion, additional surgery with lymph node dissection is required. For both sm2 tumors with sessile, superficial elevated, or depressed configuration, and sm3 lesions of any shape, surgical resection is warranted.

A more accurate estimate of lymph node metastasis can be made by combining several risk factors. Hase et al. [40] examined five histological risk factors: (i) tumor budding; (ii) poor demarcation of cancer at the invasive

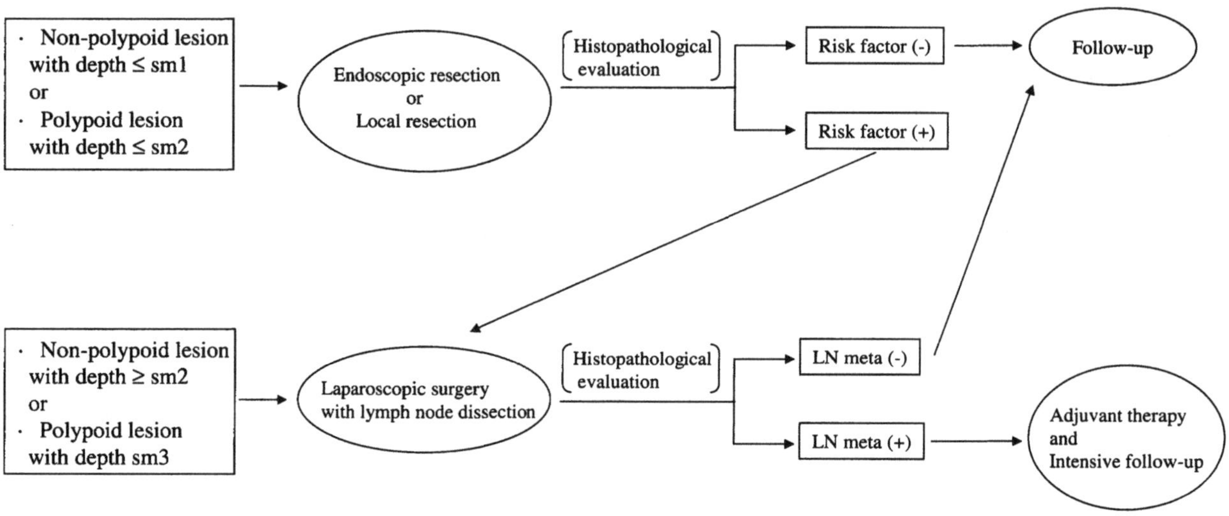

Fig. 14. Therapeutic strategy for early colorectal cancer. *Sm1*, invasion in the upper third of the submucosal layer; *Sm2*, invasion in the middle third; and *sm3*, invasion in the lower third. *Local resection* includes laparoscopic local resection of the colon as well as transanal endoscopic microsurgery, minimally invasive transanal surgery, and trans-sacral approach for rectal lesions. *Risk factor*: risk factors for lymph node metastasis including poor or moderate differentiation, lymphovascular invasion, and so forth. *LN meta*, lymph node metastasis

front; (iii) moderately and poorly differentiated histology in the submucosal invasion front; (iv) sm2 or 3 invasion depth; and (v) lymphatic invasion. They reported that tumors with fewer than four risk factors had no nodal metastasis, whereas those with four or five factors had nodal metastasis rates of 33% and 67%, respectively. The evaluation of tumor budding, however, seems to be difficult and fairly subjective, depending largely on a pathologist's experience and enthusiasm.

Surgery with lymph node dissection is indicated in 30%–50% of patients with submucosally invasive colorectal cancers, who are likely to have nodal metastasis according to the currently available risk factors. In these patients, laparoscopic resection is recommended, if technically possible, rather than conventional open surgery. This procedure is less invasive, less painful, and shows faster recovery, and does not compromise survival outcomes [46]. Dissection of the central lymph nodes, which can be achieved by experienced laparoscopic surgeons, is required only in a limited number of cases with the highest risk factors, whilst dissection up to the intermediate lymph nodes is sufficient in most patients.

3.5 Summary

The surgical strategy for early colorectal cancer is proposed in Fig. 14. Between 4% and 8% of patients develop distant metastases that cannot be prevented or treated solely with surgery. In such rare cases or in those with lymph node metastasis, comprehensive therapies including chemotherapy should be considered.

References

1. Japanese Gastric Cancer Association (1998) Japanese Classification of Gastric Carcinoma, 2nd English ed. Gastric Cancer 1:10–24
2. Lauren P (1965) The two histological main types of gastric carcinoma: diffuse and so-called intestinal-type carcinoma. An attempt at histo-clinical classification. Acta Pathol Microbiol Scand 64:31–49
3. Kurihara N, Kubota T, Otani Y, et al (1998) Lymph node metastasis of early gastric cancer with submucosal invasion. Br J Surg 85:835–839
4. Iriyama K, Asakawa T, Koike H, et al (1989) Is extensive lymph adenectomy necessary for surgical treatment of intramucosal carcinoma of the stomach? Arch Surg 124: 309–312
5. Yamao T, Shirao K, Ono H, et al (1996) Risk factors for lymph node metastasis from intramucosal gastric carcinoma. Cancer 77:602–606
6. Gotoda T, Yanagisawa A, Sasako M, et al (2000) Incidence of lymph node metastasis from early gastric cancer: estimation with a large number of cases at two large centers. Gastric Cancer 3:219–225
7. Mahara Y, Okuyama T, Oshiro T, et al (1993) Early carcinoma of the stomach. Surg Gynecol Obstet 177:593–597

8. Kim JP, Hur YS, Yang HK (1995) Lymph node metastasis as a significant prognostic factor in early gastric cancer: analysis of 1,136 early gastric cancers. Ann Surg Oncol 2: 308–313
9. Isozaki H, Tanaka N, Okajima K (1999) General and specific prognostic factors of early gastric carcinoma treated with curative surgery. Hepato-Gastroenterology 46:1800–1808
10. Inoue K, Tobe T, Kan N, et al (1991) Problems in the definition and treatment of early gastric cancer. Br J Surg 78:818–821
11. Sasako M, Kinoshita T, Maruyama K (1993) Prognosis of early gastric cancer (with English abstract). I to Cho (Stomach Intest) 28:139–146
12. Kammori M, Kaminishi M, Kobayashi K, et al (1999) Immunohistochemical analysis of PAI-2 (plasminogen activator inhibitor type 2) and p53 protein of early gastric cancer. A preliminary report. Jpn J Clin Oncol 29:187–191
13. Sowa M, Kato Y, Nishimura M et al (1989) Surgical approach to early gastric cancer with lymph node metastasis. World J Surg 13:630–636
14. Sano T, Kobori O, Muto T (1992) Lymph node metastasis from early gastric cancer: endoscopic resection of tumour. Br J Surg 79:241–244
15. Ichiyoshi Y, Toda T, Minamisono Y, et al (1990) Recurrence in early gastric cancer. Surgery 107:489–495
16. Sano T, Sasako M, Kinoshita M, et al (1993) Recurrence of early gastric cancer: follow-up of 1,474 patients and review of the Japanese literature. Cancer 72:3174–3178
17. Kaminishi M, Oohara T, Chiu ML, et al (1992) Severe gastric mucosal changes following vagotomy with duodenogastric reflux. J Clin Gastroenterol 14(suppl I): S15–S24
18. Kaminishi M, Shimizu N, Shimoyama S, et al (1995) Etiology of gastric remnant cancer with special reference to the effects of denervation of the gastric mucosa. Cancer 75:1490–1496
19. Kaminishi M, Shimizu N, Nomura S, et al (1996) Different carcinogenesis in the gastric remnant following gastrectomy for gastric cancer. Cancer 77:1646–1653
20. Maki T, Shiratori T, Hatafuku T, et al (1967) Pylorus-preserving gastrectomy as an improved operation for gastric ulcer. Surgery 61:838–845
21. Sawai K, Takahashi T, Fujioka T, et al (1995) Pylorus-preserving gastrectomy with radical lymph node dissection based on anatomical variations of the infrapyloric artery. Am J Surg 170:285–288
22. Zhang D, Shimoyama S, Kaminishi M (1998) Feasibility of pylorus-preserving gastrectomy with a wider scope of lymphadenectomy. Arch Surg 133:993–997
23. Seto Y, Ishida T, Kaminishi N, et al (2000) Vascular invasion of early gastric cancer at resection line. Int Surg 85: 216–218
24. Seto Y, Shimoyama S, Kitayama J, et al (2001) Lymph node metastasis and preoperative diagnosis of depth of invasion in early gastric cancer. Gastric Cancer 4:34–38
25. Seto Y, Yamaguchi H, Kaminishi S, et al (2001) Results of local resection with regional lymphadenectomy for early gastric cancer. Am J Surg 182:498–501
26. Japanese Society for Esophageal Diseases (1999) Guidelines for the clinical and pathologic studies on carcinoma of the esophogus, 9th edn. Kanehara, Tokyo
27. Kakegawa T, Yamana H (1995) Progress in surgical treatment for carcinoma of the intrathoracic esophagus. Jpn J Cancer Chemother 22:885–862
28. Isono K, Sato H, Nakayama K (1991) Results of nationwide study on the three-field lymph node dissection of esophageal cancer. Oncology 48:411–420
29. Baba M, Aikou T, Yoshinaka H, et al (1994) Long-term results of subtotal esophagectomy with threefield lymphadenectomy for carcinoma of the thoracic esophagus. Am Surg 219:310–316
30. Akiyama H (1993) Clinical study on adenocarcinoma of the lower esophagus and cardia. In: Esophageal cancer: toward improved results. Nakayama Institute of Cancer Research, Tokyo, pp 44–51
31. Okawa T, Tanaka M, Kita M, et al (1995) Superficial esophageal cancer: Multicenter analysis of results of definitive radiation therapy in Japan. Radiology 196:271–274
32. Sarraf AI, Martz K, Herskovic A, et al (1997) Progress report of combined chemoradiotherapy versus radiotherapy alone in patients with esophageal cancer: an Intergroup Study. J Clin Oncol 15:277–284
33. Heintz A, Morschel M, Junginger T (1998) Comparison of results after transanal endoscopic microsurgery and radical resection for T1 carcinoma of the rectum. Surg Endosc 12:1145–1148
34. Maeda K, Hashimoto M, Nakajima K, et al (1997) Transanal surgery with a new anal retractor and a stapler for tumours in the proximal rectum. Eur J Surg 163: 219–221
35. Kuramoto S, Kobayashi K, Mimura T, et al (1997) Establishing a standard for treating flat early cancers of the rectum. Jpn J Gastroenterol Surg 30:955–960
36. Hase K, Mochizuki H, Utsunomiya K, et al (1996) Management of submucosal invasive colorectal cancer in view of long-term follow-up outcome. J Jpn Surg Soc 29:1013–1021
37. Kitamura K, Taniguchi H, Yamaguchi T, et al (1997) Clinical outcome of surgical treatment for invasive early colorectal cancer in Japan. Hepato-Gastroenterology 44: 108–115
38. Okabe S, Kanenobu M, Matsumoto A, et al (1992) Controversy on therapeutic modality to early carcinomas from the viewpoint of histopathological features. J Jpn Surg Soc 93:1079–1082
39. Mainprize KS, Mortensen NJ, Warren BF (1998) Early colorectal cancer: recognition, classification and treatment. Br J Surg 85:469–476
40. Hase K, Shatney CH, Mochizuki H, et al (1995) Long-term results of curative resection of "minimally invasive" colorectal cancer. Dis Colon Rectum 38:19–26
41. Kikuchi R, Takano M, Takagi K, et al (1995) Management of early invasive colorectal cancer. Risk of recurrence and clinical guidelines. Dis Colon Rectum 38: 1286–1295

42. Kudo S, Kashida H, Nakajima T, et al (1997) Endoscopic diagnosis and treatment of early colorectal cancer. World J Surg 21:694–701
43. Matsunaga A, Mochizuki F, Fujita N, et al (1996) Diagnosis of early colorectal cancer by microscanner (MS)—evaluation of degree of submucosal carcinomatous infiltration. Gastroenterol Endosc 38:1322–1331
44. Maruyama M, Koizumi K, Kai S, et al (2000) Radiographic diagnosis of early colorectal cancer, with special reference to the superficial type of invasive carcinoma. World J Surg 24:1036–1046
45. Kodaira S, Yao T, Nakamura K, et al (1994) Audit of invasive early colorectal cancer with metastasis from the view point of submucosal layer sub-classification. Stomach Intest 29:1137–1142
46. Fazio VW, Lopez-Kostner F (2000) Role of laparoscopic surgery for treatment of early colorectal carcinoma. World J Surg 24:1056–1060

Index

MIX
Papier aus verantwortungsvollen Quellen
Paper from responsible sources
FSC® C105338

If you have any concerns about our products,
you can contact us on
ProductSafety@springernature.com

In case Publisher is established outside the EU,
the EU authorized representative is:
Springer Nature Customer Service Center GmbH
Europaplatz 3, 69115 Heidelberg, Germany

Printed by Libri Plureos GmbH
in Hamburg, Germany